Alfred Hill

The History of the Reform Movement in the Dental Profession in Great Britain during the Last Twenty Years

Alfred Hill

The History of the Reform Movement in the Dental Profession in Great Britain during the Last Twenty Years

ISBN/EAN: 9783337297190

Printed in Europe, USA, Canada, Australia, Japan

Cover: Foto ©ninafisch / pixelio.de

More available books at **www.hansebooks.com**

THE HISTORY

OF

THE REFORM MOVEMENT

IN

THE DENTAL PROFESSION

IN GREAT BRITAIN

DURING THE LAST TWENTY YEARS.

BY

ALFRED HILL,

LICENTIATE IN DENTAL SURGERY OF THE ROYAL COLLEGE OF SURGEONS OF ENGLAND;
DENTAL SURGEON TO THE DENTAL HOSPITAL OF LONDON;
AND LATE HONORARY SECRETARY TO THE MANAGING AND MEDICAL COMMITTEES
OF THAT INSTITUTION.

LONDON:
TRÜBNER & CO., LUDGATE HILL.
1877.

TO

EVERY LICENTIATE IN DENTAL SURGERY,

OF THE

ROYAL COLLEGE OF SURGEONS OF ENGLAND,

HONOURABLY PRACTISING HIS USEFUL PROFESSION,

This Work

IS RESPECTFULLY DEDICATED

BY

THE AUTHOR.

PREFACE.

THE reasons which induced me to write this work were various. The principal one was a keen sense of justice due to those whose long-sustained labours were pre-eminently the cause, the effect of which is the present organised and improved condition of the dental profession. During the twenty years which have elapsed since the first real movement in the direction of reform took place, many of the most influential and energetic men have been removed from our midst by the stern hand of death. It appeared to me an injustice to their memory to allow their names and their self-sacrificing endeavours to pass quietly into forgetfulness. We all owe them the tribute of acknowledgment and remembrance, and I conceived the present method to be, at the least, appropriate. Not only to those who have departed, but also to those who, happily, are still with us, is this simple record of their work and its successful result, due.

Moreover, it seemed to me very desirable that those who are so manifestly reaping the many solid and invaluable benefits, which are the outcome of what has been accomplished, should be not only made acquainted with the names of their benefactors, but have placed before them an outline of the way in which the many obstacles in the path of dental reform had been, one after the other, removed or surmounted. When the younger members of the profession learn what the condition of things actually was so short a time since, they will be naturally led to rejoice in their enfranchisement from so many of the disadvantages and disagreeables to which their predecessors had to submit. Also, by comparing what has been with what is, I am inclined to believe that they will more fully appreciate their present circumstances by a just estimation of the heritage thus handed to them, and seek by honourable conduct and scientific and practical attainments to uphold the dignity, and promote the further advance, of dental surgery in this country.

Another reason for the course I have taken arose from the fact that I had been closely associated with those who had so energetically worked for dental reform, and had fought, in turn, on both sides of the field. From this cause, and having held official positions in the College of Dentists of England, the Odontological Society, and the Dental Hospital of London, I was drawn into intimacy with the various movements as they took place, and with the leaders and influential members of the profession, as such, from the commencement to the present time.

I am indebted to several gentlemen for assistance offered, and, in some cases, very kindly rendered. It is but just to Mr. Tomes to say here that, nearly simultaneously with my published intention to write this book, he had determined to issue a similar notice of the work accomplished for the dentists of this country. On learning my intentions he very generously abstained from doing any more, and handed over to me, for my own use, the manuscript he had already prepared, together with documents of value. Mr. R. Hepburn kindly furnished me with copious records of the proceedings of the College of Dentists, which he had carefully preserved, and for which, with many other contributions, I have to thank him. To Mr. Rymer, also, for similar generous assistance I am indebted. Nor can I omit the name of Mr. Thomas Arnold Rogers, who from the first has been ever anxious to render me every service.

I have to thank the council of the Odontological Society for permission granted me to search the records of their proceedings: but for the restrictions with which the permission was encumbered, I should have cheerfully availed myself of the opportunity thus given. The managing committee and also the medical committee of the Dental Hospital of London freely offered me the use of their books, and I hereby return them my thanks for the privilege accorded.

The following pages have been written with the intention of gathering together such facts as would constitute a reliable history of the struggle for improvement, which has taken place, since the year 1856, in the dental profession, and the record virtually terminates with the removal of the Dental Hospital of London to its present site. I have not thought it advisable to enter into the relation of events which have occurred subsequently, such as what is known as "The Manchester Movement," &c., &c., leaving them for another and abler pen to describe at a future time. The style I have adopted is the simplest, believing such will more readily commend itself to most readers.

In conclusion, I may add, that it has afforded me the greatest satisfaction to have been permitted to contribute, in my limited degree, to the general welfare of my profession throughout the whole period here described. I have been honoured by the friendship of the chiefest and the best in our ranks, while in the humble work itself which I have done I have ever found a complete and abundant reward.

LONDON, 1876.

CONTENTS.

CHAPTER I.

Dentistry a generation since—Scarcity of scientific practitioners—Wholesale extraction of teeth—Dentifrices and their purveyors—Opportunities for the unscrupulous and ill-informed—Books and book-makers—Pamphlets and pamphleteers—Their real object and results 1

CHAPTER II.

Mr. Waite's appeal in 1841—Absence of results—The Medical Bill of 1843—Movement among dental practitioners in London thereon—Their plan for reform of the profession—Steps taken to effect it—Modification of views—Disunion and disappointment—Final abandonment of the scheme. 17

CHAPTER III.

Period of apathy and inaction—Effects upon students generally—Mr. Tomes' work on Dental Physiology and Surgery—First symptoms of reform—Mr. Rymer's letter to the "Lancet"—Its effects—Announcement of a public meeting of the profession, to be convened by Mr. Rymer—Gathering of dentists at the London Tavern—Proposal to found a Dental Institute—Dawning of difficulties—The memorial to the Royal College of Surgeons—Effect upon the profession generally—Mr. Clendon, and his opinions—Formation of the Odontological Society of London—Second public meeting of dentists—Third public meeting of the profession—Formation of the College of Dentists of England—Mr. Samuel Cartwright, first president of the Odontological Society—Mr. James Robinson, first president of the College of Dentists of England—Two ways to one goal . 32

CHAPTER IV.

The years 1856-57—"The British Journal of Dental Science"—Co-operation with the college scheme—Change of proprietorship, and altered opinions—Proposed "Quarterly Journal of Dental Science"—The medical press and the college movement—Antagonistic journalism—The objects of the Odontological Society—Statement by the president, 1857—Increased energy of the college party—Introduction of Medical Bills into Parliament—Notice to the profession thereupon by the College of Dentists—Features of the year—Diminution of party feeling—Mr. R. Reid and mediation—Meeting of Mr. Tomes and Mr. Underwood—Impression on the profession thereby . . 75

CHAPTER V.

Messrs. Tomes and Underwood as delegates—Propositions for amalgamation of opposing societies—Appointment of more delegates—Terms of union arrived at—Mr. Rogers and Mr. Robinson at the first dinner of the Odontological Society—Terms of amalgamation submitted to meeting of the College of Dentists—Their rejection—Resignation of college officials—Resolution of the Odontological Society—Law of vote by proxy at the College of Dentists—Dissension at the college meeting—Action of the Odontological Society—The College of Surgeons—Notice of the Bill of Mr. Headlam, M.P.—Petition of Odontologists to College of Surgeons—Reply—Its effect on the College of Dentist's party—Further memorialising by the Odontological Society—Further replies—Proposed clause in the Medical Bill—Secession of college members, and protest by seceders—Counter-circular by Mr. Rymer—Proposed Dental School and Hospital by the Odontological Society—Organisation of the Dental Hospital of London—Its opening—Criticism by the opposite party—Electricity in dental operations—Committee of investigation appointed—Hopes of a charter for College of Dentists—Medical legislation—Success of the Odontological Society's memorial to the College of Surgeons . . 111

CHAPTER VI.

New dental journal—Activity of the College of Dentists—Curriculum for acceptance by the council of College of Surgeons—Opinion of the "Dental Review"—Violent party spirit—Internal action of the College of Dentists—Fresh courage—Amendment of college laws—American opinion—The Metropolitan School of Dental Science organised by the College of

Dentists—The initials M.C.D.E.—Opening of the Metropolitan School of Dental Science—Legal action taken by the Medical Registration Association—Opposition by the College of Dentists—The entire profession addressed—Petition to the House of Commons. Petition for a charter for the College of Dentists—Increase of the Odontological Society—Determined opposition of the two sections of the profession . . . 143

CHAPTER VII.

Institution of Board of Examiners at Royal College of Surgeons, 1860—Protest against the College of Dentists by the Odontological Society—Counter protest by the College of Dentists—"The Lancet"—Other medical journals—Strife on the increase—First examination of candidates for the licentiateship in dental surgery—The London School of Dental Surgery instituted—Tenacity of the College of Dentists—Terms of membership with the Dental College—Education—Hope of success and assertion of strength by the "Independents"—"The Lancet" condemns the College of Dentists—Mr. Waite's reply—Inauguration of the National Dental Hospital—Mr. Makins' work on "Metallurgy"—Death of Mr. James Robinson—Presentation to Mr. Tomes—Dinner to foreign dentists—Longings for the cessation of strife 167

CHAPTER VIII.

The College of Dentists and dissolution—Extinction of hope and consequent action of Mr. Rymer—Overtures by the College of Dentists on the subject of amalgamation to the Odontological Society—Appointment of sub-committee—Result—Amalgamation considered in full meeting of Odontological Society—The "glorious minority of one"—Complete fusion—Recognition of Mr. Rymer's and Mr. Hockley's past labours—The Dental Students' Society—Proposed method of dealing with advertisers—The late Mr. Lawrence's opinions—Proposed extension of time to candidates for the licentiateship's degree—Petition to the council of Medical Education and Registration—Result—The licentiates and the "Medical Directory"—The Odonto-Chirurgical Society of Edinburgh established—Professional sympathy with Mr. Statham—Nitrous oxide—Committee of investigation—Report thereon—Testimony concerning anæsthetics—Testimony of the profession to the claims of Mr. Horace Wells—College of Surgeons' concessions to licentiates

—Proposal by Mr. Saunders to remove the Dental Hospital—
Counter proposition by Mr. W. Ash—Result—Mr. T. A.
Rogers first Dean of the Dental Hospital of London—Address
to the students 195

CHAPTER IX.

Dental Reform in Edinburgh—Dr. Smith and the Odonto-Chirurgical Society—Difficulties and defections—Determination to proceed—Result—Edinburgh Dental Dispensary—Feeble progress of the charity—Liverpool Dental Hospital—Its originator and first supporters—Progress—Increasing usefulness—Plymouth Dental Dispensary—The projectors and first workers—The value of the charity—Birmingham Dental Dispensary—Its founder and the usefulness of the institution—Spread of such centres of public and professional benefit—Prospect of recognition of all well-directed schools of dental surgery . 242

CHAPTER X.

Benefactors of the dental profession—Short notices of Mr. J. M. Arnott—Mr. S. Cartwright—Mr. De Morgan—Mr. C. J. Fox—Mr. W. A. Harrison—Mr. R. Hepburn—Mr. J. H. Parkinson—Mr. James Robinson—Mr. A. Rogers—Mr. S. L. Rymer—Mr. E. Saunders—Mr. J. Tomes—Mr. T. Underwood—Mr. E. Sercombe—Mr. A. Coleman—Mr. Kempton—Mr. Hockley Mr. T. A. Rogers—Mr. D. Hepburn—Mr. Newman—Mr. Parker—Mr. S. Bate—Mr. Belfour—Mr. Trimmer . . . 260

CHAPTER XI.

Present position of the profession—Its recognition and status—Dental literature—Journalism and professional demands—Professional conduct—Method of manipulation—Recognition of the importance of the dental profession by the medical practitioners and the public—Spread of its influence—Education—Registration—Conclusion 353

APPENDIX 385

ERRATUM 400

HISTORY OF THE REFORM IN THE DENTAL PROFESSION.

CHAPTER I.

A RETROSPECT of dentistry as it existed some thirty years ago in this country is by no means a pleasant study. From such a standpoint there is very little to encourage, and much which can only be looked upon with a feeling, to say the least, of regret. That, however, which is uncongenial, or in direct opposition to the tastes and inclinations of those concerned, has often to be accepted and dealt with as a necessity by them. No picture is complete without its background; and although the sombre shading may prove to be the least pleasant portion of the artist's work, the dashing and effective high lights would lose their brilliancy without it. So with the subject which will form the substance of the following pages. It is not only needful but imperative that the dark background formed by the ignorance, disorganisation, and empiricism of that epoch should be mentioned, in order that the bright and clear light of education, order, and progress, as they now exist, may be more effectively seen and appreciated. Really, to understand our present position legally, socially, and professionally, we must know what we then were in those respects. To value the advance made, we must see and estimate our circumstances at the point of departure. Looking back, then, to those days, it cannot fail to be observed that the dental art was exercising a fascinating power over the minds of many, and inducing considerable numbers to attempt to practise it. From the records available it could be easily seen that large proportions of those dentists (?) were ignorant of the merest rudiments of this branch of surgery, and were totally dependent upon their unblushing effrontery playing its part upon the outside public for the measure of success they hoped to attain. Nor were the men of that day different from those who had preceded them— that is, of course, those who were really ignorant. For long years before, dentistry had apparently offered tempting facilities to uneducated individuals to practise it; and, if we can trust the statements made by various writers on the subject, its characteristic was that of being hampered by the unprincipled and unscrupulous. It may be safely affirmed that, at the time when this record commences, the great bulk of dentists practising in the United Kingdom, of whom there were some hundreds, were, as a class, sadly lacking in scientific knowledge. Scattered through the cities and towns of our land were to be found those who evidently had no idea of what a profession, as such, demanded at their hands. Many had entered upon the practice of dentistry as a means of obtaining a livelihood only, and had not hesitated to combine with it a trade of some sort or other, in order to secure a larger emolument than dentistry, *per se*, would bring to them. Others, again, had abandoned their former calling for this one, under the impression that it was an easy and simple thing to be a dentist. The author has heard of those who had been milkmen, watchmakers, &c., who had no scruple in posting the words "surgeon-dentist" on their door-plates, in the hope of making the passers-by believe they were what they thus professed themselves to be. Advertisements were plentiful, and the most wonderful announcements constantly appeared in the daily press, setting forth the miraculous ability and the fascinatingly low fees of these dental magicians. Others, again, openly displayed their tradesman-like principles by keeping shops for the exhibition of anatomical preparations, casts of mouths, and metal-gilt dentures, and in some cases wrote up their names in decayed teeth. Sober-minded and really respectable men, who hoped by honourable effort and proper professional conduct to advance their position, felt it to be a reproach when called by the name of dentist. Originally drawn to this special branch of surgery by the highest motives, they found that to practise it they must be associated in the minds of the indiscriminating with those whose character and conduct they indignantly repudiated. While the large majority of practitioners, then, were to be ranked among the partially educated or absolutely ignorant, still dentistry as a composite profession, one embracing both science and art, was not without representative men. In each of these departments were to be found names which can never be mentioned without the respect that real worth, high principles, and unsullied integrity, coupled with skill, must ever command. Like lofty peaks in a mountain range, they showed clear and bright above others; but they were the great and glorious exceptions to those around them. At their base lay the broad valley of empiricism, steeped and bathed in the mists of ignorance, and claiming recognition by the noise of its own impudent pretensions alone. Here and there were to be seen those who upon the smallest amount of information were practising as dentists, some, perhaps, well content to know nothing more than the alphabet of their daily calling so long as the result, in the direction of fees, proved satisfactory; while others may have hoped to obtain knowledge sufficient to enable them to rise to a level above the unblushing rascality of so many among them. Tooth-extraction in those days appears to have been a principal source of revenue. Who has not heard of what we would fain hope was a legendary character after all, viz., the blacksmith who drew teeth for sorrowful village urchins? Barbers, for many years preceding, had enjoyed the almost prescriptive right to be considered dentists—that is, if extracting teeth constitutes a man a dentist. But in the time to which allusion is more particularly sought to be made, the extraction of teeth had gradually been relegated to the chemist, who perhaps might lay more claim to the *savoir faire* than the barber or the blacksmith. That this portion of dental practice largely obtained then there is no question or doubt whatever. The great cure for the terrible pain arising from a carious tooth was extraction. People flocked, especially the poor, to the chemist for help and deliverance from torture, and at a nominal cost to them he was prepared to operate. Wardroper in his work on tooth-drawing (1838) informs us in a foot-note (page 9) of this custom thus: "As a proof of the prevalence of tooth-drawing, I know a chemist in a large country town, who some time ago assured me that he received £200 *a year* from drawing teeth at one shilling each. On examining these teeth—the greater part of which he had preserved —I found none of the fangs in the least degree affected." If we can accept the above statement as true, we have the astonishing number of four thousand teeth removed by one man, in one town, in the course of one year. The calculation carried a little closer, and allowing fifty-two Sundays for rest—needed alike by operator and patients we should say—there yet remain twelve and a fraction of teeth to fall to the busy chemist each day during the year. Those who practised as dentists only were then in the habit of increasing their returns to a considerable extent by the sale of such accessories to the teeth as might find a place on the dressing or toilette table of their patients. This practice was not considered incompatible with the respectability or professional status of the dentist.

Although distinctly appertaining to the shopkeeper, and really claimed by the vendor of drugs as legitimately his, nevertheless, the dentists of those days made no scruple of engaging in this branch of trade. Many based upon their possession of such and such remedies a more distinct appeal to the public for their confidence in and patronage of themselves, and in their published works drew the attention of their readers unhesitatingly to the fact. The following quotation from Woofendale (1833) among others is to the point: "Dentists have in general various preparations under the title of *dentifrice, tooth-powder, electuary, &c., &c.,* which for many reasons they preserve as secrets; and each, no doubt, recommends his own. I have a preparation of that sort (*dentifrice*) peculiar to myself, which I have used for many years; and as it has always answered my utmost wishes, I hope I may stand excused recommending it for that purpose." And again, further on, "The lotion here alluded to is such as I can recommend, and is peculiar to my own practice; and as it has in the course of an extensive practice fully answered my expectations, I am enabled to offer it in this place to the public. I hope the same reasons that have been offered when treating of the *dentifrice* (p. 17), will be thought a sufficient apology for not explaining its composition."

With the merest verbal alterations to suit the articles on sale, such an announcement as the above would be admirably adapted for the flying circular of the smallest tradesman. No new trick by which apparent success could be hoped for failed to obtain a prominent place in the public announcements continually being made. The public were posted up with a remarkably systematic and ingenious regularity concerning the wonderful discovery made by this or that individual, of course, after years of laborious research and patient investigation, and at the cost of a fabulous amount of money, whereby, for a consideration, all the evident advantages thus obtained could be placed within reach of suffering humanity. Those who thus appealed to the public seemed perfectly oblivious to the fact that they thereby cut the ground on which they essayed to stand from under their own feet, and forfeited every claim to be considered professional men. They had the soul of the shopkeeper, the spirit and method of the tradesman; and although there can be, and in fact is, nothing of which any one need be ashamed in following the walk of commercial life, yet professional life is, and always will be, very distinct from it. At that time, a very heavy percentage of those who were in practice, if they could be called in the profession at all, were not at all careful to uphold its honour by their acknowledgment of and obedience to professional canons. It may also be truthfully said that many were totally devoid of that education which would enable them to properly practise at all. Dentistry, in fact, very much resembled the border warfare of feudal times. Every man was "fighting for his own hand." Any step in advance, achieved either by industry or accident, was carefully hoarded as a secret, to be used for the possessor's own benefit, and recourse was had to the Patent Office that it might become legally his personal property. Nor should the fact be omitted, that the spirit of personal advancement by questionable, if not disreputable, methods was not confined to the lowest class of practitioners. It was no uncommon thing for men of better stamp to dabble with the dubious, though they might hesitate to touch the unclean thing. We have, indeed, only to look a very little way back to see gentlemen of the highest position permitting their names to be associated with tooth-powders, &c., sold at fashionable shops in the fashionable quarters of London. It would be an interesting study, and, to those whom it most concerned, perhaps a useful and instructive one, to try and ascertain how the amount of money, directly or indirectly gained by them in this unprofessional manner, looks by the side of the loss of respect which they have sustained through such transactions in the estimate of all true practitioners. Facts in parallel columns, as a rule, are easily remembered. The press has all along been brought into frequent requisition in connection with dentists and their art. With some honourable exceptions, however, the publications which have appeared have had but one end in view, which the various writers sought, and too often with a transparent eagerness, to attain. To use the mildest terms, it may be fairly said that they were written with an eye to popular acceptance. As a rule, their contents were interlarded with medical and semi-scientific phraseology to give a spice of profundity. The dainty appeals made to parents' susceptibilities about the teeth of their children—the enumeration of difficult cases for treatment overcome by the superior skill of the author—the ample resources at hand for meeting every kind of circumstance liable to present itself—and even the "getting up" of the productions in crimson or purple covers, gilt edges, superior paper, and every other possible attraction, could not hide the real motive of the writer. In looking over some of these productions as they lie on one's table, with their coloured illustrations of "the human face divine" in one aspect, and distressingly human in another, according to the will of the beholder and the skill of the artist, the conclusion forces itself upon the mind, that if the publication did not answer the end contemplated, it failed not from want of ingenuity, trouble, or expense, not to mention another though short and expressive word. In some of these books coloured delineations of the teeth and gums with their diseases appeared. The instruments also necessary for operations upon the mouth were represented by coarse engravings, and their uses described in what must have been to the non-professional reader terribly suggestive language. A few quotations from the prefaces, introductions, or body of these books will speak for themselves; they are *verbatim et literatim* copies. The following is taken from a work which appeared under Royal patronage and was dedicated to a Prince of the blood royal :—

(1824.) "The short time allowed to individuals in this troublesome and transitory life, should induce sentiments of *Samaritan feeling* for fellow-sufferers, amidst mankind in general, and the *Medical* class in particular, who from inspections and calculations, *behind the scenes*, of the complicated *cords, pulleys*, and *levers* which keep Life's Theatre, the Human Frame, in motion, are best adapted, from reading and research, and the happy combination of Theory and Practice, to promulgate and establish most valuable additions to the general stock of useful knowledge. Under this impression, the Opinions on the Causes, Effects, and Mode of cure for TIC DOULOUREUX, herein contained, are humbly offered to the Public, and if through their perusal, and subsequent consideration, they can be found to conduce in any shape to the comfort, or amelioration of the many suffering *victims* of this *disease*, the happiness afforded to them and their relative connections, will be felt in a tenfold degree by the delighted AUTHOR."

(1826.) "Having recently obtained a double Patent for a newly-invented Instrument for extracting teeth, and also for a new and very superior method of fixing artificial teeth, I shall, after a few prefatory observations, submit to the Public, in this tract, as concise a description as possible of the two inventions above named, being fully persuaded that a simple statement of the subject will be sufficient to ensure a very extended approbation and patronage."

(1836.) "That which was at first a duty, by dwelling long and intensely on it, is gradually exalted into a pleasure ; every difficulty overcome, every error detected, every new discovery made—all are so many fresh sources of gratification, tending to attach us to that particular study, and to create a proportionate indifference to other occupations. I mention this as some excuse if I should seem to lay too great stress upon my own pursuits, or to triumph too immoderately upon the success of my efforts to found a rational system, in place of the crude and uncertain practice which has hitherto prevailed amongst the dentists. That I have succeeded, I must needs flatter myself, since I have been so informed by those who, from their high rank, are not likely to descend to compromise the truth, while their knowledge affords an ample assurance for the integrity of their judgments.

"The object of this work being to inspire confidence in a system, resulting from long experience and mature consideration, by which the beauty and health of the mouth and teeth may be established for life, it is most respectfully dedicated to the most valuable portion of Society, the Mothers of the Rising Generation, by their sincere friend and devoted servant THE AUTHOR.

"But how different is the state of things in the present day (1836): the exclusive self-complacency of the empiric is considered as disreputable as it is found ordinarily unsuccessful; and he who builds the hope of professional success on the basis of advertised self-praise, though for a brief time he may delude the ignorant or the unwary, in the end must find the level of his own merit; whilst with the more rational classes of the community, his expedient is as vain as it is dishonourable."

Whether the above deliverance of what is intended to be a pure and virtuous statement is in accordance with established fact need not be discussed. The consideration of what appears in connection with another of these works may help those who care to do so to form a conclusion. It would appear that there must have been a considerable demand for these books if we judge by the inordinate supply. As literary productions it may fairly be inferred they must have yielded no small profit. Whether or not, the following announcement, taken from the pages of the next on the list, is sufficiently significant; the little book alluded to appeared in 1837, as the second edition. Concerning the first issue, we are informed in the preface that "the sale of eleven thousand copies in this country alone, in little more than four years, with few of the ordinary aids employed in such cases," had induced the author to prepare a new and enlarged edition. A foot-note then gives what, perhaps, after all, was the real incentive to this step: "It has also been reprinted in France, Germany, and America, and has circulated extensively in each of these countries. The author has been consulted by persons from all parts of the continent of Europe, from America, from the East and West Indies, and in more than one instance from China, who had become acquainted with him through this little work in those parts of the world. He has also been informed that an edition in French has appeared, and that another is in progress, or published in German." What sort of information lay between the covers of this particular publication it is not necessary to mention, after such a circulation and reception by, up to then, an unenlightened world. If angling through the press could draw individuals to the consulting-room of the writer, and from all parts of the globe, another edition to tell the rest of suffering humanity the astounding fact is, perhaps, a sufficiently justifiable proceeding. When we arrive at the end of this second edition, and the record, consequently, of all the wonders of nature and art in this department of study, a final farewell appears in italics to the following effect: "*Casts and preparations of the cases referred to, and others, as well as models illustrative of the various methods of Restoring lost Teeth, I shall feel happy to exhibit and explain to any persons who may feel interested in the subject;*" and then, in capital letters underneath, "AT HOME FROM 11 TILL 4." How the writer of that work could escape or hope to escape from the condemnation of being an advertiser it is difficult to say; at any rate, the way to such a conclusion was open and easy. The press, we are informed, however, accepted it, and the author was lecturer on the anatomy and diseases of the teeth at one of the Metropolitan hospitals. But to take another instance: "The experience of the author for a series of years, in regulating the teeth of young persons, has been extensive. A long period is indeed necessary to make observations of the dental art. He shall be in a great measure recompensed for the years of laborious assiduity he has given to its study, if the following Treatise shall be the means of rescuing any individual from the afflictions which attend a neglected care of the teeth." This statement is brought to a close by the insertion of the writer's address also. The following is a specimen which speaks for itself, and is interesting as the deliverance of one who called himself "Consulting Dentist, &c., Member of the Royal College of Surgeons in London, and Honorary Doctor in Medicine." Its date is 1842:—

"As some persons are under an apprehension that they must be put to great pain and inconvenience by the removal of teeth or stumps, and other painful operations, before they can be supplied with artificial teeth, I feel it incumbent on me to remove this error, so far as it relates to my system, which requires no removal of teeth or stumps, or any pain or inconvenience whatever, any more than if the article in question were an ordinary piece of dress." . . . "The things called mineral, or Jews' teeth, are now plentifully manufactured of porcelain; but they always look like what they are, and can never be mistaken for teeth. Placed in front of the dark cavity of the mouth, the unnatural material has, necessarily, a very different appearance in day and candlelight, and by acting as a whetstone on any of the natural teeth it comes in contact with, soon wears them away." . . . "Long forceps, or tongs, of enormous weight, are used by non-surgical practitioners, for the purpose of tearing out molar teeth, by which the other teeth often suffer in the operation, from being made to bear the weight of the extraction as fulciment; which, together with the nature of the instrument employed, often destroys them. These irregular practitioners affect to dispense with the lancet, under pretence of stripping the gum from the tooth by pushing their forceps up; but it is sufficiently obvious that no part should either be stripped or torn that admits of being divided by the lancet." In another portion of this work the writer informs us, that "the 'London Directory' contains the names of upwards of one hundred and twenty-five individuals calling themselves surgeon-dentists, a large majority of whom are said to be Jews, while the list of the members of the Royal College of Surgeons reduces the number to seven." Another case may be instanced, where the writer, fearing to extend his rod and line to "earth's remotest bound," hopes by a happy cast among the medical men, and with an appropriate bait upon his hook, to draw out of these quieter waters a sufficient recompense for his ingenuity and trouble. The author has in his possession an autograph letter which accompanied the presentation of the gilt-edged, illustrated *brochure*, and of which the subjoined is a copy:—

. . . .
"GENTLEMEN,—I have taken the liberty of enclosing for your acceptance my Essay on the Teeth, a work treating generally on Dentistry; and beg to inform you that for some years past I have made it a practice to remit gentlemen in your profession 15 per cent. on the amount received through their recommendation. Respectfully soliciting your favours on the above terms, I am, gentlemen, your obedient servant," . . . . . .

This essentially "business man" requires no comment. His malady was chronic by his own confession, and so there is no need to further consider his case. The next instance quoted shall be the concluding one. It saw the light of day in 1854, and conveys to the reader's mind that the writer would not only increase his practice, but at the smallest amount of inconvenience and expense to himself. The italics are in the original. " The author would impress upon all who read or in any way profit by this work, that it would be *an act of kindness to present it to any friend who may require the aid of the dentist.*" These, then, are a few selected specimens of the writings put before the public in connection with the dental profession about a generation since. The veil covering them is too miserably thin to prevent the merest tyro discovering the true intentions of the writers. There is no necessity to deepen the colour of this background, or disgust the reader by alluding to the grosser sort of publications. With these the profession has been defiled and disgraced from the earliest date; and in the absence of any enactment of the legislature to prevent, by prohibition, ignorant, unprincipled, and rapacious men from practising as dentists, we dare not hope for their cessation. If those among us who hold respectable positions will persist in rushing into print with their adulterations of Hunter, Blake, Fox, or other later and celebrated authors, and succeed in their fondest hope and strongest aim, it cannot create surprise in any intelligent mind that other and less fortunate men venture before the public in the naked deformity of their own impertinent ignorance. This was the result of such practices in the days of which we speak; and the constant flow of the baser sort of announcements, which incessantly invade our letter-boxes and the domain of our kitchen-maids, proves that the effect is of the same order now. Supposing the intentions of the writers of those days to have been irreproachably disinterested, the question remains, Was writing others down ever likely to produce a proper and complete result? But the shafts of ridicule and reproach which were thus launched against them by those more pretentious writers did not darken the atmosphere enough to hide the evident selfishness which actuated so many of those apparently indignant essayists in taking up the pen.

Out of nearly fifty of these publications at hand for investigation, scarcely one can be found without a doleful lament, and in the majority of them a positive Jeremiade over the naughty men and their doings. In the bulkiest of these books, all the way down to the cheapest of them all in price, we find either protest, fiery denunciation, or scorn, &c., &c., as the fancy flies. In some instances it is really laughable to read the remarks on this head. With what plaintive printed sighs do our authors assure the public—that dear, kind, indulgent public—how gratified they will be if they " shall have corrected erroneous notions, or imparted salutary advice, so as in any degree to have arrested the progress of empiricism ! " They draw over their own ink-stained fingers the whitest of kid-gloves, and with lifted shoulders and outstretched arms implore the deluded, but patiently enduring, outside world to remember that they are the only individuals capable of taking care of its interests, so far as the teeth are concerned, at the least, and how delighted they will be to become the fortunate deliverers of the prey from the spoiler. Doubtless ! It appears that the idea never occurred to those gentlemen that example is stronger than precept. They were in ignorance of, uninterested in, or oblivious to the true principle of real reform. Charlatanism was the child of ignorance and presumption, and while those who could instruct, enlighten, and lead preferred the easier, and, to them, more remunerative method of writing works or pamphlets of indifferent merit, and thereby parading their names before the public, there could be no reasonable hope of professional pretenders taking a different course. Darkness was to be dispelled then as it is now by light taking its place, and this aspect of morality was not to be had then any more than it is now, by wishing for it on the one hand, or the mere denunciation of immorality on the other. As we endeavour to get a clear view of the state of dentistry at that time, one or two matters become conspicuous. We see gross ignorance as the general characteristic of many if not most of those who practised it. Attempts at personal recognition constantly being made, some feeble, some furious, according to the idiosyncrasy and circumstances of the parties concerned. Those who were irreproachable in character and conduct holding aloof, as by a natural law, from those who were tainted in any degree. Others who could not claim actual purity, trying to assume it, and wishing the beholder to believe it. While many who took the pen in hand could not wield it ingeniously enough to hide their thirst for greed, or disguise the (to others) distressing malady of "the first person singular on the brain," from which they were evidently suffering. The pictures they presented to the public were certainly enshrined in more decent frames and surroundings than the coarser sort appeared in, but the design was ever the same in all alike. When once these treatises had emerged from the press, the industry and ingenuity employed to circulate them was remarkable. The author has heard of one method which has the merit of boldness about it. Advantage was taken of the opportunities afforded by the carriages of the wealthy and influential stopping at the doors of the houses of well-known dentists, to scatter, during the absence of the owners, a supply of these little works through the open windows of the vehicles. This may be called the aggressive style. Another method which has come to the author's ears was the packing away, in large numbers, of copies of the work in question in cases containing other commodities destined for foreign parts. This may be termed the cautious style. But what is strangest of all is the favourable notice which was taken of some of the most inferior of these productions by the medical press, and by which a reading was gained for them in many directions where, otherwise, they would most justly have been altogether unknown. How this was obtained, whether by the reviewers' ignorance of the subject before them, or by the mere printing of the notices in question prepared by some friendly hand, or even the hand of the original writer himself, or by the subtle and strong influence of another and easily-guessed agent, it is needless now to discuss. An indiscriminating public offered temptations too strong to be resisted by the rapacious and unprincipled empiric pretending to practise what to a very large extent was considered to be a semi-mysterious art. Opportunities abounded for throwing dust in the eyes, and the occasion was diligently utilised. Under the garb of censors many appeared upon the scene, book in hand, earnestly asking the same public to consult their pages first, and, through their writings, themselves afterwards, until the profused remedy proved as bad as the disease. Looking upon the thousand and one literary efforts in connection with the dental profession of the past generation, it is only after a terribly long process of sifting and sorting that the eye rests upon that which the judgment and a sense of justice can approve. The most of them were, in fact, but the nineteenth-century version of the old notice-board lately presented to the Odontological Society of Great Britain as a curious relic of a bygone age, and of which the following is a correct copy:—

Thos. Smith Glazier, Let Blood & Draw Teeth att 3 Tea Kittels & Potts Buckels Lantrens Cups To Be Handled Heare.

CHAPTER II.

In the year 1841 Mr. Waite issued a pamphlet embodying his regrets at the then condition of the dental profession, and offering suggestions for what he conceived would tend to its amelioration and improvement. The paper was called "An Appeal to the Parliament, the Medical Profession, and the Public, on the Present State of Dental Surgery. By George Waite, Esq., Surgeon-Dentist, M.R.C.S., &c. London : Highley & Co., Fleet Street." The following are some of the writer's remarks :—" I purpose showing the necessity of the legislature and the medical profession recognising this (*i.e.*, dentistry) as a legitimate branch of the science, and that no persons be permitted hereafter to practise without having undergone examination by one or more censors of the Royal College of Surgeons. As it now is, dentistry can be considered no profession; a person, however illiterate and uneducated, may commence practice: and society being unprotected, there is no reason why he may not be consulted; in which case, there being no guarantee that he is professionally competent, he may operate on a tooth in the neighbourhood of an incipient malignant tumour, and thereby do the greatest mischief ; for it can hardly be supposed that he can know the diseases to which the jaws are liable, their intricate anatomy, and all kinds of irritability which ill-judged dental operations may give rise to."
. . . "To me it appears extraordinary that in this great capital, the most enlightened in Europe, and in this age of advanced science, such charlatanism should not directly be checked; and I have no hesitation in saying, that the ranks of the profession and the interests of

society demand legislative interference." . . . "Among dentists, at present, no cordiality exists; first-rate science has been confined to a limited few; no new and essential theories on practice have been suggested under fear of piracy; narrow feelings entertained towards each other; and the practice of the one, however perfect, depreciated by the other to answer his own selfish views." . . . "The College of Surgeons might easily nominate a board of officers from dentists, members of their college, who might issue diplomas to such dentists as undergo competent examinations, and act as censors appointed for that purpose; and hereby they would place an important branch of the profession on a high footing, which would contribute materially to the welfare and health of the community. Dentists likewise would enjoy many advantages under such regulations; for it is but fair to state that many are not properly remunerated under the present system. This would not be the case did a better understanding exist generally."
. . . . "That it may not be thought I am adverse to the practice of many dentists in our metropolis, I beg most distinctly to assert that I wish by no means that changes should be made unacceptable to the regular and present respectable members of our profession, whether recognised or not by any scientific body. It is but justice to remark, that among their number are men who, although unprivileged by diplomas, are of high honour and respectability." . . . . "Accordingly, with all this evidence before us, it is manifest that the interposition of the legislature is demanded to place dentistry, which is *de facto* a branch of surgery, on a legitimate footing. The interests of the medical profession and the public alike support the appeal which I have thus, perhaps imperfectly, submitted. But perhaps I might subjoin a view of the system of education which I should recommend a dentist to pursue. Mathematics and mechanical philosophy should form the groundwork of his education. I would urge that it

ought to be imperatively demanded by the Medical Reform Bill that he pursue a system of work for three years at least, to gain a steadiness of hand and a thorough knowledge of instruments." .... "I would have every dentist well versed in chemistry, have attended three courses of lectures on anatomy, physiology, and surgery, and also have pursued hospital practice. This should qualify him for examination. His licence to practise, or his diploma, should be given to him on his qualifications being proved, and his pupils afterwards always apprenticed to and examined by a board of officers. There might exist a reserved clause that all dentists being established at this time should be examined as to their qualifications, and their age noticed; and wherever gross abuse has existed, and can be proved, the licence should be refused." These were some of the more salient points in the pamphlet, and are interesting when read under present circumstances, indicating as they do the existence of a strong desire for professional reform, and giving evidence of embryonic or fœtal life, prepared to make itself manifest in the direction of scientific progress. What was the result of this publication it is not possible to say. Whether it was ever extensively distributed it would be difficult to assert. But, assuming that it was largely circulated, and thoroughly considered, it could only claim to be classified with other and similar isolated attempts at improvement. Although a highly respectable, and, from the surgeon's point of view, a qualified practitioner, Mr. Waite appears not to have possessed sufficient influence among dentists generally to induce them to respond to his desires; or else the dogged selfishness and want of cordiality of which he complained was too deep-seated to give way before his individual "appeal." At any rate, the dark waters of ignorance and prejudice of that day seemed to flow on untroubled as before, and no light was yet on the horizon.

Whether influenced by Mr. Waite's appeal or not, or, if influenced by it at all, to what extent, it is not easy to say; nevertheless, during the year 1842, Mr. James Robinson, whose name will be more freely mentioned in the course of this work, endeavoured to raise the profession by means of a dental society. His idea was in the direction of organisation first, and, when that was effected, then education, with its upraising power, was to be introduced and energetically worked. Mr. Robinson was a man of such remarkable activity and energy, that it looked very much as though his proposal would succeed from this cause alone, yet, on trial, the terrible apathy and the strong jealousies which prevailed were too powerful for him, and his scheme unfortunately had to be abandoned.

Further than this there does not appear to have been any particular manifestation made in the direction of progress. At any rate, a sort of calm prevailed. The essential quality of ripeness or readiness for definite action had not been attained, or, if it actually existed, no person appeared on the scene to take advantage of it. Those who have had to hold a prominent position in any such matters have given testimony to the fact, that reform in any class needs not only able leaders, but an assurance, more or less certain, that, at their signal to advance, there should be a sufficient number of followers to obey their word. The fitting moment was likewise to be evident to them. In the early part of the year 1843 a Bill was being laid before the House of Parliament, in which, at the instigation of many provincial surgeons, certain clauses were sought to be introduced, whereby the charter of the Royal College of Surgeons would be materially altered, and, as the petitioners considered, improved. The college authorities were in the dark as to the general scope and tenor of the Bill, which was known as Sir James Graham's Bill, and had only been consulted upon several clauses, and at the last moment. The opportunity, however, seemed convenient to the minds of some of the leading dental practitioners for an effort to be made to introduce the claims of dentists to have the profession included in the measure. At a meeting held at the house of Mr. Arnold Rogers in Regent Street, March 4, 1843, the following gentlemen being present, namely, Messrs. Nasmyth, Tomes, Saunders, Stokes, Parkinson, Morell, and A. Rogers (chair), it was resolved that two of their number, Mr. Rogers and Mr. Stokes, should wait upon the president of the Royal College of Surgeons, and ascertain from him whether this Bill did or would include dentists in its provisions.

On the following day, Sunday, March 5, 1843, the deputation saw the president of the Royal College of Surgeons (Mr. White), who appears to have been exceedingly cautious in his answers, and gave his opinion with what looks now like tartness. He considered that "the members of the college practising exclusively the dental profession were, in strictness, *seceders*," and even asked the deputation whether, "in the event of a case being brought to them, they would set a limb, or reduce a dislocation." With the proper prudence which becomes the head of this learned and important body, Mr. White also "seemed desirous to know if they contemplated a participation in the government of the college." This aim the deputation instantly disavowed. The president was then informed that it was the intention of the respectable body of dentists to memorialise the college and Sir James Graham. He begged they would not memorialise the college, but address a letter as members of the body of surgeons—those who held diplomas—and procure as many accompanying notes as they could from gentlemen practising as dentists, but not possessing diplomas, stating their regret that, at the time they became professors of the art, there was no compulsory law in existence. He further advised them to obtain all the facts possible, and lose no time in doing so. The conclusion of this interview was an assurance that the application should have his support, although he as much as feared there would be some who would object to the proposal they sought to make. One or two things may be noticed here. The first is the construction placed by the president of the Royal College of Surgeons on the practice of dentistry by any member of that college. Whoever did so, according to Mr. White's opinion, had thereby *seceded*, which, if it means anything, means *retrograded,* or, in simple phraseology, the individual had lost caste. This idea has been, all along, very pronounced, and it has not yet become extinct. Then, again, we have a very clear evidence of the jealousy with which the sacred table of the governing body in Lincoln's Inn Fields was guarded. Had there been on the part of this deputation the slightest trace of such a desire as that mentioned, no doubt the interview would have been abruptly terminated. Furthermore there is the information, politely enough offered, it is true, that the college authorities could only be appropriately addressed through members of the college. Men who were not *diplomé*, however high their acknowledged professional standing might be, could only appear as train-bearers, and words of regret at their unfortunate position are kindly put into their mouths by the president. Allusion is thus made to this condition of things here, as it will help to explain the difficulties which had to be overcome further on. It is useless to disguise the fact, that a stiffness of demeanour has always, more or less, characterised the members of the College of Surgeons in their intercourse with dentists as such. That such should be so is not surprising. If there is an advantage, both social and professional, in being able to write M.R.C.S.E. after one's name, those who cannot do so need not wonder at the assumption of a superiority by those who can. Whether the exhibition of this in a marked manner and measure has been politic, not to say polite, is a doubtful question. Certain it is that its reiteration has not made respect for the degree, or the holders of it either, any easier than formerly. Especially so when the profession has seen so many painfully evident proofs that the membership of the Royal College of Surgeons did not confer upon its possessors the power rightly to understand or practise dentistry. Another meeting took place at the house of Mr. Nasmyth, March 10, 1843. On that occasion Mr. Nasmyth occupied the chair, and Messrs. Cartwright, G. Parkinson, Tomes, Saunders, Morell, Rogers, Stokes, Bigg, Harrison, J. W. Parkinson, F. Parkinson, and Hyde (solicitor) formed the committee or meeting. The number attending was considerably increased, and the gathering, no doubt, was considered representative of the profession. It is evident these gentlemen were in earnest in the matter before them. Mr. Rogers reported the result of the interview he and Mr. Stokes had had with the president of the Royal College of Surgeons, but he had not been contented with resting things there. Between the two meetings he had made use of the advantage which a professional acquaintance with Major Graham, brother of Sir James Graham, afforded him. He had enlisted that gentleman's interest in the subject they were considering, and had secured his promise to assist them by presenting their stated views to his brother. No time had been lost, for a rough draft of a memorial had been already prepared by Mr. Rogers, Mr. Stokes, and Mr. Tomes, and was there for the consideration of the meeting. The document was read to the meeting by Mr. Tomes. A discussion then ensued concerning the form of the memorial, which eventuated in its being submitted to the revision of Messrs. Nasmyth, Rogers, Stokes, Tomes, and Hyde. These gentlemen were to meet two days further on (12th instant) at Mr. Rogers', for that purpose. Another important matter was discussed, namely, the propriety of *all* memorialising the Council of the College of Surgeons. It resulted in the determination to communicate with the college. The liberty to bring any friend was accorded to each gentleman on the occasion of the next meeting, which was fixed to take place at Mr. Cartwright's house on the 15th instant. Considering who had taken part in these meetings, and the peculiarly exclusive views held by some, it is not very surprising to find a different tone adopted, and a very different condition of things evidenced, when the time came round for the next convention. As appointed, a meeting was held on the 12th, for the revision of the memorial to the College, but one gentleman of importance failed to attend. A little word, of three letters only, which had been introduced into the resolution which brought this meeting together, looks ominously significant as the reason for Mr. Nasmyth absenting himself. That little word is "all." From subsequent correspondence it will be abundantly manifest whether the author is right in his conclusions or wrong. At any rate, when Messrs. Rogers, Stokes, Tomes, and the solicitor (Hyde) met, the first thing to be done was to read a letter from Mr. Nasmyth, stating his reasons for not attending the meeting, or continuing his assistance towards the intended object. Furthermore, on discussing the form which the proposed memorial should take, it was agreed by those present that the following suggestions should be submitted to the next meeting:—"That the best way in which the intended representation could be made to the minister, would be rather by private communication, by way of letter, expressing the opinions of those only who signed it, than by a formal petition or memorial; for it appeared to them that the gentlemen who had hitherto taken part in the proceedings could not be considered to represent the body of dentists, and could not speak in their collective name without a public meeting were first called, and they were by such meeting empowered formally to address the minister; that they were of opinion that such a step would be attended with numerous difficulties, and that the object to be obtained would be more easily or likely to be accomplished by a private communication in the form of a letter to be signed by the parties who should attend the next meeting."

Perhaps it was the influence of the "legal" mind in the person of Mr. Hyde that superinduced the dawning of the truth as to the real position and the validity of action of these evident well-wishers to the dental profession. Their aim and object was laudable, their energy was indisputable ; but their gatherings together were private, and entirely devoid of authority. The mass of dentists outside their circle was by no means an inviting object for contemplation, or that which courted their co-operation in the direction of improvement, and any attempt to maintain and improve the respectability of the dental profession, where it did exist, was entitled to the thanks of every honourable practitioner. The thing to be lamented in this effort is that it did not rest on the right foundation. Those who thus met were truly representative in the sense of their acquirements and scientific and practical knowledge generally ; but no one had commissioned them to act, even beneficially, as they imagined and desired, and therefore in that sense their *representative* character was simply *nil*. While such men as Mr. Nasmyth gathered with them they had internal as well as external difficulties to deal with. The severe spirit of caste and exclusiveness was often painfully manifest, and proved over and again an obstructive to progress in the right direction. Such as he had to learn the difficult lesson that no practical sympathy can be displayed anywhere without a forgetfulness of self. However, when the next meeting came to assemble, with Mr. Cartwright in the chair, the following letter was adopted ; and after the solicitor had called upon Messrs. Bigg, Morell, Sherwin, and Oswin to obtain those gentlemen's signatures, it was forwarded the next day by Mr. Rogers to Major Graham, to be delivered to Sir James Graham for consideration :—

"32 Old Burlington Street, *March* 15, 1843.

"Sir,—We, the undersigned, having heard of your Bill for the better regulation of the medical colleges, would most respectfully suggest for your consideration that part of the profession practised by dentists, and would also present to you an opinion. We earnestly believe that much benefit would be gained by the public were a legislative enactment made which should oblige parties purposing to practise as dentists to pursue a course of education similar to that followed by those intending to practise surgery, and to gain for themselves a similar diploma. Evidence of patients suffering from the ignorance of parties who have not received any professional education, and yet practise as dentists, and who through advertisements delude the public by quackery and fraud, are constantly presenting themselves to our notice. Such gross imposition could not be practised by educated men, as all must be who are qualified as surgeons. We confidently believe that such an enactment would meet with the approbation of the public at large, and of all the respectable members of our branch of the profession. That other nations have considered this subject of importance may be inferred from the enactments of France, Germany, Austria, and America, where those who practise as dentists are required to possess a certificate of qualification, given after examination by an authorised medical body. In England no qualification is imperative; yet the importance of a proper knowledge upon the subject can hardly be doubted when England's greatest surgeon (Hunter) thought the subject worthy of a place in his mind; and that he gave time and thought to it may be seen by referring to his work upon the teeth, their diseases and treatment. With these facts strongly impressed upon our minds, we have considered it our duty thus to address you, and have the honour to be, sir, your very obedient and humble servants,

"Samuel Cartwright, 32 Old Burlington Street.
G. H. Parkinson, Raquet Court, Fleet Street.
J. H. Parkinson, 36 Sackville Street.
Arnold Rogers, 296 Regent Street.
Edwin Saunders, 16 Argyle Street.
W. A. Harrison, 34 Keppel Street, Russell Square.
Charles Stokes, 65 Brook Street, Hanover Square.
John Tomes, 41 Mortimer Street, Cavendish Square.
Frank Sherwin, 14 Bruton Street, Berkeley Square.
Charles Oswin, 72 Harley Street.
Dominique Morell, 1 Langham Place.

"To the Right Hon. Sir James Graham, Secretary of State for the Home Department."

With the general scope and purport of this petition no fault can be found, although exception may be taken to that portion of it where the inference is drawn that the possession of a diploma would prevent empiricism. The history of the medical profession, and in fact every other also, refutes this idea. One thing is noticeable also in connection with this document, that all signing it omitted inserting their qualifications. It is not remarkable, therefore, that Mr. Nasmyth's name was not appended. That gentleman was present when it was resolved that this petition should go forth, and even withdrew his letter, but he was the only objecting party to the resolution. The polite letter by Mr. Rogers which accompanied it elicited from Major Graham the annexed satisfactory reply:—

"GENERAL REGISTER OFFICE, SOMERSET HOUSE,
17th March 1843.

"MY DEAR SIR,—I will with pleasure take a good opportunity of giving to Sir Jas. Graham the letter you have intrusted to my care.—Very faithfully yours, GEORGE GRAHAM.

"To ARNOLD ROGERS, Esq."

It is thus seen that the original position and proposals of these gentlemen—who must be considered true friends to their profession, and as such deserving its thanks— had become considerably modified. Instead of assuming the place and power of dictators to their brethren, they had contented themselves with modestly signifying to the proper minister in parliament what their "opinion" was with regard to the educational necessities of future dentists. True, this opinion thus expressed only bore the signatures of eleven members of the profession, but still several of the names that were appended were those of men of influence, who could claim the unfeigned respect of their brethren throughout the three kingdoms. One gentleman, who, on the score of the authority which his scientific writings alone gave him, Mr. Thomas Bell, does not appear personally to have attended the meetings which led up to the result thus attained. What amount of influence, if any, he may have indirectly used, the author is unable to say. His inflexible adherence to surgical ideas, and rigid severity in insisting upon all dentists receiving a medical education, and possessing a medical degree, can easily account for his abstention from any connection with this movement, or the projectors of it either. Educated as a surgeon, he imbibed such strong sentiments as to the imperative necessity of all men having to do with any department of surgery passing through the college, that all who did not do so called down upon themselves his contempt. This peculiarity has clung to him throughout his entire career. All honour must be accorded to him for his excellent contributions to the scientific literature of our profession, and by which his name is not only known, but justly celebrated; but he cannot claim to have been helpful in the practical reform which has taken place; and this is to be traced to the exclusiveness of his ideas on what constitutes professional fellowship or brotherhood. What his hearty co-operation might have produced is a problem; but, seeing it was not given, there is no need to speculate concerning it. The gentlemen who had been thus endeavouring to bring about an amelioration of the evils which flourished through ignorance, and sought to introduce a higher régime, and offer inducements for the students in dentistry to submit themselves to it, certainly demand the recognition of the profession for their desires to do good, although they could not be commended for the method they adopted of giving them effect. It will be well here to correct the impression which these meetings generally made when the fact of their having been held became known. They were characterised, if not actually stigmatised, as mere occasions of eating and drinking, when, after all, though the social features were not absent, they were really true business meetings. The subjects were formally introduced, discussed, rejected, or adopted, according to all recognised rules, and therefore it is neither just nor true to say that they were simply festive occasions. The document which had been thus forwarded to the state authority was followed up by one addressed to the college as follows :—

"To Anthony White, Esq., President, and to the Council of the Royal College of Surgeons.

"GENTLEMEN,—The attention of the legislature being now distinctly and ostensibly directed to the subject of medical reform, every individual member of the profession, in whatever branch and of whatever rank, is naturally led to inquire into his present position and future prospects; and the profession looks with peculiar confidence to the high character of the present council of the College of Surgeons, so to carry out the projected changes as to leave no branch of the surgical practice unprovided with the means of gradual improvement in knowledge, and of elevation of professional character. Considering, however, the small number of persons recognised by the college who practise the branch of surgery to which we have directed ourselves, and knowing also the limited opportunities generally possessed of appreciating the circumstances and relations of that department of practice, we trust that our testimony in regard to its actual condition, and our advocacy of its claims to your consideration, may not be thought misplaced at this moment. The indispensable importance of this branch of practice to the community at large, and the necessity there seems to be to encourage enlightened views on the subject, may be judged of from the fact, that at present there are no less than about $\frac{1}{10}$th part of the whole aggregate number of practitioners in London occupied exclusively in the real or pretended practice of dental surgery, viz., about 200 out of 2000; but of these 200, twelve only are associated with any of the corporate bodies which preside over medicine, and those are members of the College of Surgeons. We are far from wishing to insinuate that amongst the number whom we have stated to be unconnected with the college there are not many whose high personal character and general knowledge of their profession entitle them to respect and consideration, but as our present object relates exclusively to the projected changes in the constitution of the college, it is only with reference to the few who are of its members that we now by permission approach its council. We are convinced that it must be wholly unnecessary to point out to the gentlemen whom we have the honour to address the intimate connection between the diseases of the teeth and the various organs in immediate relation to them as affecting many of the most important local and constitutional derangements of the human frame; the practice of every surgeon affords him daily proofs of this, and the council must therefore be sensible of the high importance of encouraging this department of surgical science by all the advantages likely to result from the education necessary to become a member of your learned and distinguished body, and it is only by your recognition of this principle that we can hope to have our branch of the profession rescued from the obloquy which has of late been too frequently cast upon it by the malpractices of ignorant and empirical pretenders. Under these circumstances it is to you, the influential and ruling body of our college, that we naturally appeal at this important epoch, and most respectfully yet earnestly submit not only our individual claims, but also the claims of those few others who, being with ourselves members of your college, devote themselves to our branch of the profession, as not unworthy to be recognised in the arrangements now in progress, and to have secured to us that character and that rank to which we believe the regularly-educated surgeon-dentist legitimately entitled. A prominent feature we understand in the projected reform of our college is to consist in the creation of a new grade amongst its members to be called Fellows, and with whom the elective franchise of the governing body is to reside. Now, surely the fact of a member devoting the whole of his time and attention to the study and improvement, and bringing all his professional skill and acquirements to the produce of our art, or any other peculiar branch of the healing art, or to any other given class of diseases, ought to operate as no disqualification for that contemplated and distinguished order, and we do earnestly solicit for ourselves and others practising as surgeon-dentists, that we may not by this projected alteration be left on a footing below gentlemen with whom some of us have been long before the public, connected together either as professional associates or official colleagues. Earnestly confiding our claims to your protection, and relying on your appreciation of the justice thereon, we have the honour to be, gentlemen,

"Your most obedient and faithful servants."

The names of those who signed this document do not appear on the copies of the transaction which Mr. Tomes has placed in the writer's hands, and therefore cannot be inserted; but it is probable that those who appended their signatures to the preceding one did not withhold them from this. At the present time, however, it is not of much importance to attempt to ascertain the certainty, and it therefore may be left in the region of conjecture. Here, also, all record of these meetings ceases. From the present standpoint it is interesting to look back upon and register this attempt to improve the status of the dental profession, and note the opinions which then prevailed, at least with those concerned, as to how it could be best accomplished. The leaning was evidently towards affiliation with the Royal College of Surgeons, a tendency in the minds of those of the survivors which has not undergone alteration in the efforts with which they have been subsequently engaged.

From many causes at that time in operation, which, when regarded as a whole, doubtless left the impression on the minds of the gentlemen who had thus far acted in this matter that the attempt to better their profession was impracticable, the scheme, which had been devised with the best intentions, and pushed forward with considerable energy, was very reluctantly but altogether abandoned.

CHAPTER III.

AFTER the failure of the effort just recorded, for a decade onwards, at least, the profession was in a state of accepted quietude. The falling through of the project was in itself of a discouraging tendency. Either the time or the disposition again to make any further endeavour was evidently wanting. Such practitioners as were worthy of the name felt, or appeared to feel, the hoplessness of real advance, except as might be attained by their own careful and consistent conduct as scientific men. Their example, perhaps, might slowly achieve what the Royal College of Surgeons was unable or unwilling to accord to them. Without a common centre or bond of union, the dentists of that time practised exclusively and primarily for their own individual interests. It must not be understood, however, that the good men and true were callous and indifferent concerning the future of the profession. The position they held had been arrived at after long effort, nobly sustained, and by close and patient study, while the conduct of their practices absorbed their whole time. The habits of the uninitiated around them were, as they ever must be, repulsive to men of unimpeached integrity; and the indisposition or inability of the legislature and the College of Surgeons to carry out their ideas may, together, be accepted as sufficient reasons for no further attempt at advance being made. But while this is easy to understand it is also to be lamented. There were many young and highly respectable men being educated as surgeons, with the ulterior object of practising as dentists. There were others, also, who were serving their articles under those who were practising dentistry upon a very scanty knowledge of its true requirements, but who, they hoped, might impart a sufficiency of practical instruction to them. To such as these the whole aspect and outlook of the profession was very gloomy. The published works to which they had access were by no means numerous, and their technicalities and general scientific terminology were hindrances rather than aids to all who had not commenced their studies in a thoroughly medical school. However, they clung to their books, looked earnestly for opportunities for further information, valued every scrap of it when it was obtained, and were thrown back in dependence on their own courage and patience of hope. Such was the disconnected and estranged condition of the profession, that very few except the parties immediately concerned were aware of the effort which had been made to secure an improved status generally. Even among those who had been so zealously at work there was no particular tie, and it cannot be wondered at that, when that which had brought them together for a time collapsed, they should be content to accept the inevitable, and each retire, as it were, to his own individual and private sphere. A select few occasionally met at each others' houses for social intercourse, but no new plan was talked of, and the profession remained unaltered, and apparently unalterable. Those were dull times and weary days to the young men at their studies. The general hospitals afforded them the only opportunity for gaining experience in operative dental surgery, and it was not all of these valuable institutions that had a strictly dental department. Where, indeed, this was the case, it was but on certain days in each week, and then but for a very limited time, and with comparatively few cases before him, that the dental student might hope to improve himself in that important branch of his profession. Patient plodding on was the only method of procedure open to him. No journal represented him or his interests either. What he wished to know or make known concerning dentistry had to be sought for, or made public through the columns of the ordinary medical press. If he looked to the influential members of his profession, he found them at a great distance from him, and became disheartened by a feeling of isolation; if he turned to the opposite side, he could but be disgusted. If circumstances such as these tended to develop the manly virtues of honest effort and determination, they were none the less disagreeable to those who had to accept them; and not a few felt that anything but dentistry, as a professional pursuit, would be a welcome change. Among those who most keenly felt the failure of the late project, in connection with the Royal College of Surgeons, were Mr. Arnold Rogers and Mr. Tomes. Whether the latter gentleman sympathised with the young men of that day in their disadvantageous circumstances or not, one thing is certain, that about that time, or perhaps a little further on, he devoted himself to the preparation of a course of carefully-considered lectures, which, in his capacity as dental-surgeon to the Middlesex Hospital, he proposed to deliver to the students there. In due course they were given, and not unfrequently to very sparse audiences, in itself another evidence of the indifference to dental matters which then prevailed. Mr. Tomes had largely availed himself of the use of the microscope in his researches, and the result of his labours was a compendium of most valuable information. Many ideas which had been held by other writers of repute who had preceded him were brought out in a new light altogether, and many new and most important theories were given to the profession when these lectures were published. Their reception by the profession generally, and by the younger members in particular, was a very cordial one; and not only in this country, but upon the Continent, and also in America, Mr. Tomes' work on Dental Physiology and Surgery was acknowledged to be a well-advanced and carefully-written standard book of reference. It certainly gave a quiet but strong stimulus to scientific investigation on the subjects treated, and must be considered as a valuable contribution in the direction of true professional progress. The whole scope and tendency of the work was remarkable as a contrast to the trashy productions which were so unblushingly scattered far and wide. Young men found in it a safe and reliable basis on which to work for themselves, while the more difficult points were so treated as to render their comprehension by the student comparatively easy. Apart from the new facts which histological research had enabled the author to bring forward, the distinct advantages arising from the use of " the adapted forceps " which Mr. Tomes had designed, were set forth both in the text, and by means of well-executed illustrations. These same forceps had been the subject of a sharp wordy conflict between Mr. Tomes and the late Mr. Clendon, the latter gentleman having asserted a priority of claim to the design, which, however, eventually but signally failed in proof. The publication of Mr. Tomes' work was, perhaps, the most prominent event in the profession between the years 1848 and 1854. It very acceptably disturbed the ominous quietude of the profession at that time, and gave evidence that in one at least there was a determination to render real service to the cause of progress, by making use of the best, and the then only, method which remained available, viz., instruction. It can be well seen now that had others, fully competent to impart knowledge, occupied their spare moments in giving the results of their accumulated experience to their co-practitioners, or those who were in training for dental practice, instead of standing aloof from the profession as a whole, and to so large an extent from one another, the result would have been a clearing away of many obstacles which lay upon the path of progress. Whether the gentlemen who had endeavoured to rouse the College of

Surgeons to give them the assistance they had sought at their hands on behalf of the profession were watching the course of events, and prepared to act at any moment, is difficult to say. One thing is known, that year after year rolled peaceably on without a sign from high or low, educated and ignorant alike.

While the dentists of this country were thus slumbering, or at any rate inactive, their brethren in America had been organising Dental Colleges for the purpose of properly educating the students who proposed applying themselves to the practice of dentistry proper. The progress which these institutions had already made was noticeable, and doubtlessly noticed by many on this side of the Atlantic. It does not fall within the purpose of this work to give even a *résumé* of the rise and advance of the profession in that country. What had been accomplished there was tolerably well known in England through the medium of the press, although it would be scarcely correct to say that this acquaintance with Transatlantic dentistry generally permeated the profession in Britain. What feeling was shown in the matter was more of a scornful character than otherwise. Very little of the amicable spirit manifested itself, and that possibly arose from insufficient knowledge of the persons themselves, their principles, or their practices. Still, when these same Dental Colleges in America were considered at all, it was only a very natural thing to expect that a wistful, semi-envious feeling, especially among young men, should arise. The question would force itself on the mind, " If these things can be done there, why not similar things in our own style and after our own method here?" At the best, however, these were but mental exercises. No one seemed to care to take the initiative, even if any one had a scheme to propose, and consequently the same monotonous condition of things continued to prevail. Upon the authority of Mr. Rymer, of Croydon, the statement was made in a pamphlet published by him in the year 1857, that during the year 1854–55 "the profession appeared to recognise the importance of organisation, and a general desire seemed prevalent that some means of intercommunication of ideas should be established." There is no doubt that Mr. Rymer had come to know that such was the fact from safe and reliable sources, but it may be safely asserted that the information he had obtained was by no means general or even largely diffused. The great bulk of the profession at that date was, so far as union even in sentiment was concerned, as far from it as it had ever been. Nothing of importance appeared to break the long, straight line of the leaden horizon, and "each for himself" was more or less the motto of that epoch. Whatever may have been the purposes and plans in any individual instance, or whatever great transitions may have been in embryo, it was not until the 25th of August 1855 that any sign of advance was given, or any sound of progress was heard. The first pulsation originated with a letter which Mr. Rymer addressed to the editor of the "Lancet," and published in the columns of that journal. As that letter was the dawn of brighter days, it is but just to transcribe it.

NECESSITY FOR A COLLEGE OF DENTAL SURGERY.
To the Editor of the " Lancet."

SIR,—There are few medical practitioners who have not had come under their notice cases exhibiting the serious consequences resulting from a recourse to the inducements so pertinaciously pressed into public notice by the host of ignorant charlatans practising the *specialities* of surgery and medicine. In these free-trade days it is not for any particular class of men to claim protection for *themselves* in the exercise of their vocation, even though they be fitted through great sacrifice of time, trouble, and expense, to alleviate the sufferings and conduce to the comfort of humanity; yet, when they witness, as the general medical practitioner in common with the properly qualified *special* practitioner commonly *do* witness, such calamities as an eye rendered sightless through the maltreatment of a so-called oculist; the frightful and sometimes irremediable condition of the victim of the quack cancer-doctor; the total deafness occasioned through the pokings and dressings of the puffing aurist ; the suffering and loss (both in teeth and pocket) from the ignorance and extortion of the supposed dentist ; and other distressing evils too numerous to mention, having their sole origin in the ignorance of impudent pretenders,—when, I say, such calamities are witnessed by duly informed and qualified persons, it becomes at once their duty and interest to raise a warning voice, to admonish the *public at large* on the danger of placing themselves in the power of unprincipled and ignorant men. But experience has proved the difficulty of arousing the public mind on so important a subject ; too often the warnings of professional men, be they never so wisely given, are disregarded, perhaps from a suspicion that they are prompted by interested motives, whilst the victimised suffering members of society are not willing to expose those by whom they have been duped, for this would involve the necessity of an *exposé* of their folly in being taken in by the promises of impossibilities held out by charlatanism, as well as discovering to their friends and to the world the fact of their being troubled with corns, or of wearing false teeth. I can speak from experience as to the roguery (for that is not too strong a word) of a very large number of men who call themselves dentists, but who, in reality, are wholly ignorant of the surgical anatomy of the mouth and parts adjacent, as well as of the principles (to say nothing of the practice) of mechanism as applied to dentistry. No wonder such men are the origin of so much disappointment, pain, and, as I believe, death. Now, the question arises, How are the public to be saved from the effects of disreputable practices ? It has been seen that professional remonstrance does not, as a general rule, avail, and that *mauvaise honte* seldom permits the victim of the charlatan to expose him. In the United States of America, Colleges of Dental Surgery are established, wherein the students receive a thorough professional education ; and in that country, unless a practitioner has been through the prescribed course of study in one of these colleges, he cannot be looked upon as an orthodox dentist.

Some few years ago an attempt was made in this country to follow the example of our brethren in America, and to establish a seminary wherein the pupils would have the opportunity of acquiring such knowledge as would entitle them to certificates of qualification ; but, owing to some unfortunate misunderstanding amongst the projectors, this excellent scheme was abandoned. If the College of Surgeons were to appoint a properly-constituted board of examiners, whose duty should be to hold periodical examinations of such candidates as were desirous of obtaining such a distinction, for instance, as might well be termed "Licentiate in Dentistry," I believe that, on the one hand, the public would be spared a vast amount of injury, and that, on the other, dental surgery would take its just position by the side of other liberal professions. The adoption of such a course would in no way interfere with the establishment of a Dental College; on the contrary, such an institution would become almost necessary; for although the certificate of apprenticeship to a recognised practitioner for at least three years might, perhaps, be deemed sufficient to entitle a pupil to present himself for examination, yet in all cases it would be desirable that a few months should be spent at college. I cannot but think that the question now sought to be brought under the notice of the constituted medical authorities will receive the attentive consideration it so eminently deserves. —I am, sir, yours, &c., SAMUEL LEE RYMER.

This, then, was the stone cast by the hand of a true friend to the profession into the silent if not stagnant waters, the widening circles from which have not yet ceased to expand in the direction of genuine reform. The then effects which this letter produced were of a double nature. Among the majority of the profession it was most favourably received; the only hesitation on the part of those who were gladdened by it arose from the feeling that the prospect held out by it was too bright to be realised. This was to be attributed to the fact that so little was mutually known of the instincts, as they may be called, of the profession, that mistrust had ample room to work upon the minds of even the most enthusiastic. The mischievous effects of isolation and estrangement were at that moment most keenly and deeply realised by every genuine practitioner. On the other hand, there were those who, considering themselves to be the heads of the profession, could not but feel the stimulating effect of Mr. Rymer's letter, and were aroused sufficiently by it to take action in the matter. The position and influence which these gentlemen claimed were points which were generally admitted, and most justly so too; therefore they were not matters at all likely to be the subjects of dispute. Numbers, in fact, had, as a matter of course, been quietly and hopefully expecting them to assume the position to which, by their acknowledged attainments, they were most fully entitled. If, indeed, the feeling of the mass of the profession could have been then ascertained, there can be no doubt that it would have taken the form of disappointment that the signal for advance had not emanated from them. Had they but instituted some public method of obtaining the opinion of the bulk of their *confrères*, there is not the least question as to the result being a willingness, aye, even an eagerness, respectfully to listen to any proposition they might have thought it prudent to make for the general benefit. Unfortunately a spirit obtained amongst them which inclined them to separate, if not exclusive, action. This can be accounted for by the general demoralisation which existed in the profession. It was no easy thing to lay aside prejudice, and practise self-sacrifice. Apart from this, also, there was the fact that these gentlemen had their own views as to the method by which reform should be essayed. They were, perhaps, fully informed as to the probable difficulties to be encountered, not only from within but also outside the ranks, and it is but reasonable and just to accord to them full credit for a strong desire to see a proper status given to the profession they were themselves practising with so much success. It must never be forgotten that in England the spirit of "caste" is sufficiently pronounced. There is, and always has been, a certain amount of friction when broadcloth and fustian are brought into even momentary contact. A due consideration of these and other circumstances, as they then existed, may well account for the position which these gentlemen eventually assumed. That there were difficulties, in whatever aspect the position of things was viewed, will be fully demonstrated further on. Looking back now upon the step which eighteen of these dentists thought proper then to take, a feeling of regret as to the plan employed is unavoidable. Many amongst themselves have doubtless felt that, if the end which has since been attained could have been secured by a public and open appeal to the profession, it would have been infinitely better than the method they pursued. However, it is very easy to be wise after the event. Mr. Rymer being pre-eminently a man of energy and action, proceeded to make use of the columns of the "British Journal of Dental Science"* to reiterate his views concerning the establishment of a society of dentists for educational purposes. In the second number of that periodical we find him saying, "I would suggest the immediate organisation of a society of dentists, to meet periodically for the discussion of professional matters generally, but with particular regard to raising the dignity of our body by the establishment of a Dental College." He inserted in the following number of that journal an advertisement, informing all whom it might concern, that he intended to call a public meeting of the profession. The date of this meeting was September 22d, 1856, and the London Tavern, Bishopsgate Street, was selected as the most central locality. As may be readily imagined, such an announcement produced many replies. The condition of the profession was well typified in this correspondence. Some writers caught at the opportunity thus afforded them eagerly. Others wished the effort success, but had grave doubts concerning the issue. There were those who thought the state of things, professionally considered, hopeless; and some, again, were opposed to the project. It need not be added, that many from whom Mr. Rymer might fairly have looked for an opinion did not think it worth while even to notice his proposal. Like a wise administrator, he therefore classified his correspondents, and selecting the men whose ideas, as expressed in their replies, seemed to be most congruous and reliable, he requested their attendance at a preliminary meeting at the London Tavern, two days prior to the advertised gathering. This process of weeding out the faint-hearted and the despairing, left Mr. Rymer, on the occasion in question, face to face with the following :—Messrs James Bate, Bradshaw, Brindley, A. Hill, Hockley, W. Perkins, and C. Smith. The

* First published July 1856.

number was not imposing, but there was in it resolution enough and to spare to form a nucleus for the arrangement of the meeting on the 22d. After the formality which always encumbers the first moments, when men who have been hitherto strangers to each other meet for the first time, had passed off, Mr. Perkins was called to the chair, he being the senior ; and the business of that quiet little meeting in the City was proceeded with in such a systematic but cordial manner, that all present felt it to be a sort of foreshadowing of success. The description given of it in the "Quarterly Journal of Dental Science"—a publication of which some account will be given in the proper place—is correct. It says, "Those gentlemen, then, who formed this little convention, had ample cause for congratulation; for although in itself unostentatious enough, it was the *first stone* in the high wall of isolation loosened and thrown down—the *germ* of brotherly feelings, which was destined in its growth to eradicate the ancient spirit of jealousy and distinction which so highly coloured and completely pervaded the dental profession." When the day of meeting arrived, and the large room at the well-known hostlery was filled, it was curious to see the looks of inquiry as to who this and that individual could be, which spoke from the various countenances with silent but unmistakable evidences. It was indeed necessary that the feeling of separation, which had up to that time all but universally obtained, should cease, and that men should henceforth have ample opportunity of knowing and being known to each other. Mr. Rymer had succeeded in inducing Mr. Alfred Carpenter, M.B., to consent to be present. This gentleman, on Mr Rymer's proposition, was unanimously elected to the chair. And here the question may be asked, "How was it that no leading practitioner took advantage of this evident opportunity for guiding the future destiny of the dental profession?" It has been asked many times since then, and never without great significance. The materials for manipulation were never more plastic than at that time; and had some well-known dentist come to the front, he would not have lacked willing and respectful followers. One, perhaps, more than any besides, could have rendered great and imperishable service at this critical moment; that one was Mr. Thomas Bell. Had he been invited? He had. A letter from him, however, was read, in which he declined to take any part in the evening's engagements. The presidency of the meeting was offered him, but he refused. True, some light showed itself in letters of concurrence from a few men of position. That which, at that time, had the greatest weight was from Mr. E. Saunders. His letter, however, contained a proviso that certain "men who have leisure and zeal as well as ability" should be got as a nucleus and basis. "This," Mr. Saunders said, "you have probably done; and if so, I shall very willingly give it all the aid and support in my power." It was very evident that what was thought necessary to be done would have to be accomplished by those present, in conjunction with others who had only been prevented attending the meeting by circumstances beyond their control, but on whose sympathy and support reliance might be placed. The preliminary meeting which has been mentioned came to an agreement that the three following resolutions should be submitted to the general meeting, viz. :—

First, "That it is the opinion of this meeting that the formation of a society of dentists would, by providing opportunities for intercommunication of ideas on matters of professional interest, prove the means of promoting the advancement of dental science in an eminent degree, and also of establishing feelings of brotherly concord amongst members of the profession, and that, therefore, immediate steps should be taken to organise such a society."

Second, "That this meeting, believing that the interests of the public as well as of the profession demand that an authorised system of professional education and examination should be established, is of opinion that energetic measures should at once be adopted to secure the means necessary to provide these requirements."

Third, "That a committee be now appointed to consider the best means to carry into effect the foregoing resolutions, and to report thereon at a future general meeting of the profession."

After the chairman's address, Mr. Rymer, who was enthusiastically received, and deservedly so, explained the motives by which he had been actuated in thus inviting the profession to assemble together, and set forth in a clear and lucid manner his personal opinions as to what would best meet the exigencies of the body of dentists at large. His observations unmistakably proved the sincerity of his desire for reform, and the confidence he had concerning the success of the enterprise. In a very business-like manner the resolutions were then considered. The first was proposed by (the late) Mr. R. Thomson, seconded by Mr. P. Matthews, and supported by Mr. W. Perkins, and, despite some few dispiriting remarks from Mr. Coker, when put to the meeting was carried unanimously. The second resolution was proposed by Mr. D. Mackenzie, seconded by Mr. A. Hill. It was at this moment a surprise was given to the meeting by a statement made by Mr. A. Coleman, who said that he believed "several leading members of the profession were more generally interested in the question than was supposed. Several of these, feeling the necessity for a special course of lectures for dentists, had laid the matter before the College of Surgeons, and he believed that body was giving their best attention to the subject." This announcement, which was received with astonishment, created in the minds of all present a degree of irritation which appeared ready at one time to develop into a vote of indignation. A spirit was quickly manifested that secret and quietly-coercive measures, from whomsoever originated, would not be tolerated. The step which had thus been privately taken by an unauthorised few was felt to be so unconstitutional and ill-advised that the anticipation of its being realised seemed too feeble to be seriously thought of. The resolution before the meeting was then put, and agreed to enthusiastically. Mr. A. Hockley moved and Mr. W. Perkins seconded the third resolution ; and the result was that the following gentlemen were appointed as an executive committee provisionally :—

Jas. Bate, Brighton.	D. Mackenzie, London.
R. Bradshaw, Camden Town.	P. Matthews, ,,
T. Coker, Taunton.	W. Perkins, ,,
C. Davey, Lewes.	C. Rogers, ,,
C. J. Fox, London.	E. Saunders, ,,
W. Harnett, ,,	C. Stokes, ,,
A. Hill, ,,	E. H. Tweed, ,,
A. Hockley, ,,	R. Thomson, Camberwell.
H. L. Jacob, Bridgewater.	C. Vasey, London.
J. Jones, London.	G. J. Watt, Chelsea.
A. Lows, Carlisle.	R. White, Norwich.

With power to add to their number.

S. L. Rymer and A. Hill, Honorary Secretaries.

It is just to record that at this period of the evening's engagements there was manifested a desire still to have the co-operation of Mr. Thomas Bell in the movement about to be made, and although the wish was expressed by one gentleman present, it was reciprocated by all. So much was this evident, that Mr. Rymer was constrained to read the following letter from that gentleman to prove the inutility of hoping for his assistance:—

"17 New Broad Street,
"*September* 12, 1856.

"My Dear Sir,—Although I assure you I do not underrate the importance of the object you have in view, I feel that the same reasons which led me to decline to take the chair at the proposed meeting would render my attendance at it equally inconsistent. Permit me to add, that the tone of your letter and the sentiment it expresses make me the more regret that it is not in my power to co-operate with a gentleman whose feelings and motives I must highly appreciate.—Believe me, dear sir, faithfully yours, Thomas Bell."

This note was of course final. After the usual formalities the meeting separated, with the feeling that there was a real prospect of genuine reform opening out before them. Although a sense of disappointment at the abstention of those who could have rendered powerful assistance had been experienced, yet those who sincerely desired to see the condition of the profession advanced were by no means daunted, much less dismayed. Here was an opportunity for the manifestation and exercise of what money cannot buy, namely, whole-heartedness, with its inevitable sacrifices. There were sturdy spirits in that meeting; and it was an unspeakable pleasure to them to know that the enterprise did not lean for success on the unstable props of patronage or purse. Had it been so, there would have been the usual patting which generally accompanies the distribution of the surplusage of influential people, or the crude overflow of some plethoric pocket opened, the owner of which desired a little cheap popularity. As it was, the building up of the profession rested on broader bases than bank-notes, or any amount of them. Nothing less than self-denial, energy, tact, prolonged activity, and thorough devotion, and these, too, not in spasms, but in nobly-sustained, disinterested effort, could by any means avail to secure the desired end. The question of that hour was, Could these qualities be found? and if so, were they to be had in sufficient quantity to be made available to meet the necessities of the case? Fortunately this question in its double aspect was answerable, and answered immediately, in the affirmative. The demand having been announced, the supply was secured in the first office-bearers, who, as a whole, met with a firm determination to prosecute their labours with uncompromising consecration. This proved no empty boast, as has been frequently admitted by those who were opposed from the first to their method of procedure. The difficulties in their way were indeed formidable. Shunned by those who could

have given both direction and impetus to the thus
expressed desire of a large body of dentists for a system
of education, they had to push forward as best they
could, in what is understood as "the cold shade."
Having to manipulate the *disjecta membra* of a profession
noble in itself, but at that time suffering from empiricism and ignorance to a terrible degree, they were called
upon to exercise largely tact coupled with conciliation
and firmness. Conflicting opinions among the respectable practitioners had to be delicately weighed, due
consideration being given to all. And amongst many
other impediments stood out prominently the novelty of
the movement which in itself constituted a grave and
serious obstacle. The national characteristic of slowness
to adopt any new idea manifested itself very plainly, and
the more so then as in this case the idea had such far-
reaching, if not actually revolutionising, tendencies.
Add again to these things the opposition which had
been silently and suddenly organised in high places, and
connect this with the sluggishness in the minds of some
men, ranked as supporters, and the work which lay
before this executive committee was by no means contemptible for its quality or amount. It must be
recorded to the honour of these gentlemen, that looking
at it so as to embrace it in its entirety, they were not
discomfited, but coolly settled down to their task with
animation and hope. In Mr. Rymer the committee
found one who had thoroughly familiarised himself with
the scheme as proposed; and his unbounded faith in
ultimate triumph greatly, if not absolutely, disarmed the
fear of failure which might have been, and probably
was, secretly working in the minds of his colleagues
who had thought less upon the subject. The characteristic necessary to constitute a leader in any cause,
namely, the courage of his convictions, he possessed. It
is casting no indignity upon Mr. Rymer to say that up
to this time he was generally unknown. The fact of
his having been so is a mortifying proof of the injury

isolation had been inflicting for so long upon the profession. Those who had met him for the first time at that epoch were pleased to find a brother practitioner whose transparent candour was only equalled by his ardent desire to help forward a thoroughly good cause; and those who still know him have not had one reason for withdrawing or altering their good opinion concerning him. To him belongs the credit of giving the signal for dental reform to be attempted in such a way as always .commends itself to Englishmen. In a public and thoroughly constitutional manner he had invited the dental profession to come together and discuss the subject of progress by means of acknowledged educational measures, the gist of which by long consideration he was prepared to submit to them. The recognition of all who called themselves dentists, in a matter which concerned the body as such, seemed to him not so much a necessity, perhaps, as a simple, self-evident piece of justice and common sense. That it commended itself to so many cannot be therefore a subject of surprise. The obverse of the medal is · also true. It cannot be too distinctly understood and remembered that no individual, however exalted his position and great his attainments, has not thereby a prescriptive right to frame laws or cause them to be enacted, however beneficent they may be in their conception or effects, without the sanction and approval of his co-practitioners. As a matter of course, the same rule applies to parties, when they are only of numerical strength enough to form a clique or coterie. No amount of influence can justify dictation surreptitiously arrived at, neither can titles and degrees be accepted as an excuse for clandestine legislation. The spirit of openness and fair play is happily ingrafted in, or rather forms part of, our national life, and he or they who seek to ignore or violate this principle cannot escape the due measure of reproach which must follow in such cases as by an inevitable natural law. The thorough recognition and adoption of this principle in his procedure fully accounts for the reception of Mr. Rymer, and his plan by the meeting at the London Tavern. There were other members of the profession, however, who chose to set it aside, and these gentlemen have since then been styled "The Memorialists." There can be no doubt that Mr. Rymer's correspondence in the public journals had led to the awakening to the need of reform in the minds of these practitioners. In December 1855 they met in private conference, drew up the celebrated "Memorial," appended their signatures and despatched it to Lincoln's Inn Fields, while their brethren all around, qualified and unqualified alike, were allowed to know nothing of their proceeding.

The following is a copy of the notable document, with its preface, when it was sent forth publicly:—

"LONDON, *October* 1856.

"The expediency of forming a 'British Institute of Dental Science,' being at present under consideration amongst certain members of the dental profession,—for the furtherance of their project, and for the support of their professional brethren, it has been thought desirable that it should be made generally known that the following 'Memorial' has been addressed to the Royal College of Surgeons, the answer to which has not been given:

"TO THE PRESIDENT AND COUNCIL OF THE ROYAL COLLEGE OF SURGEONS, LONDON.

"GENTLEMEN,—We, the undersigned, feeling that the department of dental surgery in England, in the absence of any recognised qualification, is wanting in that character and position which its importance merits, have consulted together to devise some means whereby a standard of qualification may be established. Of those who practise dentistry, some have made themselves members of the College of Surgeons, some have obtained the medical degree at the University of London, while others possess that of Edinburgh. But a strictly medical or surgical degree cannot in itself prove that the possessor is familiar with the practice of dental surgery. Yet the student, feeling the necessity of some sort of recognised qualification, devotes that time to a strictly medical education which should have been shared in acquiring a practical knowledge of dental surgery; hence it happens that men enter upon their professional career having yet to learn those practical details so essential to their legitimate success. Very many, however, practise without any medical degree, and among them may be found some of the most eminent of our practitioners, who, nevertheless, are equally anxious that some standard of qualification should be established. In America the necessity of a special course of study was felt, and this led to the establishment of Dental Colleges, where the subjects necessary for the education of a dentist are taught, and the student, at the end of his pupilage, is examined, and if found competent, receives a diploma in testimony of his fitness to practise. These institutions send forth into the world year by year numbers of qualified dentists who, in virtue of their diplomas, assume a superiority over all other practitioners, and are consequently regarded with confidence by the public, who reasonably look upon a special qualification as an indication of superior professional merit. Feeling that the time has arrived when it is imperative that some educational course should be instituted, and that an acquaintance with the general principles of surgery, anatomy, and physiology, and an intimate knowledge of such parts of those subjects as relate to the region of the mouth, are absolutely necessary to the duly qualified practitioner, we, the undersigned, beg to submit to the president and council of the College of Surgeons, whether an examination in the department of dental surgery, as in midwifery, might not be instituted. The adoption of such a course would, we are sure, prove a great boon to practitioners, and would, at the same time, secure a manifest advantage to the public.

"(Signed) SAMUEL CARTWRIGHT, F.R.S.
JOHN H. PARKINSON.
JOHN H. PARKINSON, Jun., M.R.C.S.
EDWIN SAUNDERS, F.R.C.S.
WILLIAM M. BIGG.
SAMUEL CARTWRIGHT, Jun., M.R.C.S.
G. A. IBBETSON, M.R.C.S.
JAMES PARKINSON.
JOHN TOMES, F.R.S.
H. L. FEATHERSTONE.
ALFRED CANTON, M.R.C.S.
ROBERT NASMYTH, M.D., M.R.C.S.
J. L. CRAIGIE, F.R.C.S.
T. BARRETT, M.R.C.S.
ARNOLD ROGERS, F.R.C.S.
THOMAS A. ROGERS, M.R.C.S.
HUBERT SHELLEY, M.B., London, M.R.C.S.
S. JAMES A. SALTER, M.B., M.R.C.S., F.L.S."

A very divided opinion prevailed when this statement

became known, as to the intentions of those who dispatched it. Some asserted that it was evidently meant for the whole profession, and, therefore, each member might hope to receive a copy, if he had not already had one. Others, and by far the larger number, inclined to believe that it was sent to a few, and to them only as a sort of safety-valve to the credit of openness, at last, of the memorialists. Whatever may have been the intention, it is certain that many members of the profession were not in possession of it, and in fact came to know of its existence only when it was mentioned at the public meeting summoned by Mr. Rymer, as has already been stated. In his official capacity the author had, of course, to meet with a very large number of dentists, and he is not aware of a single one to whom he wrote or spoke that had a good word to say of this particular action. Even those who were members of the College of Surgeons stigmatised it as an impertinence, they never having been consulted; while the fact that there were names of unqualified men attached to the document made the ignoring of those outside who were qualified a still more annoying injustice to bear. Amongst those who, at that time, expressed their strong disapprobation, the late Mr. C. Clendon was, perhaps, the most prominent. In a letter addressed to the editor of the "Medical Circular," dated November 1856, that gentleman undertook to review the agitation which had been produced by the attempts on the part of the promoters of the Dental College, and the signitaries of this obnoxious memorial to the College of Surgeons. He wrote incisively, and, as some felt, with dogmatic sourness; not that he had ever done more to advance the true interests of the profession than others, or was even better known than they. Beyond practising quietly as an educated dentist, Mr. Clendon had no particular claim to be heard by his brethren. However, at this epoch, letter-writing to the medical and other journals prevailed, and this correspondent ventilated his views, although he took no steps to identify himself with either of these movements, or to suggest a really practical issue to the matter in hand. He simply contented himself with pulling both men and things to pieces. (The late) Mr. Cartwright " had long been a most able and successful practitioner, but he never had any professional training." (The late) Mr. A. Rogers, F.R.C.S., was "a most successful practitioner, a worthy man and universally respected; but there," says Mr. Clendon, " I must stop: I never heard of anything *he* had done to advance science, to extend knowledge, or to further the interests of his profession." This was "damning with faint praise." But the College of Dentists in embryo, with its provisional committee quietly performing its appointed work in preparing a report to be submitted to the next proposed meeting of the profession, was not animadverted upon so much in this letter of Mr. Clendon's as the proposed Odontological Society. As has already been stated, the memorial of the eighteen practitioners had been sent in to the Royal College of Surgeons in December 1855. This document was taken charge of and presented formally by Mr. James Moncrieff Arnott. Through the influence of Mr. Tomes, the interest of this gentleman had been enlisted in the direction of forming a dental department of the College of Surgeons, and his powerful influence and advocacy were from time to time brought to bear in ventilating the views of those who advanced the opinion of the necessity of such a union between surgery and dentistry as one of its specialties. Mr. Arnott well knew the immense difficulties of the case, and gave his intimate friend, Mr. Tomes, to understand that no speedy solution favourable to his views could be consistently hoped for; but, as time and opportunity served, he courageously advanced the subject from his own place at the council table. Altogether this was a very fortunate occurrence for that portion of the profession who, for the sake of distinction, may be called the "orthodox" party. Mr. Arnott's quiet sagacity enabled him to deal in a masterly manner with the complexities of the subject; his experience had also led him to see the desirability of having really capable men to practise this branch of surgery; and while his predilections leaned to an unostentatious but distinct step in the direction of professional improvement, his exalted rank among surgeons and acknowledged worth gave him the most excellent opportunities of trying to secure all the advantages which would be sure to accrue through well-directed educational measures. The result of Mr. Arnott's introducing the subject at Lincoln's Inn Fields had been the "Memorial" with the names of the eighteen signitaries attached. While this paper was lying at the College of Surgeons, the memorialists agreed to constitute themselves into a scientific society. This, however, was not done without much cogitation and many meetings, all of which maintained their original character of privacy. At length a notice appeared from Mr. Rymer in the public press that the second meeting of the profession, to be publicly convened as before, would be held on Tuesday, November 11th, 1856; and on the day when this was announced, the profession was made aware that the day previous (November 10th) the Odontological Society was formed. The significant fact that this society was born just one day (by date) prior to that when the effort being made to organise the profession, by a publicly instituted educational method, was advertised to take form, created mingled feelings of surprise and mirth in the minds of numbers of the profession, while others saw in it a stroke of diplomacy, brought about by the increasing pressure of those steps which had been taken in the broad light of day. In Mr. Clendon's communication to the journals of the day, he stated both institutions to be composed of "heterogeneous materials." The idea of a Dental College was condemned as "of American origin"—as though, forsooth, that would be utter obloquy; and then a sarcastic remark or two concerning the "colleges," "professors," and "degrees" of our Transatlantic brethren. "The Transactions of the Baltimore College of Dental Surgeons" came in for their share of opprobrium, being stigmatised as unsatisfactory both in their scientific and literary aspects. So far as the proposed institute or college was concerned, all sorts of dark clouds and unpropitious circumstances—according to this writer's opinion—attended it. It was begun at an improper time of the year. Some names of eminent men were stated as connected with it, but these were soon withdrawn. Difficulties were already thick upon its path as to what constituted respectability, &c., &c.; uncanonical conduct was analysed, and then defined as a matter of taste, rather than morals; and, in fact, out of the attempts to improve the profession, Mr. Clendon was unable to extract a single grain of hope. Allowing the naturalness of the desire on the part of the great majority of dentists who were without legal qualification to have a college where "they could severally display their profound anatomical knowledge and announce their physiological discoveries," he proceeded to assume the prophet's garb and vocation concerning it. An analysis of the difficulties attending the fitness for membership followed, and a sharp stroke about respectability. Comparing the poor but worthy practitioner with his richer brethren, he confessed that if the latter should enter into judgment with the former, the "*tu quoque*" could be appropriately uttered. Speaking of the advertiser, Mr. Clendon said, "He may instance magnates and the 'Morning Post,' and eminent practitioners, with their shilling and sixpenny 'Five Minutes' Advice' indiscriminately distributed." The imminence of failure which hung over the College of Dentists extorts a sigh of regret; and with a hint, merely, of that which might be done, if certain men could be got to do certain things, which human nature has generally found to be very difficult, it was dismissed. But with regard to the Odontological Society Mr.

Clendon had much more to say. Its founders were "the remnant of former dinner-parties;" their method of commencing it was culpable; the pretence set forth in the prospectus was "a false one." The president was chosen "at the private meeting of a few friends," &c. Mr. Clendon also prophesied about this society thus: "Of this I am quite sure, a society commenced so insidiously, not to say under false pretences, and founded on injustice, can never prosper; foes will spring up within as well as without." The promoters of it were even made to soliloquise after the following fashion: "We, who have memorialised the College of Surgeons, praying for education and a diploma, on the pretext that we were representing the *general feeling* of the profession, proceed to form ourselves into a *private* society, to elect ourselves its officers, and admit whom we please. And, although our plan of secret organisation, and admission of none but personal friends to conferences, by which we are seeking to govern our whole fraternity, may appear '*somewhat invidious,*' we are too well aware that we are outraging rather than representing general feeling to hope for success by any other means." With such remarks he filled up a very long letter, casting on every side criticisms of the keenest kind, sparing none, and producing in the minds of the readers generally the very disagreeable idea that they were reading the sentiments of a self-inflated but sour-tempered man, who was out of humour with everyone else but himself. Mr. Clendon was very vexed with the promoters of the Odontological—or, as he termed it, "the dinner-party"—Society, and, indeed, said so in the following unmistakable terms: "I had already expressed much indignation on learning these proceedings from private sources, but after this public avowal I felt it my duty publicly and most emphatically to protest against them." In the matter of protest, as has already been said, this writer was by no means alone, although, perhaps, few endorsed all the sentiments he expressed.

His opinions were framed upon those of such men as Mr. Bell and the late Mr. Nasmyth, and therefore it was no strange thing to hear him advocating the necessity of every dentist becoming a full surgeon. He himself was a member of the Royal College of Surgeons, and lecturer on dental surgery at the Westminster Hospital. It was but natural, therefore, that he should speak highly of his *alma mater*. Eventually Mr. Clendon collected his letters, together with the correspondence they had produced, and published the whole in the form of a pamphlet, entitled, " Letters and Papers on the recent Dental Movement, with Remarks upon the Present anomalous State of the Dental Profession."* His remarks, however, produced no effect beyond that which was felt to be true of others besides himself at that juncture of affairs, namely, that it was easier to criticise than create. The tide of feeling ran strongly in various channels on one basilar subject—the proper proficiency to practise. Some advocated the full curriculum of the College of Surgeons; others, that the amount of knowledge necessary to constitute membership with the College of Surgeons was over and above that which dentists, as such, required. The importance of sound mechanical instruction—on the score of dentists being art-practitioners—was insisted upon in one direction; and the separation of the mechanical from the surgical or operative portion of dental practice in another. The combination of the two departments constituted the perfection of dentistry in some men's estimation; while the mention of the laboratory appeared to be positive defilement with others. To those gentlemen who, with a very legitimate pleasure and pride, laid stress upon the addition of M.R.C.S. to their names, was opposed the fact that in numberless instances surgeons made shameful blunders in the treatment of diseases of the teeth and oral cavity. Such were some of the difficulties besetting and obstructing reform at that

* Webster & Co., Piccadilly, 1857.

time; to mention them all would simply extend the present volume to an unnecessary length. To summarise, then, we find that at the close of the year 1856, a determination had been displayed in two different directions to seek to elevate the dental profession by educational measures. With the larger body of practitioners engaging in the work, the result was sought for through the instrumentality of open public meetings, to which the entire profession was invited to come. With the smaller but more influential body, the adoption of the private and exclusive course was taken. The former maintained the necessity and greater usefulness of an independent institution; the latter asked for an incorporation with and consequent dependence upon the Royal College of Surgeons. The profession had at last been stirred throughout the three kingdoms, and an opportunity having thus been afforded for the free expression of opinions on the important matter of dental reform, this was eagerly caught at by men of all ranks, the result being mental conflict and collision to a very considerable degree. Although the two main parties were prominent all through, the confusion of strife was the more palpable from the division and subdivision of opinion upon many subjects which, as a whole, formed the general idea of progress. It needed cool heads and experienced hands to direct matters, and so manipulate the material as to bring order and harmony out of the chaos that then abounded. The provisional committee appointed at the first public meeting of the profession for considering the best method of practically carrying out the resolutions which had then been passed had, for a period extending to some six weeks, assiduously prosecuted their labours. They were prepared to make their report on the 11th of November 1856, and, accordingly, due notice was given to the profession that a public meeting—this time to be held at the Freemasons' Tavern—would be convened on the evening of that day. The memorialists, too, had not been idle, for they had so arranged their affairs as to be able to announce the formation of the Odontological Society, as has been seen, on the 10th of the same month. As chronology is an important feature in this history, precedence must therefore be accorded to the newly-formed society. The following is the text of the announcement concerning

The Odontological Society.

At a meeting, held November 10th, 1856, a society for the encouragement of knowledge in dental surgery, entitled the "Odontological Society," was formed, and the following officers and council were appointed. The meetings, for the discussion of professional subjects and the election of members, will be held on the first Monday in each month, excepting September and October. The first meeting will be held in January next; the hour and place of meeting will be duly advertised.

President—SAMUEL CARTWRIGHT, Esq., F.R.S.

Vice-Presidents—J. H. PARKINSON, Esq.; ARNOLD ROGERS, Esq., F.R.C.S.

Treasurer—EDWIN SAUNDERS, Esq., F.R.C.S.

Council—H. J. BARRETT, Esq., M.R.C.S.; WILLIAM M. BIGG, Esq.; ALFRED CANTON, Esq., M.R.C.S.; G. A. IBBETSON, Esq., M.R.C.S.; R. NASMYTH, M.D., M.R.C.S.; JAMES PARKINSON, Esq.; JOHN H. PARKINSON, Esq., M.R.C.S.; S. JAMES SALTER, Esq., M.B., M.R.C.S.; HUBERT SHELLEY, Esq., M.B., M.R.C.S.

Honorary Secretaries—SAMUEL CARTWRIGHT, Jun., Esq., M.R.C.S.; JOHN TOMES, F.R.S.; THOMAS A. ROGERS, Esq., M.R.C.S.

In accordance with the general feeling of the profession that a society of dentists should be formed, capable of supporting itself on an equality with other learned societies in this country, a meeting was convened in November 1855. It was then proposed by the undersigned members of the profession to memorialise the Royal College of Surgeons on the necessity which existed for some recognised qualification for those practising this specialty of surgery. This suggestion was carried into effect; and on 11th December 1855, an appeal to the College was made, stating the great benefit the public would receive, and the advantage which would accrue to the profession generally, if a diploma were granted to those who passed an examination in this branch of the medical science. This important measure being thus in abeyance, it was deemed by the memorialists desirable to commence, without further delay, the operations of the society. At a meeting held for this purpose in November 1855, the bye-laws for the society were framed on the model of those of existing medical societies; it was also determined that invitations should be sent to those members of the profession who were either personally known to the memorialists or were deemed anxious to promote the well-being of the society. This plan of selecting from among so many who are eligible would appear somewhat invidious, but the absolute necessity of securing at the outset a working body, the feeling of which would be unanimous, seemed to demand that certain limits should be placed upon the selection. It is believed that, by the means adopted, a nucleus will be formed, including the names of many gentlemen well known in the profession, capable of embracing ultimately within its circle all those who may desire to devote their attention to the objects comprehended by the society.

(Signed)   SAMUEL CARTWRIGHT, F.R.S.
JOHN H. PARKINSON.
JOHN H. PARKINSON, Jun., M.R.C.S.
EDWIN SAUNDERS, F.R.C.S.
WILLIAM M. BIGG.
SAMUEL CARTWRIGHT, Jun., M.R.C.S.
G. A. IBBETSON, M.R.C.S.
JAMES PARKINSON.
JOHN TOMES, F.R.S.
H. J. FEATHERSTONE.
ALFRED CANTON, M.R.C.S.
ROBERT NASMYTH, M.D., M.R.C.S.
J. L. CRAIGIE, F.R.C.S.
H. J. BARRETT, M.R.C.S.
ARNOLD ROGERS, F.R.C.S.
THOMAS A. ROGERS, M.R.C.S.
HUBERT SHELLEY, M.B., London, M.R.C.S.
S. JAMES A. SALTER, M.B., M.R.C.S., F.L.S.

The laws by which the society was to be regulated were printed, and a copy of them appeared in the "British Journal of Dental Science," in the number for December 1856. The statement thus made public did not tend to allay the irritation which had been very generally produced. To a large number of highly respectable practitioners the step taken by the gentlemen who had been the promoters of the society appeared both selfish and unjust. There was literally no valid reason why certain picked and selected dentists should combine and institute this or any other society in such an absolutely private and clandestine manner. There were practitioners, members of the Royal College of Surgeons, occupying excellent positions in the profession, who had never been consulted in this important matter, who felt keenly the affront to them by their non-recognition, qualified as they assuredly were to give an opinion or act upon the staff. In more than one instance the author had, subsequently, to listen to expressions of the deepest indignation concerning this transparent partiality. The originators of the Odontological Society had evidently felt the injustice of the position they had assumed towards this class of their "*confrères*," and admitted it in their circular, but the apology there offered was insufficient to appease the irritation. There was another class of practitioners who, although not *diplomé*, had nevertheless earned for themselves an undeniable position, and seeing that the signitaries of the celebrated circular were not all holders of medical degrees, they also had just cause for feeling aggrieved. Many excellent dentists asked the question, and justly enough, why they had been passed over, and their existence as dental practitioners totally ignored? In their case, as well as the former, the idea of "selecting," as adopted by the founders of the society, pressed unjustly and with hardness. Seeing they with many others had never been consulted or even permitted to know of what was going forward, the excuse of the projectors that they wished to commence the society with unanimity of feeling and opinion was simply invalid. The plan which had been adopted had evidently been founded in a serious mistrust of the profession generally. Those who had thus united were more or less personally known to each other, and the accord which they sought for and arrived at was purchased at a very heavy price. The general mass of dentists, while they could not have expected to be taken into the inner chamber of confidence of the magnates of the profession, had nevertheless an undoubted right to expect to be treated in a way which would ensure their recognition. They accordingly did not fail to grumble both publicly and privately, and in general condemned the action of the Odontologists as unconstitutional and un-English, as indeed it was. Whatever had been the course of reasoning which led up to the decision of exclusive action, the result on the minds of the large majority of dentists was certainly a very distinct disapproval of the same.

The first meeting of the Odontological Society was held on January 5th, 1857, at the house of Mr. Saunders, No. 32A George Street, Hanover Square. Up to then, although it had found for itself "a name," it had not secured, as a permanency, "a local habitation." In the opening address of Mr. Cartwright, the president, as was, of course, to be expected, allusion was made to the reasons which had actuated the gentlemen who had originated it. The following are the words employed touching the celebrated "Memorial," which may be termed the foundation-stone of the entire proceeding: "It was not thought necessary by those who prepared this memorial to procure to it the signatures of *all* the leading members of the profession, as the memorial contained only a *suggestion* for the consideration of the members of the council of the College, which, if entertained by them, will be submitted for the approval of our profession. Circumstances, however, connected with medical politics have hitherto prevented the College of Surgeons from giving a definite reply to this requisition; but I believe I may say that the subject is favourably entertained by many, if not by most, of the members of the council. No other feeling guided those who prepared and signed this memorial than an earnest desire to benefit their profession, and a sincere conviction that a recognised connection with the College of Surgeons is best calculated to raise the status of the dentist to an equality with other medical practitioners, and rescue our profession from the anomalous position it has hitherto held." In explanation of how the society had come to be originated, Mr. Cartwright said—" The members of the dental profession have hitherto kept aloof from one another, and retained in exclusiveness the modes and peculiarities of private practice. The want of a point of union among its members, where subjects interesting to the whole body of educated practitioners might be introduced and freely discussed for the mutual benefit of all, and through which the contributions to dental literature at present scattered through the pages of medical journals, and often lost to those to whom they are most interesting, might be collected so as to form an instructive and available library for reference, has long been felt. The necessity of such a union, generally acknowledged, but never carried out, has given rise to the formation of the Odontological Society. Founded on the basis of other scientific societies, it, like them, originated with one or two, and has been organised by several—the gentlemen applied to to form it being those who had signed the memorial to the College of Surgeons. These formed themselves into a society, and out of their number appointed officers and a council for the first year. Having arranged the bye-laws for the governance of the society, it was then determined to invite a limited number of town and country practitioners to join it, so as to secure, from the first, a sufficient number of members for the purpose of carrying out the objects of the society, previous to throwing it open to the profession at large for admission in the ordinary mode by ballot—a plan borne out by the early history of every society on the model of which the present is based. Such limitation of invited members was found absolutely necessary, and was made without the slightest intention of creating any invidious distinction, it being evident that the names selected could not be considered as representing *all* the gentlemen who rank high in the profession, there being many not included who are equally respected, as intelligent practitioners, as any among those to whom the invitation to join the society was sent." This official announcement was such a lame apology, that if it did not actually increase and intensify the annoyance so generally prevalent, certainly gave satisfaction to none but the few who composed the society itself. Thus, however, was the Odontological Society started. It emanated from the decision of eighteen dental practitioners, first to memorialise the Royal College of Surgeons to take action in the direction of professional reform by organising a dental department in connection with it; and while this important subject was being considered by the council of the College, these same gentlemen met at each others' houses, as occasion offered, and proceeded to form a scientific society bearing the above name. There has never been a doubt as to the deep interest which the memorialists took in regard to the profession, and the sincerity of their motives in thus taking action in the matter. None could have felt more painfully than they the condition of the profession they were practising. It might, perhaps, be advanced, none so much, considering the position of several of them in it. But what made this step so unpalatable to the general body was the secrecy which had characterised the entire undertaking, and the painfully invidious distinctions they had ventured to make between men of equal eminence with themselves. Even the success, which, as a rule, has attended the society, has not been sufficient to obliterate the remembrance of the unauthorised and sudden patronage which it was felt had been extended to the mass of practitioners of dentistry, not only in London, but throughout the provinces of the three kingdoms. It is not to be wondered at that many letters appeared denouncing, not so much the scheme itself, as the method employed to consummate it; and that more verbal expressions—to be likened to "curses not loud but deep"—were heard from time to time as the meetings of dentists gave opportunity for utterance. It must not be forgotten, however, that a very large number of practitioners objected to connection with the College of Surgeons "*toto cœlo.*" To the steps taken by these gentlemen—whose name, in comparison with the handful comprising the Odontological Society, was "legion"—we must now return. The dentists who were willing to follow the leadership of Mr. Rymer, together with the profession generally, received a public notice of the preparedness of the provisional committee, instituted at the first general meeting, to deliver their report. The meeting for this purpose, as has been stated, was summoned for the 11th of November 1856, at the Freemasons' Tavern. In the interval which had elapsed since the first gathering of the profession, the provisional committee had drawn up a code of regulations which they called "suggested rules," and a copy of these was forwarded to every known member of the profession, accompanied by a circular signed by the two honorary secretaries, Mr. Rymer and Mr. Alfred Hill, and which contained the following questions: "First, Do the resolutions, of which the enclosed is a copy, meet your approval? Second, Are the rules suggested in accordance with your views? and if so, Should it be determined at a future general meeting of the profession to form the society to which they have reference, would you be a supporter of it?" A very large response was the result of this, many of the replies containing suggestions of considerable value. The committee duly consulted over the whole correspondence, and drew up for presentation at the forthcoming meeting a set of "amended suggested rules."* In anticipation of the meeting, the writer had been deputed to obtain a chairman. He visited during two whole days several members of the profession for this purpose, but was unsuccessful in every instance. Many cogent reasons were adduced by these gentlemen for

* See Appendix A.

their non-acceptance of the post. Such, indeed, was the then condition of things, that a most disheartening unwillingness to venture into anything like a prominent position seemed to prevail universally. Last upon the list of the names which had been selected was that of Mr. James Robinson of Gower Street, Bedford Square. The interview, which took place in the presence of Mr. Robinson's partner, Mr. Thomas Underwood, was marked by great courtesy by both those gentlemen, but the former quickly perceived "the situation," and he duly estimated the position in which he had been placed by being asked in this matter last of all. It was evident to him that the failures hitherto made in the attempt to secure the services of a chairman for the forthcoming meeting had produced a crisis. The question in his mind was, "Was there any sufficient reason existing why he should be made use of for the solution of the difficulty?" He thought there was not, and said so. Although Mr. Robinson's refusal was distinct, it was not final. At the earnest solicitation of the writer he consented to think the subject over, and gave permission for another interview. This was to have taken place on the following day, but, through the pressure of Mr. Robinson's engagements, it could not be effected. The pen was called into requisition where the person could not avail. An appointment was given, the interview took place, and after a considerable struggle Mr. Robinson at length agreed to take the chair, in answer to the committee's request. It was very essential that this post should be occupied by a gentleman of position and influence among his brother practitioners, and these two necessary qualifications Mr. Robinson possessed. In the conversations which had taken place, the objects and aims of Mr. Rymer's movement were fully stated to him, and he not only grasped them in their scope and entirety, but they seemed very completely to meet his own views in the direction of dental reform. When the committee met to arrange for the public meeting, there was a very considerable amount of gratification evinced in the result obtained with Mr. Robinson. A very large number of the profession, some two hundred or more, assembled at the Freemasons' Tavern on the 11th of November. The announcement of the chairman's name by Mr. Rymer elicited loud applause. His opening speech was practical, humorous, and to the point. The "amended suggested rules" formulated by the provisional committee were discussed *seriatim* with business-like zeal, and in their altered form agreed upon; the committee, by a unanimous vote, being empowered to proceed to form a society, according to the resolutions which had been passed. At this stage of the proceedings it was determined, mainly through the suggestions of Mr. Robinson, that provisions should be made for dentists' assistants in the society or institute, so that this important department might be made partaker of the benefits to arise from the union and consolidation of the profession. To this end a circular was addressed to them, of which the following is a copy:—

"To Dentists' Assistants.

"Gentlemen,—From circumstances which have transpired, the committee at present organising a Dental Society or Institute consider it a duty to so large and respectable a body that the advantages of membership with this society should be laid before them. It is proposed, then, that all gentlemen now acting as assistants to dentists be received as associate members at half the entrance fee and half the annual subscription of full members; that such membership shall entitle them to *all the uses and privileges of full membership*, except that of voting for the election of council or the admission or introduction of full members; that as soon as such associates commence practice upon their own account they be eligible for admission as full members. Under these circumstances, the undersigned will be glad to receive names at once—the list closing 13th day of December next.

"Charles James Fox,
"Alfred Hill,   } Honorary Secretaries."
"Samuel Lee Rymer,

This step was a manifest evidence of the desire which the committee felt to make the Dental Institute as comprehensive as possible in its foundation and design, and was a strong contrast to the sentiments, so far as they had been made known, of the Odontological Society. The result of this appeal was a large and acquiescent reply. The next public meeting was convened at the Freemasons' Tavern on the 16th of December to receive the report of the committee, who in the meantime had been diligently proceeding with their labours, and had drawn up a code of regulations called "laws and constitutions."* The chair on this occasion was occupied by Mr. Donaldson Mackenzie. The objects of the meeting, which was again numerously attended, were set forth in the chairman's address; and Mr. Rymer, who felt strongly on the matter of open discussion at all times, constantly maintaining its necessity, explained that, although the committee had been empowered to frame the society's laws, they had resolved to submit those which they had drawn up to the consideration of the meeting, to ensure a full expression from the gentlemen present. Each law was therefore discussed *seriatim*, and after the free expression of those who chose to offer opinions or suggest alterations, the whole were adopted. The following is a list of the officer-bearers elected on the occasion :—

President—JAMES ROBINSON, Esq.
Vice-Presidents—ANDREW CLARK, Esq., London; SAMUEL CORBETT, Esq., Dublin; F. B. IMLACK, Esq., Edinburgh; NORMAN KING, Esq., Exeter; JAMES LOUIS OXLEY, Esq., Leeds; ROBERT REID, Esq., Edinburgh; F. H. THOMSON, Esq., Glasgow; SOMERSET TIBBS, Esq., Cheltenham.
Council—WM. CRAMPTEN, Esq.; W. L. CANTON, Esq.; JAMES HARLEY, Esq.; ROBERT HEPBURN, Esq.; WILLIAM HUNT, Esq., Yeovil; HENRY LONG JACOB, Esq., Bridgewater; W. H. LINTOTT, Esq.; DONALDSON MACKENZIE, Esq.; JAMES MERRYWEATHER, Esq.; J. W. MITCHELL, Esq.; J. B. MURPHY, Esq., Derby; ADAM THOMSON, Esq.; THOMAS UNDERWOOD, Esq.
Treasurer—PETER MATTHEWS, Esq.
Honorary Secretaries—CHARLES JAMES FOX, Esq.; ALFRED HILL, Esq.; SAMUEL LEE RYMER, Esq.

* See Appendix, B.

The duties of the three Honorary Secretaries were thus apportioned:

Mr. Fox—*Library and Museum.*
Mr. Hill—*General Correspondence on College Business.*
Mr. Rymer—*Communications in reference to the Council.*

Under the title of the College of Dentists of England, then, an amalgamated society of dentists practising in the three kingdoms was founded. The idea of such an institution originated with Mr. Rymer; and that gentleman having surrounded himself with many of his brother practitioners, had, with their assistance, in a very practical and always open and public manner, thus formed a nucleus from which expansion and advance could most fairly be anticipated. The result thus attained gave very great satisfaction to a large majority of town and provincial dentists; and numbers, who had either never had hope of unity in the profession, or having felt it had suffered it to die, now looked forward to the future with eager anticipation. It is difficult for the present generation of dentists, especially the younger members, to realise the sentiments which had thus been produced. From a state of disorganisation and estrangement, the profession had by a double effort, very like a spasm, emerged into a condition of plasticity and preparation for improvement beneath the manipulative administration of men of mark on the one hand, or of such who, though less known, were chosen from and by themselves, and intrusted with the powers of leadership and direction. The two institutions aimed at one object, namely, the elevation of the dental profession to its proper position among kindred scientific bodies. The instrumentalities proposed to be used were the same in each instance, and may be summed up in one word—Education. Only in the matter of its source and application did they differ; but this difference was of so radical a character as to keep the two institutions apart from each other, not only by a sharp, well-defined line of separation, but by a considerable distance also. It was evident that rivalry would become the order of the day, and this expectation was fully and speedily realised. While the Odontological Society leaned towards and depended upon the influence which name and position usually supply, and had demonstrated their trust in this direction by secret action in the establishment of their society, the College of Dentists of England looked to overwhelming numbers rather than name, and from the very first courted publicity, shrinking from any and everything which savoured of the clandestine or suggested a *ruse*.

In the first president of the Odontological Society was seen a gentleman who, by natural gifts of a very high order, had elevated himself to the pinnacle of his profession, and was conducting a large and exceedingly lucrative practice. The name of Cartwright had been for many years, perhaps, the best-known name, not only in England, but in Europe. His great skill as a dentist had earned for him an enormous fame; and although not a member of the Royal College of Surgeons, he had obtained the coveted prize of Fellow of the Royal Society, than which no higher scientific distinction in this country exists.

Given to hospitality, and able to dispense it in a princely style, Mr. Cartwright had been long in the habit of surrounding himself with the celebrities in literature, science, and art; and at his *ré-unions*, the greatest and most illustrious men in these departments were to be seen. The noble and wealthy flocked to his consulting-room to seek his advice and skill, and his name and reputation had been and still were very great. At the time of his accepting the presidency of the new society, Mr. Cartwright was not entirely in active professional life, his health requiring repose; but he was fully prepared to give all the time and energy he could command to the promulgation of such measures as this society hoped to advance—he being fully cognisant of the great advantages which would accrue to the future dentist by a course of well-chosen, appropriate, and systematic education—while the name of Cartwright was in itself a tower of strength.

The choice of such a gentleman as the first president of the Odontological Society reflected great wisdom on the part of those connected with it, and was a proper tribute of esteem to one who had earned for himself so much respect, both in and out of the profession, and in the world at large.

The president of the College of Dentists was an example in himself of what untiring energy, coupled with ability, can attempt and attain. Mr. Robinson was a man of exceedingly strong will and determined spirit. When a project lay before him with which he was connected, either as friend or foe, his dark eye would glance fire as he brought his fist vehemently down into the palm of his other hand, indicative of his resolution to take action in the matter. It needed not his expressive, "I'll do it! you shall see!" which he frequently made use of, to prove to the bystander that his mind was made up. Many times, as might be expected, his impetuous nature overruled his judgment, and led him into what he subsequently admitted to be mistakes. But the fiery courage which he possessed so abundantly was a most valuable characteristic at this time, if properly used and controlled. The author had had occasion to speak to many kindly-hearted men, to many amiable and genial-spirited men, and to many more who may have, and doubtless did possess, determination of character, the manifestation of which, however, they did not permit him to see. But when face to face with James Robinson, and he seeing his way clear for taking up a certain line of action, there was no doubt on the mind possible as to the rapid, practical, and resolute manner in which he would proceed. Promptitude, if not precision, was his notable characteristic. He ever leaned towards action. A restless spirit, he found solace and support in energy and hard work where most men only find exhaustion. From close and frequent observation of him, he appeared to the writer to partake of the character of the double-handed broadswords-man rather than the skilled fencer with the foil. Whenever and wherever his blade fell it made an ugly wound, although, at times, it missed its mark, and left his antagonist in possession of a momentary advantage. With such predilections, so strongly demonstrated, a new difficulty was experienced. This was to harness and then guide his impetuous will, so that it might subserve the end his friends and colleagues had in view. His keen susceptibility, his almost instinctive discovery of anything like the curb-rein, made this still more difficult.

With regard to the presidency of the college, which had thus been offered to and accepted by him, the committee had felt the matter to be a critical one, Mr. Robinson having been—without any intention, however, on their part—a sort of *dernier ressort*. Simple justice to his memory demands that it should be put on record that no lower motive than the strong desire to be useful to the struggling members of the profession actuated him. By his own indomitable perseverance he had risen to an acknowledged position as a dentist, and was conducting a very large practice which fully absorbed his time and attention. It would have been a very easy thing, therefore, for him to have met the request made with a negative, as so many others had done. Without attempting to critically analyse the reasons which induced him to accept office at this juncture, it may be safely asserted that a spirit of daring, if not of defiance, was in active operation. *Because* others had been timid, he determined to show that fear had no control over him.

To one of such a temperament there was also a certain amount of fascination in the post. It offered ample opportunities for the display of generalship in guiding the affairs of the institution itself; and every now and then the *élan* of such a character and disposition might produce marked and lasting results. At any rate, there would be sure to be found a certain amount of activity and excitement which were alike congenial to his natural tastes. As to the honour of the position, that seemed to have no effect upon such a mind as Mr. Robinson possessed. The apparent satisfaction which he drew from it was that there would be plenty of work, a certainty of conflict with apathy, pride, and indifference, with just a chance of a happy hit or two in directions which had hitherto been sealed against him. Full of energy and hot blood, ready for the fray, and rejoicing in the expectation that battle would end in blessing, he quietly put all other considerations of self-interest into his pocket, and determined to serve heartily in what he sincerely believed to be a righteous cause. His remark to the writer at the time of his making his decision was, "Remember, if I draw the sword, I fling away the scabbard." Henceforth, therefore, there was to be war in earnest, if not actually *à outrance*. So far as Mr. Rymer's views had been promulgated, Mr. Robinson accepted and endorsed them. He thoroughly felt the importance and necessity of educating the coming generation of dentists. He, moreover, most thoroughly believed in the wished-for reform springing up from within rather than from without the profession, and considered that the means being taken to ensure an independent position was a step conducive to the benefit of all.

It is easy, therefore, to understand that the measures taken by the memorialists, both in petitioning the College of Surgeons for patronage and in secretly forming the Odontological Society, met with no stronger reprobation and fiercer opposition than fell from him. Although Mr. Robinson was not a member of the Royal College of Surgeons, he did not despise such a medical degree, but held that its possession by no means guaranteed a proficiency to practise dentistry; and, therefore, maintained that it should be subordinate, and not supreme, as a mark of qualification to the dental surgeon. The College of Dentists had no firmer believer in the ability of dental practitioners, as such, to educate and examine the younger members of the body, than their first president ever proved himself to be. He vehemently opposed the idea of submission to or dependence upon the Royal College of Surgeons; and was, therefore, a thorough representative of the views held by those who had publicly formed the College of Dentists of England.

Thus, then, it may be said, that at the close of the year 1856 two important institutions had been organised, each affecting in the closest possible manner the deepest and dearest interests of the dental profession. The unhappy part of considering them as they stood forth prominently, lay in the fact that they were in antagonism one to the other, and that the animosity was both bitter and undisguised. When, however, the circumstances which had led up to their formation were remembered, together with the method proposed by each society for carrying out its object, there is not much room for surprise at the opposing elements, as such, or the intensity of feeling which prevailed. However, there they stood, having in their birth and organisation created an amount of excitement through the ranks of the dentists in the three kingdoms such as had never been realised before; and, henceforth, it was apparent that everything necessary to enlist the sympathy and support of those who up to this time were non-adherents would be done, so as to prove inherent power of development, and, on the part of those who were guiding the affairs of each institution, wisdom and aptitude; that so, in due time, results beneficial to the body of practitioners at large might happily be achieved.

The Odontological Society at this time could not, perhaps, count fifty members on its list; the College of Dentists appeared upon the scene with more than three times that number of supporters. The following published statement sets forth the objects and the proposals which the founders of the latter institution then had in view.

"The objects for which the College of Dentists of England is established are to unite members of the dental profession into a recognised and INDEPENDENT body, and to provide means of professional education and examination. The manner in which it is intended to seek the attainment of these objects is to invite all dentists practising as such, *exclusively* and *legitimately*, to become members of the college.

"This invitation is extended to the 31st of December 1857; after which period it is proposed to provide means whereby the competency of each candidate for membership must be satisfactorily proved by examination.

"The large number of practitioners who have already enrolled their names as members, with the approbation of the council, would appear to prove that the constitutional principles upon which the college is founded must prevail in bringing the profession together as a body, before the lapse of many months, when it is hoped a charter of incorporation will be obtained, so that the public may be effectually protected from the serious effects of charlatanism, and every duly-qualified practitioner be enabled to maintain his position with dignity."

CHAPTER IV.

ALLUSION has been made to dental journalism, and the present work would be incomplete without direct reference to and mention of this important feature in the general advance of the profession. The year 1856 must ever be memorable in the annals of dentistry in this country from more causes than one. The first, however, in the order of time, was the establishment and appearance of a monthly journal to represent the profession. It was launched as the enterprise and property of a Mr. Walter Blundell, and bore the name of "The British Journal of Dental Science," the publisher being the well-known (late) John Churchill, of New Burlington Street.

The dentists of that day did not concern themselves about the motives which had operated with the proprietor of this journal in inducing him to institute such a medium of communication throughout their ranks. They were content with the fact that a proper opportunity was thus given for literary and scientific intercourse. The announcement that a monthly journal devoted to their interests was about to appear, gladdened them. In the opening number, issued in the month of July, the editor, in his address, assured his readers that "the columns of 'The British Journal of Dental Science' were open for free discussion, unfettered by cliqueism, and at the disposal of any and every member of the profession requiring a medium for the extension of accumulated knowledge, let it be ever so fragmentary or varied in degree of excellence." After stating the general intent and scope of the periodical, the concluding paragraph ran thus : " Finally, we beg for mutual aid in this common interest, which we fervently hope will unite us in the most friendly intercourse, and prove a lasting source of gratification and advantage." The contents in general were most encouraging as a specimen of what the future numbers would be. The "getting up," was all that could be desired, and, consequently, this new friend received a very cordial if not enthusiastic reception. It gave rise to a hope in many plodding but worthy men's minds of the beginning of better things. At any rate, it could not fail of becoming the medium whereby the isolation throughout the profession might be altered, if not transformed into union among its many members. Through its columns men could fairly expect not only to receive but contribute valuable information, and thus, in the best possible way, become more fully known the one to the other. There were so many facts constantly occurring in every one's practice which could be chronicled with advantage to the entire body, that the wonder now is why a special journal for the profession had not been thought of before.

The appearance of this periodical at the moment when the profession was being aroused from its dormant condition was to be considered fortunate, especially as the editor, in the second number, advocated in an unmistakable manner the necessity for organisation and education by means of a Dental College. It is highly probable that the writer of the article in question had, with many others, felt the force and justice of the remarks Mr. Rymer had made exactly one year previous in his letter published in the "Lancet." Whether this was the source of his inspiration or not, the editor of the new journal warmly espoused Mr. Rymer's views, for, in the number for September 1856, the month when the latter gentleman called a public meeting of the profession, we find him writing thus: "To style ourselves 'surgeon-dentists,' therefore, is clearly an error. Even those who possess the diploma of the College of Surgeons, and now confine themselves to the speciality of dentistry, are no better off than the most ignorant of the profession, who can equally assume the above title. The College of Surgeons, in common with the medical colleges, looks with an eye of little favour on 'speciality' of any kind, and to demand of them an acknowledgment of our own would be utterly absurd. It follows, then, that any code of laws which may be framed for the proposed institute or college, should not be *retrospective;* that is, that those existing practitioners, who can fairly show an honest proficiency in their art, should not be debarred the rights and privileges which such an institution would secure to them as a class." The gentlemen, therefore, who met at the London Tavern, with this very purpose in view, had every reason to congratulate themselves upon the prospect of having their ideas to this end fostered and encouraged by the editor of the "Dental Journal." This hope was further strengthened when the next monthly number saw the light, for there was commendation in that enough and to spare. In remarking upon that meeting, the editor observed, "A more business-like and practical set of men could not well have assembled; for each seemed to be imbued with the spirit that he was striving for an object which, if attained, would not only ameliorate and raise his own position, but hand him down to future generations as a benefactor of a useful and honourable profession. They had, in fact, something to do, and they did it offhand, and, rather singularly, without the interruption from any of those crotchety pests who generally haunt public meetings. The painstaking gentleman who had summoned them together set before them at once three very lucid and practical propositions, which, with very few words, were adopted unanimously. *Tarde scd tute* must be their motto, and they must succeed. Chosen by a fair representative body of their profession, they possess its entire confidence." Nothing could have been more animating than such expressions as these, and they were undoubtedly appreciated at that critical time. The next month's issue brought with it a statement, in the usual place devoted to editorial deliveries, which might, for the sentiments expressed, have been written even by a member of the College of Dentists itself. While assuring the gentlemen who were assiduously working at the open organisation of the profession that they should not fail to find a cordial helper in the "British Journal of Dental Science," the writer of the article proceeds to draw the attention of the magnates in the dental body to the necessity for their co-operation thus:—" Once more we say to the more prosperous members of the profession, a great responsibility rests upon you; your brethren are aspiring for an organisation that shall improve their social position and increase their public usefulness. Will you help them in this arduous effort? Will you extend a hand to land them safe on firm ground, or will you stand complacently by while they work their way with many struggles through the rough waters? Once ashore they will not want your help, and depend upon it they will bestow the honours of success only on those who deserve them. We hope, then, that these gentlemen will exhibit a generous spirit, and set an example of union by at once enrolling their names on the register of the proposed society." It was evident that the writer of these words was ignorant of the separative spirit which actuated that class to whom he had appealed, and either did not know, or, knowing, did not put any credence in the statement which had been made at the public meeting convened by Mr. Rymer, that several leading men had taken action in the matter, and had petitioned the Royal College of Surgeons for identification in some sort with them. Under whatever circumstances it was written, the editor was beside the mark; and if the party under Mr. Rymer's leadership had been inclined to trust for support to the only journal which represented dentistry, there would have been but a short time for that trust to remain unchecked, if not absolutely broken. As it proved, there was left but one more month of favourable notice for the toiling men who had been appointed to the task of setting matters straight in the dental profession by the meeting of September 22d.

With the closing of the year 1856 came the conclusion of journalistic encouragement. Whether the undertaking was too onerous and expensive for the proprietor of the "British Journal of Dental Science" to carry it on need not be discussed; but the result, from whatever cause it originated, was important just then. The journal having been offered to the committee under Mr. Rymer for a certain sum of money, the offer was refused, and it eventually became the property of some gentlemen in the profession, all of whom had either openly or tacitly espoused the Odontological Society. It is not necessary to quote the leading articles under the new régime. Little by little the difference of spirit and tone was made apparent, until the "British Journal of Dental Science," in a few months, was seen flying the flag of bitter opposition. From a friend it had become a foe. But journalism was not a thing upon which Mr. Rymer and his committee placed absolute reliance, although he and they were sensible of its many and distinct advantages. This defection, therefore, had no other effect than that of a healthy stimulant upon those who were making such praiseworthy efforts. With unabated vigour they prosecuted their difficult task. In a circular, signed by the Honorary Corresponding Secretary, the Council of the College of Dentists informed every member of the institution of the circumstances concerning the offer made to it of the purchase of the journal—these circumstances including unreasonable demands, accompanied by statements which looked very much like a threat, if the terms stipulated for were not acceded to; and announced that "as it appeared indispensable that the transactions of the college should be reported, and its claims fairly advocated by an independent publication, it had every reason to believe that very shortly a periodical would appear for that purpose, wherein would be found matter abundantly interesting and useful to every member of the college and the profession at large." This prophecy was eventually fulfilled by the publication of the "Quarterly Journal of Dental Science," under a proprietary of gentlemen practising as dentists. As the "British Journal of Dental Science" had fallen into the hands of those who were members of the Odontological Society, so the new Quarterly belonged to gentlemen who were members of the College of Dentists. The undertaking was promulgated by Mr. Robinson, who, with his usual spirit of determination, resolved that the college enterprise should not be written down or snuffed out without an earnest effort to prevent it. He cheerfully aided it by becoming a co-proprietor, and with his purse and pen helped it forward to the best of his power. The first number appeared in April 1857, and the contents reflected credit on all concerned.

There was sufficient matter at that epoch to fill many of its pages, supplied by the college and its work alone. A regular staff of lecturers had already been appointed for the instruction of the members—the names of the lecturers, together with the subjects of their teachings, being as under, and commenced February 19th:—

JOHN STEGGALL, M.D., &c. Subject: Descriptive Anatomy of Bones, Muscles, Vessels, and Nerves of the Head and Face, embracing Physiology and Therapeutics.

JABEZ HOGG, M.R.C.S., &c. Subject: Histological Anatomy; its value to the Student—The Microscope—Historical Introduction—Optical Arrangement—Appliances—Preparation of Objects —Histology of Cell Development—General Characters and Development of Tissues—Hard Structure and Tooth Structure in particular—Histological and Comparative Anatomy of Teeth—Diseases of the Dental Tissues—Dental Caries, &c.

G. SIMPSON, F.R.C.S., &c. Subject: General Anatomy—Special Anatomy.

DR. GLADSTONE, F.R.S. Subject: Bone Enamel, and the Metals used in Dentistry.

ALFRED CARPENTER, M.B., &c. Subject: Principles of General Surgery.

As these lectures were delivered the "Quarterly Journal" published them, together with the account of the various meetings and transactions of the college as they occurred. It also contained much matter of general interest on many subjects, among which may be mentioned extracts from a new work on dentistry by Mr. Robinson, with illustrations. The wood-engraver's art was liberally introduced into the pages of the new college journal, and Mr. Purland added his quota by sending the whims and oddities of dental advertisements as they appeared in the publications a century or so back. The projectors of the "Quarterly" left nothing undone to provide dental literature for its readers, while they availed themselves of the medium thus in their own hands to push the principles of the institution they had established, by advocating and advancing its claims upon the great body of practitioners at large, giving full reports of the meetings and transactions of the college, and showing a bold and uncompromising front to their equally resolute adversary. The two sides of the dental question had thus organs of their own, and the various aspects of the movement were fully discussed, as from time to time necessity arose, from the opposite points of view. It has been often said "The pen is sharper than the sword," and the truth of the *dictum* was fairly proved in the keenness of the correspondence which appeared on the all-absorbing subject in hand. While speaking of dental literature, it may be as well to mention the opinions which the medical press held concerning the efforts at organisation being made. The "Lancet," of 21st February 1857, makes the following statement :—

"The ground which the dentists take is now clearly laid out, and its limits are distinctly defined. The intention, it appears, is to create a new body, separate and apart from any existing college. In a word, the dentists aim at being a distinct corporate body. . . . We hope, notwithstanding the criminal apathy of the council of the College of Surgeons, that the members of that college will not sanction such a proposal. . . . Surgery is a most important department of that science (medicine), and dental surgery is one of the most important branches of that department. We cannot follow the council of the College of Surgeons as guides on this occasion, and we protest strongly and urgently against permitting the legitimate practitioners of surgery to be robbed of one of the chief sources of emolument in the profession, and the public to be deprived of the benefits which the proper cultivators of that branch of surgery known as dentistry is calculated to afford. Where are these divisions to terminate? Are we to have colleges of dentists, colleges of oculists, colleges of aurists, colleges of cuppers, and colleges of chiropedists? The idea is monstrous enough. Amongst the dentists of the present day there are men of distinguished ability, who are legally qualified members of the Royal Colleges of Surgeons of England, Ireland, and Scotland. Amongst the gentlemen who practise dentistry, but who are *not* members of any medical college whatever, there are also men—to their honour be it spoken—who have acquired high reputation, and who have made large fortunes. Why, then, if there be a desire to obtain for dental surgery that distinction which its importance and utility so fully warrant, do not these gentlemen unite and take part in forming an institution, wherein they may associate, cultivate friendly feelings, and combine in promoting their professional and the public interests? Why not endeavour to obtain a charter for a Royal Dental Institute, admitting during the present year the existing practitioners of dental surgery, but making it an unbending law *afterwards* that not any person shall be received as a member of the Royal Dental Institute who is not a member or fellow of one of the Royal Colleges of Surgeons? . . . . Dental surgery, founded on the science of surgery, is a beautiful art, and the benefits that it has conferred upon the public are but as the merest trifles in comparison with what it can really accomplish. As it is not likely that the council of the College of Surgeons will be awakened to a sense of its duty on this subject unless the voice of the profession be loudly sounded, we trust that, before the next annual election at the college, the feelings of the members will be expressed on this question in a manner that cannot be misunderstood."

This was strong and suggestive writing. Plans on paper are, however, much more easily drawn than carried out in actual practice. Here was a proposition which involved both an impossibility and an improbability. It would have been impossible to include every dental practitioner in such an institution, from the simple fact that the better class and legitimate dentists would have refused to be "levelled down" by associating with impudent empirics and fraudulent quacks. And it was highly improbable that, even if such a heterogeneous mass could have been coaxed into combination, a charter could have been obtained and the institution established within the proposed time, so as to permit the free working of the suggested law of future exclusion. The idea of this writer had some affinity to the views held by the promoters of the college, inasmuch as it looked towards an institute, but with the essential difference of affiliation with the College of Surgeons. In a subsequent number (March 14th) the "Lancet," having scolded the council of the Royal College of Surgeons for not replying to the twice repeated application of the memorialists, although a period of fifteen months had elapsed since the celebrated petition was first presented, reverts to the attempt of Mr. Rymer in the following language :—

"In the meantime, dissensions have occurred amongst the dentists, heart-sick at the deferred hope which it seems to have been the policy of the college to maintain. Hence the machinery of the Dentists' College has been independently arranged. Such an institution is in every way objectionable. It gives no status like that which a connection with the College of Surgeons would have conferred on a body of men whose occupation demands much skill, knowledge, and judgment—whose mission is so eminently the relief of one of the least endurable kinds of human suffering, that only the most narrow and selfish policy could exclude them from association with the profession."

The "Pharmaceutical Journal," after indulging in some satirical remarks upon the gentlemen elected to the office of lecturers at the College of Dentists, proceeded to say in its number for March 4, 1857 :—

"It would, therefore, be premature to pass judgment upon the curriculum of dental education at present; but we may safely predicate that the premises of the new college do not afford accommodation for entering into competition with the medical schools; and that if the college is to stand or fall according to its efficiency as an educating body, the privilege of an independent existence will be purchased by its members at the expense of professional status, and the occupation of a dentist will be reduced to a craft, instead of being an integral part of a profession."

It is unnecessary to criticise too closely or even at all the logic of such statements as these. Whether it was the avowed intention of the promoters of the College of Dentists so to arrange their scheme as to be able, at once, to enter into competition with the various medical schools was not, perhaps, worth this writer's while to consider more than problematical. However, it was evident that this journal was not favourable to independent existence and action among the dentists as a body. On the other hand, the "Medical Circular," under date February 25, 1857, observes :—

"The new Dentists' College is, it appears, to pass through the fiery furnace of controversy before it shall be proved pure and genuine metal. A certain section of the profession seem to think that the College of Surgeons should examine men as to the most scientific way of taking moulds of ill-conditioned jaws, and of making false teeth from elephants' tusks. In that case Lawrence must commence an apprenticeship at the bench, and Stanley take a turn at the lathe. We have no objection to this, only that we should soon make a demand for a new College of Surgeons. Let the friends of the College of Dentists persevere, never minding the petulant twaddle of their adversaries."

These quotations are sufficient to show the influence the attempt at organisation and education had made, not only amongst those immediately concerned, but in the ranks of the medical profession generally. It was also an unmistakable evidence of the difficulties which would beset the path of reform, and a proof that opposition was likely to spring up in many different directions. In the meantime, while the medical press condescended to comment, according to the various views held by the writers in its journals, upon the struggle being maintained between the two parties into which the dental profession was divided, the "British Journal" and the "Quarterly" did not fail to use their respective influences on every occasion.

From the commencement of the year 1857, the attitude of the Odontological Society may be described as patiently expectant. The eyes of its council were intently directed towards the College of Surgeons, in the hope of seeing some evidence manifested of action being taken by the authorities at Lincoln's Inn Fields with regard to the petition which had been presented there. At that time the society could do no more than rely upon the claims which it undoubtedly had, on the score of name and fame of so many of its members, to the rest of the profession. It existed as a scientific society. As such it was a great boon, for there was need enough of more frequent opportunities being given for the reading and discussion of papers upon scientific subjects touching the theory and practice of dental art. Its promoters, however, were not without their plans concerning the future, which, when in the process of time they were made known, reflected credit both for the sagacity with which they had been formulated, and clearly demonstrated the deep interest felt by all concerned in the permanent and increasing welfare of the profession. If the Royal College of Surgeons could be induced to institute a dental department whereby the profession would be properly recognised, it would then become the immediate duty of those through whom this step had been achieved to found a dental school, in order that the curriculum, which would, of course, be imposed, might be carried out by those students who thought proper to pass through it. This again involved another necessity, namely, the providing ample opportunity for a full and practical education to be imparted to those entering such a school. These important measures, though, from the nature of the case, still in embryo, were doubtless the subject of reflection and due consideration. However, the main object of the Odontological Society was clearly expressed in its first byelaw, viz.: "This Society is instituted for the encouragement and diffusion of knowledge of dental surgery, and for the promotion of intercourse among members of the dental profession." This purpose was being assiduously kept, and from the position and qualifications of many connected with it, gave promise of unwavering and unbroken benefit in this most important direction. The following remarks of the president—the late S. Cartwright, Esq.—on the occasion of the first general meeting of the society, held at 32A George Street, Hanover Square, January 5th, 1857, were no doubt in accordance with the sentiments of those then assembled:—"But while, in a large class of practitioners, the educational acquirements are all that can be desired, it cannot but be felt that in another, and a large class too, the standard of education is calculated to form merely a successful artisan; and, consequently, there are two distinct bodies of practitioners—the one practising dentistry as a profession, the other carrying it on as a trade or business. It cannot be doubted that a liberal education is of the greatest advantage to those engaged in practice; and the more education is extended in all ranks of society, the more it becomes necessary that the members of our profession qualify themselves as highly as they can; for those who employ the services of the dentist in these days have a right to look, and do look, to the qualifications of the mind as well as to the mechanical adroitness of the fingers." However much a large portion of the profession may have taken exception to the manner in which the Odontological Society had been instituted, every well-wisher throughout the dental ranks must have felt that through it, as a medium, a great and invaluable benefit would accrue generally, by the distribution of intellectual wealth, hitherto locked up in the minds of its possessors. On the other hand, the College of Dentists was gathering together all its strength for active and energetic work, taking its stand with regard to the future upon its second law, viz. : " The objects for which the College is established are to unite members of the dental profession into a recognised and independent body, and to provide means of professional education and examination." With such a programme before it, there was no room for idleness or indifference, and the council palpably felt the importance of utilising all the material it could command. Had there been no counter-movement in existence, the task they had allotted to themselves would have been onerous enough, but with their staff thinned as it was by the abstention of many gentlemen of influence, and actually opposed by these, the labour to be got through was simply enormous. The silence of the council of the Royal College of Surgeons was deemed by many both in and out of the Dental College as favourable to the designs of the latter. Yet, after all, that silence might at any moment be broken, and in a manner which could not but leave another and formidable obstacle, if not an actually insurmountable one, in their path. They resolved, however, prudently enough, not to ante-date their difficulties. In the arrangements for carrying out the projected college they found abundant opportunities for the absorption of their time and attention, while as yet there remained a very large number of practitioners who had given neither sign nor sound as to what course they would eventually take. From calculations which the writer had officially to make, there were at that time, as nearly as could be ascertained, some 1300 or 1400 dentists practising throughout the three kingdoms. Putting the number of those who were connected with both institutions together, the aggregate did not amount to more than about one-fifth, or thereabouts, of the whole body. Various motives had, no doubt, actuated these dentists in not becoming associated either with the Odontological Society or the Dental College. It is highly probable that the isolation and estrangement which for so many years had characterised the profession were operating still as against union. From whatever cause, however, the fact remained; and this became a stimulus to exertion on the part of the council of the College of Dentists. It was most important to give evidence to what was then called "the outsider" that the party operating with Mr. Robinson and Mr. Rymer was providing an institution which would meet the many requirements of the profession at large. The attempt in itself was a very bold bid for professional favour. Independence was a strong and wide-reaching word. Whatever had been done by our Transatlantic brethren, and however the system of separate institutions had succeeded in America, the experiment was a novel one in this country. The differences in the social as well as professional habits and characteristics of the two peoples constituted, in itself, a subject of the gravest consideration—to say nothing of the inherent objection which so many would most probably feel in becoming copyists of those who were nationally their juniors. There was not a single step which could be taken at that time but was upon new ground. The process of cohesion was in itself but in its infancy. Men were only just beginning, even remotely, to know each other; and the more intimately they became connected and acquainted, the more freely and firmly might their prejudices and predilections be expected to display themselves. There was but one thing upon which the reformers on either side could with any security rely—namely, the desire, expressed or implied, for something in the shape of reform to be set in operation. In the firm belief that the course of procedure adopted by those who had publicly solicited the opinions of the dentists as a body, was that which would most generally accord with the feeling of the mass of the profession, the council of the College of Dentists prosecuted their work. It may be truly said that in Mr. Rymer's conclusions, based upon what had been already accomplished by means of public acquiescence in his views, there lay much force. He felt that he had hit upon the proper mode of procedure; and in a pamphlet which he published in February of that year we find him concluding with the following remarks:—

"An INDEPENDENT existence is, however, demanded by the profession; and it is in obedience to this demand that the College of Dentists of England has been established. It were heartily to be wished that fruitless opposition should now cease, and that *all* should unite to hasten the time—which must inevitably arrive—when the college shall become a national institution, and when no man will be recognised as a qualified dentist unless he has received authority to practise as such from its faculty. The government of the college is in safe and efficient hands—a most important point at the outset. *Organisation* is in steady course of accomplishment, a correct system of education will follow; and the consummation of all will be seen in the elevation of the character of the dental profession by the authority granted to the College of Dentists of England as an INCORPORATED BODY."

From the general tone of this pamphlet it was evident that whoever might entertain doubts as to the necessity for and eventual success of the institution in question, the writer himself had none. So many assurances of aquiescence and support had been given, that, with the faith which is a necessary basis and constant accompaniment of the efforts of projectors, as a rule, added thereto, it was not a matter of surprise that such strong confidence in the ultimate issue of the undertaking should be evinced. One out of many encouragements to proceed with the work may be properly mentioned. Towards the end of 1856, in the November of that year, when the project had become thoroughly known, a general meeting of dentists was called at the Literary and Philosophical Institution, Cheltenham, for

* The Dental Profession : its Present Position and Future Prospects, considered in relation to the recent Reformatory Movement. By Samuel Lee Rymer. Walton & Maberly, 28 Upper Gower Street.

considering the scheme. Mr. Somerset Tibbs occupied the chair, when the subject, as it touched the dental practitioners in that town, was discussed. The result was that the following address was agreed to, and forwarded to the Committee of Organisation in London :—

"CHELTENHAM, *November 24th,* 1856.
"*To the Committee of the Dental Association.*

"GENTLEMEN,—We most cordially agree with you as to the desirability—we might almost say *absolute necessity*—of an Association of Dentists, not only for the protection of the unprincipled, but also for placing the members of an honourable and useful profession in their proper position. We fully acknowledge that such an association, to be successful in the present day, must be established on a broad and liberal basis; and while we feel the great difficulty you must have to contend with in deciding who should be admitted members of such an association, yet, as a line must be drawn somewhere, we would suggest it should be drawn so as to exclude those only, at the formation of the society, who combine any kind of business with the dental profession, and those who issue puffing advertisements, with a 'scale of fees.'

"Should you find it practicable to carry out these suggestions, we beg to offer ourselves as members and associates.

Members—
    ALEX. MONTAGUE.
    CULLIS GEO. HENRY.
    CUNNINGAM, M. G.
    PENNEY, G. S., M.R.C.S.
    ROBERTSON, JAMES.
    TIBBS, SOMERSET.

Associates—
    LEATHERBY, WILLIAM SINTHALL.
    COLLINS, JAMES FRANCIS.
    FOX, J. JOHN.
    ROBERTSON, WILLIAM."

These suggestions had already been acted upon, as a reference to the laws will show; but from such assurances of interest as this, and others from individual members of the profession which had all along been received, the council derived the encouragement to persevere in the due development of the college. It was a time not only of great activity, but of careful and earnest thought. With their opponents watching each step that was taken, and with augmenting criticism in the editorials and general correspondence in the "British Journal of Dental Science," the utmost prudence was necessary. Meetings of councils, committees, and sub-committees abounded. Under the energetic presidency of Mr. Robinson in connection with the first-named the business was systematically gone through. The president was noted for his punctuality, and any member of council arriving after the prescribed time was sure to be reminded of the fact. His leadership of these meetings was, if anything, rigidly severe. The slightest departure from the subject, the merest tendency to conversation, brought the ivory hammer upon the table with no small vehemence, while his quick glance and call to "Business, gentlemen!" would speedily rally the defaulters in attention to the work before them. Those who were then engaged as the representatives of the college felt that it was no child's play to occupy the post to which they had been called by the voice of their brethren. There was much to be done in the direction of internal arrangement. A museum and library had to be formed. Valuable contributions in these departments were received, in response to the appeals made, the president being one of the most liberal donors, Mr. Fox acting as librarian and curator. The appointment of lecturers on the subjects necessary for the purposes of education was attended with no small difficulty, but by the direct personal influence of the president the majority of these was secured, and the arrangements for the delivery of the lectures accomplished, as has been already stated. The conduct of the affairs of the council grew daily in its importance, being directed by Mr. Rymer, and it soon became evident that the general correspondence would become so great as to leave no leisure at the command of him assigned to that particular duty. About this time a Parliamentary measure affecting the medical profession closely, and involving the interests of the dentists, was under the consideration of the Royal College of Surgeons. It was known as Mr. Headlam's Medical Bill. Another measure, known as Lord Elcho's Medical Bill, was simultaneously before Parliament. The scope and tenor of these proposed legal enactments may be gathered from the following circular, which was issued by the College of Dentists of England concerning them:—

"5 CAVENDISH SQUARE, *January* 5, 1857.

"SIR,—I beg to draw your attention to the proposed Medical Bills now before Parliament. No person can be registered under either of these Acts, unless a member of some medical or surgical college or corporation. Again, none but a registered person can perform any surgical operation, or act in a medical capacity. Also, none but a registered person can recover any charges for surgical operations or medical advice. This latter clause will at once affect existing dental practitioners, and deprive them of that protection the law has hitherto afforded them. A petition, praying the House of Commons to add a clause exempting the dentists from the operation of the Act, lies for signature at the College of Dentists, No. 5 Cavendish Square. Your signature to the same is earnestly requested. Your answer by return of post is requested, as the petition must be presented early next week.—I am, sir, yours faithfully,

"ALFRED HILL, *Hon. Sec.*"

The clause in Mr. Headlam's Bill, No. 31, and in Lord Elcho's Bill, No. 42, reads as follows, and, it will be easily seen, was threatening enough to the dentists situated as above:—" After the passing of this Act, no person shall be entitled to recover any charge in any court of law for any medical or surgical advice, attendance, or for the performance of any operation, or for any medicine prescribed, administered, or supplied by him to his own patients, unless he shall prove upon the trial that he is registered under this Act." At an ordinary meeting of the college, then, which was held June 2, 1857, Mr. Underwood drew the attention of the members to this clause, and proposed "that a general meeting of the college be held on Thursday, the 4th of June, to adopt a petition to the House of Commons, praying that House to insert a clause into both Bills, exempting dentists from the operation of the Act, and to invite all dentists throughout the country, whether members of the Dental College or not, to append their names to the same." The necessity of such a step was very evident; and the proposition eventuated, after unanimous adoption, in a petition drawn up by the council, to be presented at the proper time to Parliament. The following is a copy:—

"*To the Honourable the Commons of the United Kingdom of Great Britain and Ireland, in Parliament assembled.*

"The humble petition of the undersigned dentists showeth:—

"That your petitioners humbly beg to represent to your Honourable House the great injustice they conceive would be done to them, and especially to those who at any future time may enter into practice as dentists by either of the Medical Bills now before Parliament, should it pass into a law. That of the existing number of dental practitioners in the United Kingdom but very few are members of any medical colleges or corporations. That none but members of such colleges or corporations can be registered under these Acts, and none but registered persons can perform surgical operations or act in a medical capacity, thus deterring the future dentist from following his professional calling, unless he become a member of one of the said colleges or corporations. That this, your petitioners would humbly submit, will be a great hardship on those who have entered on their pupilage without supposing such a step should become necessary. Again, no person, unless registered under either of the Acts, can, after its passing, recover in a court of law any charges for surgical operations or medical advice. This, your petitioners would humbly represent, will at once affect existing dental practitioners, and deprive them of that protection the law has hitherto afforded them in the legitimate exercise of their calling.

"Your petitioners submit that the following clause be added to the Bill :—' Nothing in this Act contained shall extend, or be considered to extend to prejudice, or in any way to affect the lawful occupation, profession, trade, or business of dentists.'

"Your petitioners, therefore, humbly pray your honourable House that the said Bills may not pass into a law as they now stand, but that they may have such relief in the premises as to your Honourable House shall seem meet. And your petitioners will ever pray," &c.

The president was enabled to state, when the meeting on the 4th of June had assembled, that he together with Mr. Hepburn and Mr. Underwood had elicited a promise from Mr. Headlam and Lord Elcho alike to insert in their respective Bills a clause to exempt dentists. Mr. Underwood also stated that he had had an interview with Lord Elcho, and that his Lordship had undertaken to present the petition framed by the College of Dentists to the House. The activity of the college on this eventful occasion was most praiseworthy; and the influence of that institution was likewise manifested by the result of their solicitations of the dentists generally to append their signatures to the petition. It was very numerously signed; and many of the signataries considered it worth the trouble of travelling long distances to do so. Thus while the Odontological Society had been pressing the Council of the Royal College of Surgeons on the subject of the introduction of a clause into the Medical Bills which would, if assented to, empower that body to institute a curriculum of education, together with an examining board for the purpose of certifying to the fitness to practise of such as passed the ordeal successfully; so also the College of Dentists had been displaying a commendable alacrity in seeking to protect both present and future dentists from the operation of what would have been a most restrictive enactment. The workings of both these institutions were producing very favourable results. Although divided in opinion as to the method of progress, the profession was certainly more united than it had ever been before in the general desire for improvement. Its pulse was beating more vigorously, and while many yet remained on what may be termed neutral ground, there was a greater facility in ascertaining the feeling throughout the entire mass than had hitherto obtained. Provincial practitioners, whether leaning to this side or to that, were watching with the greatest interest the course events were taking in the metropolis, and this alone was to be considered a matter of considerable congratulation. The great obstacle in the past had been the universal apathy which pervaded the profession. Within one short year this indifference had passed away, if not entirely, certainly to a very great extent, and was replaced at this time by an unmistakable desire to use such opportunities as circumstances produced or developed for the bettering of the dental status. Meeting after meeting was held in quick succession at the College of Dentists. Certaintly what was thought necessary to be done there by the council was accomplished in the most punctual and business-like way. Circulars were constantly being issued to the members and the profession at large, giving every information of what was either being done, or proposed to be achieved, with astonishing rapidity. Something like an idea of the amount of correspondence which was taking place at this time may be formed from the fact that the author in the short space of twelve months from the establishment of the college received at his private house nearly two thousand letters from town and country dentists, each communication requiring a specific and separate answer. The printed circulars which he had to despatch were so numerous that they more than filled up the pillar letter-box placed by the Government to receive such, and had to be carried by his servant in huge bundles to other places. The council of the college considerately offered the assistance of a paid clerk, but on trial this individual not only did not give any appreciable help, but required so much instruction that his services were soon dispensed with, and the work carried on as before. The truth is, that the department was one which demanded expedition, and admitted of no blundering. Those who have had to fill similar offices will understand how the common saying, "If you want a thing to be done do it yourself," applied here. It was while thus engaged in the summer of this year (1857) that the writer, having sat at his table until half-past four o'clock in the morning, and had concluded his work by filling to the full the pillar letter-box which was hard by his own door, that he determined to watch the effect produced upon the faithful postman who in another half-hour was to come for its contents. In the quiet of the beautiful summer morning the messenger came whistling unsuspectingly along. On arriving at his destination, the key to the door of the box was applied, the door itself thrown carelessly wide open, and, as the result, the astonished postman surrounded, well nigh to his knees, by a perfect deluge of envelopes. The poor fellow lifted his cap from his head, rubbed his forehead, adjusted the red-bordered covering, and with an exclamation which needs no repetition, cast his big bag on the pavement, and commenced filling it up to the brim. It was a little diversion to the writer to watch quietly, and unseen, from his bedroom window, what may be called "this embarrassment of a man of letters." One thing was certain to both alike, there was more than he could carry with him, and so, while he replaced the redundancy and cruel overflow, the originators of all the trouble retired to his rest. But this is a digresion, for which forgiveness is asked. The occupation of Mr. Rymer as Hon. Sec. to the council involved a very large amount of time and trouble. Nothing, however, seemed to daunt, much less dismay him, and although each meeting in Cavendish Square, where the college was located, demanded his coming from Croydon to London, there was scarcely, if indeed ever, an occasion when he was not present and at his post. Mr. Fox, also, was unremitting in his department, and under his care the library and museum grew in order and development. Nor must Mr. Peter Matthews' name be omitted, for, as treasurer to the college, the members and council alike felt that they had a careful, trustworthy, and energetic friend. Such, indeed, he proved himself to be; his accounts were a perfect pattern of correctness and complete system, the pages of his books being absolutely without error, erasure, or blot. The writer can testify to the excellent feeling which had all along pervaded the council. As the executive, they individually and collectively worked cheerfully in their various offices, each vieing with the other in the effort to conduct the affairs of the institution to a successful issue. The distinct influence exerted upon the profession by the establishment of the Dental College was shown by the fact that at the close of its first session, in June 1857, the number of its members was 218, while nearly twenty more were candidates for membership in the following month, July. The council had been exercising its power in the direction of purifying the profession from the disgraceful habit of advertising; and in order that there should be no room for controversy on this head, had framed a form of declaration to be signed by all candidates for membership. The following is a copy of the document itself:—

"*Declaration.*

"In consideration of my being admitted a member of the College of Dentists of England, I hereby undertake and agree never to insert any advertisement or advertisements (except such as may be approved of by the council of the college) in any paper ; nor to circulate handbills, exhibit showcases, boards, or placards, or to follow any other profession, business, or calling, whilst practising as a dentist, or to do anything that may be in opposition to the 8th and 10th laws of the said college ; and in the event of my departing from this agreement, I authorise the council of the said college to advertise my name in the public papers as being no longer a member of the College of Dentists of England, immediately upon which I agree that my subscription or subscriptions shall become forfeited to the college."

The subjoined circular was to be sent to any offending member :—

"College of Dentists of England,
"5 Cavendish Square, W.

"Sir,—The attention of the council having been called to your mode of practice, I am desired to inform you that, inasmuch as they consider such to be in opposition to the 8th and 10th laws of the college, they wish to know whether you are ready to sign the enclosed declaration, as by these laws all members pursuing a similar course are no longer eligible to be members of the college. Awaiting your reply, I am, sir, yours faithfully,

* * *

"*Hon. Corresponding Sec.*

"*P.S.*—Should you not return an answer to the above within a fortnight from this date, the council will consider that you decline to sign the declaration."

Nor was this a mere document to be spoken of or formally alluded to on rare occasions; it was a veritable instrument for curbing the unruly, whether the delinquent was in office or only a simple member of the college. One case of the former kind did occur, and the result was a verification of these remarks. At the monthly meetings which had been held in March, April, May, and June, the following papers had been read and discussed :—" On the Production of Mineral Teeth," by Mr. D. Mackenzie; " On Diseased Pulp," by Mr. T. Underwood; " On Dental Caries," by (the late) Mr. A. Thomson; " On Pivoting Teeth," by Mr. W. Perkins.

The meetings on these occasions were well attended, and unanimity of sentiment was stimulated by professional intercourse. The council was watchful over the interests of the profession in general and its members in particular; and those who were in connection with the college, at least, felt that it required but cautious perseverance to procure many great and durable benefits for themselves and others. The opposition from the other side appeared ineffectual to prohibit advance, and was accepted as useful in superinducing increasing caution and diligence on the part of the college executive.

The Medical Bill which has been spoken of was creating a very considerable amount of interest, not only in the medical but in the dental profession also.

It proposed very great alterations in the existing state of things, and may be thus summarised:—It sought to prevent the evils which arose from the division of authority that obtained by the independent medical corporations of the United Kingdom. It proposed a general council formed from the various corporate bodies in the persons of chosen delegates from those bodies, together with a certain number of practitioners selected by the Crown. This general council would be intrusted with the power to determine the minutiæ and general arrangements for future medical education, together with the issuing of diplomas, save and except such as pertained to physicians. The proposal included the abolition of the Apothecaries' Company. Those candidates for a diploma—which in effect was similar to that then granted by the Royal College of Surgeons and the Apothecaries' Company—would have to submit to an examination in medicine and pharmacy by a board composed conjointly of members of the College of Physicians and the Apothecaries' Company. In midwifery they would be examined by a board of members of the College of Physicians and College of Surgeons; and in anatomy, physiology, and surgery by the College of Surgeons. The examinations would have to be passed in the above order. A system of registration was also included in the measure, but very little was known or made public concerning this important item. Looked at thus, the action proposed to be taken evinced an acknowledgment on the part of the corporate bodies of the general desire and necessity for the union of the then divided powers into a central and supreme authority. As such, the circumstance appeared to be exceedingly opportune to those who held that dental surgery was a branch of general surgery, and, therefore, should not be severed from it, but recognised and associated with the parent stock. While the Odontological Society had much to say, and many cogent reasons to support their ideas on this subject, there was yet a large number of the medical profession who were not content to admit the force of their arguments. There was a certain amount of what may be, perhaps, called jealousy lest the recognition of dentists by the College of Surgeons, and the granting of certificates after examination to them, should be construed into meaning equality with those who possessed the membership of the college. From whatever cause the difference of opinion arose, many medical practitioners held with the College of Dentists of England that it was far more preferable that dentists should be an independent body, and look to their own college or institute for a certificate or diploma guaranteeing the fitness of the several members to practise. The agitation which pervaded the dental profession was, therefore, not confined to it, but was largely shared in by the practitioners of general surgery. It is not, therefore, a matter of surprise to know that the College of Dentists felt itself fortified in its efforts for an independent existence by the sentiments which were held by many general practitioners, and endorsing its own. The two dental journals received very copious matter for their columns under the head of "Correspondence," the writers of these letters in many instances, and on both sides, expressing themselves with a vehemence amounting to invective. Such contributions, wherever they appeared—and the medical journals had a considerable share of them—only fanned the flame of discord, and made the direction of affairs far more difficult for the executive on either side. Statements and counter-statements were unpleasantly frequent; but one thing was made apparent, and that was the determination of the parties concerned to avow their opinions lustily, and maintain their views and course of action with the greatest pertinacity. A glance at the journals of that period will give abundant proof of this. Yet throughout all the confusion and strife of words the two institutions were aiming steadily at but one object. How to attain it, however, was the difficult point. Upon the subject of the proposed dental department at the Royal College of Surgeons, both sides of the profession had come to a tacit understanding, viz., that those gentlemen who would form the examining board should not be simply surgeons. Although the idea had never been promulgated by the Odontological Society that only members of the College of Surgeons practising as such should be the examiners, a very general notion obtained that such was indeed the intention, and it was, therefore, a matter of congratulation that this misconception had materially died away. The true basis for advance could only be hoped for in the gradual formation of a definite opinion as to what would really prove a permanent benefit to the future dentist. There had been and still were fiery spirits connected with these two movements; but there were those also who, possessing a calmer mind, were content to allow time to do its own specific work. A feeling among some of the more influential members of the College of Dentists was manifesting itself in the direction of united action with the Odontological Society, if that were possible, characterised by the publication of conflicting opinions concerning the workings and ultimate issue of the two rival bodies. As soon as the opportunity of expressing ideas offered itself, the same was eagerly taken advantage of. Among the many writers who, either with their own names or otherwise, indited letters to the profession on the all-important subject before it, Mr. W. Perkins and Mr. D. Mackenzie were prominent on the college side of the question. Of course, their correspondence met with prompt replies from the opposing ranks, Mr. Spence Bate among others being conspicuously to the fore. As the year grew, however, the animus which had been formerly so painfully evident appeared to be moderated, and many looked hopefully towards the prospect of a blending of the divided energy of those who were so untiringly working one against another. With a considerable number of those gentlemen who had to this time been so actively engaged in the matter of reform, the possibility of an amalgamation became a subject of the highest importance. Their minds would involuntarily revert to it, and their whole conduct was in itself a proof that, if the thing could be accomplished, they would certainly assist to bring it about. Contrasting their indefatigable efforts with the supineness of the large number of dentists who had made no sign to indicate the direction of their individual proclivities, it was only a fair conclusion to arrive at that so difficult and decided a result would alone be obtained by those already in the field of conflict. Whether odontologists or college supporters, they had alike displayed resolution enough to carry out such a measure. One of the evidences of the tendency towards united action appeared in a letter addressed by Mr. Perkins to the editor of the "British Journal of Dental Science," under date August 4, 1857, where that writer, who was one of Mr. Rymer's most ardent supporters, says—

"I might just observe, that since writing the letter which appeared in the 'Lancet,' in 1855, Mr. Rymer's views have undergone some alteration in regard to what might be considered a necessary examination. An examination of the kind there mentioned would certainly have been better than *none at all;* but it has occurred to him, as well as to many others, that such an examination would of necessity be incomplete, inasmuch as it would relate to surgery *only;* and it was with a view to the complete instruction and subsequent examination of all pupils intended to become dentists, that the establishment of the College of Dentists was first resolved on; and as this object appears to be sincerely the aim of both parties into which the dentists are divided, I cannot help reiterating my regret that they do not work together to bring about so desirable a result; for I repeat, that together they would easily obtain all they want, while, acting separately, they do but neutralise each other. They are, in fact, in the one case $1-1=0$, in the other they would be $1+1=2$."

Every step towards a fusion of action on the basis of a common interest and professional elevation was fraught with difficulty. The proposer of any idea to this end was weighed in the balances as to his own standing or the probable influence he might be expected to exert. Such, indeed, was the highly-wrought sensitiveness of that day that the motives of the leading men themselves were subjected to the keenest and most critical analysis and dissection. Of course the editorial departments of both dental journals were regarded as the most reliable quarters to look for information. In turning to the pages of the "British Journal of Dental Science," we note the following as indicative of the feelings pervading the Odontological Society, whose organ it was. In the number for October 1857, the following remarks appear in the usual leaded type:—

"It is quite true that the College (of Dentists) has not announced formally that the examination for the dental diploma may be given at the College of Surgeons, but this step is proposed in the October number of the journal, originated by members of the council of the College of Dentists, and published as the acknowledged organ of the college. Now, if the college is prepared to adopt the proposal respecting the mixed board of examiners at the College of Surgeons, it will in fact have embraced in all the essential particulars the course which has been consistently held by the Odontological Society. Such being the case, the views entertained by the two societies have so few points of essential difference, that they may be said not only to be working towards the same end, but that they seek to gain that end by the same path. It is suggested that mutual concession must be made by the Dental College and the Odontological Society; but we do not see what the latter body has to concede. Its views on the educational question are adopted by the College of Dentists, and they are received by the College of Surgeons: so much so, indeed, that the latter body is virtually pledged to act upon them. As respects the fusion of the college and the society into one body, we confess we do not see either the necessity, or even the expediency of such a measure. Let the college be maintained as an educational body, like in character to King's College or University College; while the society will hold to the dental profession a similar position to that which the Medical and Chirurgical Society holds to the medical profession; each institution may perform its own part more effectually than though it were encumbered with the other, while the majority of the members of the one will also be connected with the other. Let one be strictly subservient to the education of the students, and the other to the discussion of professional subjects by those whose education has been completed. The third body—the board of examiners—must be altogether independent both of the society and the college. Let these arrangements be carried out, and the organisation of the dental will be similar to, and upon an equality with, that of the general body of the medical profession. Those already in practice cannot be influenced directly by the proceedings either of the society, the college, or the dental department of the College of Surgeons. Honours given where they are not merited reflect discredit equally both upon the givers and upon the receivers. A title indicating acquirements which are not possessed only exposes its bearer to ridicule. An opportunity of raising the professional status of the future surgeon-dentist exists: let it be shown that neither ignorance, bigotry, or selfishness shall prevent our seizing the opportunity."

The views of the College party were given in an editorial article in the "Quarterly Journal of Dental Science," in the number for October 1857, thus—

"Before these pages can be submitted to our readers, the members of the College of Dentists of England will have received a code of propositions, the result of deliberations which have been going on between the councils of the College of Dentists of England and the Odontological Society on the all-important subject of amalgamating the two societies. We congratulate the profession most sincerely, that thus far there is every probability of its being represented by a united body of practitioners, and that hereafter we may hope to see enrolled beneath one standard every respectable dentist in the three kingdoms. The College of Dentists was instituted with the intention of offering the means of education to the younger members of the profession—to be, in fact, the recognised medium for obtaining that knowledge which was felt by all to be necessary in order that the future dentist might become a thoroughly qualified person; and we are gratified to find that whatever changes are proposed, this *vital, fundamental principle* remains unaltered. We trust that the members of the college will attend the meeting to be called on the 8th of January next, with a full determination to give the subject their most serious attention, and decide upon the measures with the strictest impartiality. Let us not forget that on the occasion in question an opportunity will be offered to cement the interests of the profession by a common tie, and that such an event will most probably not occur again. Those who have laboured so indefatigably in connection with either society cannot reasonably be regarded as likely to continue their labours *ad infinitum*, and we feel bound to conclude, that should these proposals be dealt with in any other than the most liberal way, there will be a declension on the part of many, whose services and aid the profession should strive to retain. For obvious reasons we do not specify these propositions in detail, but we sincerely trust that shortly after the date of this meeting, the dentists of Great Britain and Ireland may be represented by one institution, let it be called by whatever name it may."

Onwards, then, to the close of the year the idea of reform was carried, with more or less of variation in the views of the parties concerned, but the general feeling evidently gravitated towards a great effort at reconciling conflicting sentiment, and securing unity of action for the future. While thus looking back on the year 1857 as a whole, it will be necessary to consider it somewhat more in detail, or at any rate to summarise its workings as they bore upon the profession at large. So far as the College of Dentists was concerned, its executive had been unceasingly at their posts, and unwearied in their efforts to consolidate and utilise it as an institution. Meetings had been systematically held each month. The promised papers, together with others, had been given with due regularity, and thorough discussion of the various subjects treated of had taken place. That the essays delivered were important the following list of them will prove :—

"On the Production of Mineral Teeth," by Mr. D. MACKENZIE.
"On Diseased Pulp," by Mr. UNDERWOOD.
"On Dental Caries," by Mr. A. THOMSON.
"On Pivoting Teeth," by Mr. W. PERKINS.
"On the Electric Cautery," by Mr. T. HARDING.
"On the Alveolar Hemorrhage Compress," and the "Dentition of the Lilliputian Aztecs," by Mr. R. REID.
"On Refining and Assaying Gold," by Mr. W. G. BENNETT.
"On Mechanical Dentistry," by Mr. A. HOCKLEY.

The appointed lecturers had given excellent lectures to the students on the following subjects, viz. :—

"Descriptive Anatomy," by Dr. STEGGALL.
"Histological Anatomy, the use of the Microscope," by JABEZ HOGG.

"On the Skeleton," by G. SIMPSON.
"On Dental Surgery," by A. CARPENTER.
"On Substances used in Dentistry—1. Bone enamel; 2. Metals in Dental use," by Dr. GLADSTONE.

The library and museum had each received a very large amount of contributions, and could be considered excellent as storehouses of great value for the students, either for mental or material reference. The number of adherents steadily increased as the institution and its claims became better known through the influence of its own members, and the published account of its proceedings by means of the "Quarterly Journal of Dental Science;" while the growing confidence in its essential usefulness and ultimate success, both within its walls and without, constituted it a most important subject for consideration, and object of wide-spread notice. There was no disguising the fact that, as a rival of and opponent to the Odontological Society, it not only held its ground tenaciously, but made steady advance in its own proposed direction. During this year it had very carefully drawn up the laws and constitution, together with a code of byelaws, of the institution, and included therein the means whereby the diploma of the college could alone be obtained.

On the other hand, the Odontological Society had been steadily pursuing its course, its supporters constantly availing themselves of every opportunity to promote its interests and progress. Its affairs were systematically published in the "British Journal of Dental Science," which, as its own organ, did not fail to push forward its claims for acceptance by the profession at large. Papers, of which the following is a list, were read at its meetings, and altogether its establishment had become considerably consolidated:—

"On the Reduction of Limaille," by Mr. ARNOLD ROGERS.
"On Absorption of the Roots of Temporary Teeth," by Mr. SPENCE BATE.
"On the Best Method of Excluding Moisture from Teeth during the Operation of Plugging," by Mr. JOHN TOMES.

"On Dental Exostosis," by Mr. HUBERT SHELLEY.
"On the Removal of the Four Permanent First Molars, at an Early Period, in Overcrowding Arches," by Mr. SAMUEL MACLEAN.
"On Improvements in Operating Chairs," by Mr. J. BARRETT.
"On Cleft Palate," by Mr. E. SERCOMBE.
"On the Cause of the Early Destruction of the Teeth," by Mr. ROBERTSON.
"On Capping Exposed Nerve," by Mr. T. A. ROGERS.
"On an Improved Dentist's Lathe," by Mr. G. OWEN.
"On Gutta-Percha as a Permanent Stopping," by Mr. H. L. JACOB.
"On the Materials used by Dentists," by Mr. G. A. M. DUFF.
"On the Method of Taking Impressions of Cleft Palate," by Mr. E. SERCOMBE.
"On Plate Casting," by Mr. J. H. STATHAM.

With such a catalogue of efforts made on both sides as have thus been recorded, it was abundantly evident that the latent energies of the profession were thoroughly astir. One other matter, however, must be mentioned before closing this chapter.

Shortly after the middle of this year, memorable in the history of dentistry, a circumstance occurred which, simple in itself, operated materially upon the future course of events. It was an illustration of the principle acknowledged by all, and not unfrequently demonstrated, that apparently insignificant causes produce large and important results. Mr. Reid, of Edinburgh, was the actor, and, at the request of the author, has furnished him with a succinct account of the circumstance, which will be best given in his own words. Mr. Reid says:—" In passing through London during the summer of 1857, I met with several of my professional brethren, with whom the all-absorbing subject of the division of the profession into two rival bodies formed the topic of conversation. From what I heard, I became impressed with the feeling that a considerable misconception existed in the minds of the Odontologicals I came across, as to the views and the honest working of those of the college, who in a straightforward way sought to advance the status of the profession, and give it position as a learned body. That impression was strengthened and afterwards confirmed by what passed during an interview I had with my old and valued friend Mr. Tomes. On thinking over all I had heard, the question arose within me, Could not a better understanding be effected between the two sections who, although estranged, were travelling in parallel lines while worthily working to attain the same end? But how was that to be accomplished? The only way that occurred to me was, to devise the means of bringing the motor powers, as it were, of each section together, so that, in coming to know each other, their views might be better understood, and misconception thereby dispelled. Acting upon this, perhaps impulsive, idea—my stay in town being but short, and having a strong desire to place matters on a friendly footing ere I left, if at all in my power—I penned a letter to Mr. Tomes, feeling the while that I was treading on dangerous ground on entering on such a delicate undertaking. I cannot do better than give you that document *in extenso*, from the copy I kept. It is as follows :—

"'MY DEAR SIR,—Casting over in my mind what passed between us during the interview I had the pleasure of having with you to-day, I feel strongly impressed with the idea that a great deal of misapprehension exists between the two bodies at present representing the dental profession. I cannot express the concern it gives me that members of the same family, as it were, should thus be at enmity. Surely something might be done to end such an unseemly state of things. My time in town is limited, as I propose leaving on Monday; and could I in any way be instrumental in bringing about a meeting betwixt individual members of each body, I need not assure you what pleasure it would afford me. I am now about to make a suggestion, which, believe me, comes entirely from myself, and which, if listened to on your part, will, I feel confident, be as readily responded to by the party I am about to name. Will you afford me an opportunity of introducing you and Mr. Underwood to each other as individual professionals? If agreeable, I would propose that you meet on neutral ground—that is, in my apartments, No. 5 Duke Street, Portland Place, and that on Monday, at whatever hour you may find most

convenient. As I have already stated, I leave on Monday evening, and no other chance is left me of mediating in this matter. An acquiescence on your part can be but regarded as a graceful act by every generous-minded man, and every well-wisher of our profession. Need I then say I feel hopeful—nay, confident, you will accede to my proposition. I shall call on you at half-past ten on Monday. If you can spare me two minutes I shall be glad. If engaged, will you kindly leave for me a note, saying how this is received. Believe me, my dear sir, ever yours most sincerely, ROBERT REID,
'1st August 1857. 5 DUKE STREET, PORTLAND PLACE.'

" As intimated, I called on Mr. Tomes on the Monday morning—found him very far from well; nevertheless, he said he would be happy to meet Mr. Underwood, if he would kindly waive ceremony by coming along to Cavendish Square, as he was too unwell to leave his room that day to get to my apartments. To this proposal I could give no other answer than to say I would carry it immediately to Mr. Underwood. This I did, and having, with certain misgivings, acquainted the latter of what I had done at my own hand—of Mr. Tomes' inability to meet him on the proposed 'neutral ground' owing to illness, and at the same time delivering his message of invitation to meet him, by accompanying me to Cavendish Square, Mr. Underwood in the circumstance promptly acquiesced. On being shown into Mr. Tomes' apartment I introduced the two plenipotentiaries in these terms: 'Gentlemen, you know each other, and need no introduction.' The frank and friendly way in which they met, assured me there was a mutual desire to know and be known, so that misconception might be dispelled, and a right understanding arrived at of the views of those who were in truth, each after their own fashion, working to effect one common good. After a few commonplaces an amusing little colloquial passage-at-arms took place, thrust and parry following each other in quick succession; the good-natured bantering give-and-take ending in merriment, and the hearty hand-grasp at parting, while evincing mutual esteem, raised in me a feeling of gratification that amply repaid the disquiet and the misgivings I had experienced as to the issue of my unauthorised attempts at mediation."

It was a happy idea which occurred to Mr. Reid thus to bring together two such truly representative men, and his management of the whole affair reflects the greatest credit on his generosity of mind, and also on his excellent tact. There was in it all through *la finesse* of diplomacy. The proposed "neutral ground," the carefulness as to the introduction, alike proved that Mr. Reid not only understood the amount of sensitiveness which had been produced by the conflict of opposing sentiments, but demonstrated also his capital ability to deal with it under the circumstances. The effect of that interview was in itself admirable, and its results leave the profession indebted to the originator of it in no insignificant degree. It must be remembered that Mr. Underwood had from the first warmly espoused the College of Dentists' scheme, and tenaciously adhered to it as the most beneficial method which could be employed to elevate the profession. With excellent effect he had publicly spoken in advocacy of that system, and was well fitted to advance and discuss its merits in the presence of such a defender of the opposite plan as Mr. Tomes. No one who knows the latter gentleman could doubt for a moment the ability with which the principles and plan of the Odontological Society would be dealt with when such a close reasoner and acute thinker, as Mr. Tomes has ever proved himself to be, undertook to explain and enforce them. They were, in fact, "foemen worthy of each other's steel." By this interview an important barrier in the way of union was, so far, removed. The difficulty of effecting such intercommunion, and the apparent danger of failure, were painful evidences of the estrangement which had been prevailing throughout the profession, and when the feat—for it was nothing less—had been accomplished, every right-minded man felt not only a sense of relief, but could justly entertain a brighter hope concerning the future.

CHAPTER V.

MATTERS having worked up to this point, it was a happy augury that such men as Mr. Tomes and Mr. Underwood could come together and calmly discuss the subject in hand. The circumstance, of course, became known to both institutions, and this eventuated in the resolution that Mr. Tomes should act in the capacity of the appointed delegate from the Odontological Society, and Mr. Underwood as the appointed delegate from the College of Dentists, to confer together upon the subject of an amalgamation of the two bodies. Armed with this official authority, these two gentlemen accordingly met, and the result of their conference was the following:—

"The parties delegated by the respective councils of the Odontological Society and the College of Dentists of England to confer upon the propriety of adopting a common course of procedure in respect to the organisation of the dental profession, beg to recommend to their respective councils the adoption of the following conclusions:—

"1. That a definite course of education shall be provided for those who may in future enter upon the practice of dental surgery.

"2. That those subjects which are taught at the existing medical schools, a knowledge of which is necessary to the dentist, shall be learnt at such schools.

"3. That those subjects which specially relate to dental surgery shall be taught at a school established for that purpose.

"4. That a dental diploma shall be granted after an examination, and that the examination shall be conducted at the College of Surgeons by a board composed of surgeons and dentists in equal numbers.

"5. That, in order to carry into effect the foregoing propositions, a committee shall be formed, consisting of three members of each of the respective councils, namely, the College of Dentists and the Odontological Society.

(Signed)   "THOMAS UNDERWOOD.
"JOHN TOMES.

"*November* 24, 1857."

This preliminary step met with the approval of both institutions, and the consequence was that it was determined that the subject should be further considered; and to this end three members of the council of each body were delegated for that purpose. After mature deliberation, the annexed propositions were mutually agreed upon by these gentlemen :—

"*Proposed Terms of Amalgamation between the College of Dentists of England and the Odontological Society, December* 19, 1857.

"1. That the two bodies shall be merged into one, and that the name shall be 'The Institute of British Dentists'—to consist of a president, vice-presidents, council, officers, members, and associates.

"2. That, in the event of the amalgamation taking place, the united body pledges itself that it shall press upon the College of Surgeons the necessity of granting, within a reasonable time, special dental diplomas on the following terms.

"3. That the court of examiners at the College of Surgeons of candidates for the dental diploma shall consist of surgeons and dentists in equal numbers.

"4. That the dental portion of the court of examiners at the College of Surgeons of candidates for the dental diploma shall be chosen by the amalgamated body of dentists; and that it shall not be essential that the dentists on such court shall hold the diploma of the College of Surgeons.

"5. That in the event of the College of Surgeons declining to grant the above-specified dental diplomas, the Odontological Society and the College of Dentists of England, in thus uniting, pledge themselves that the united dental body shall grant its own diploma.

"6. That the united Dental Society shall be the chief educational body in all subjects connected with dental surgery and mechanics.

"7. That the council shall consist of eighteen members, six only of whom shall be country members; and that the mode of nominating the first council shall be, that the council of the Odontological Society shall choose nine members from the present office-bearers of the College of Dentists of England, and that the council of the College of Dentists of England shall choose nine members from the present office-bearers of the Odontological Society.

"8. That the above council shall nominate a president.

"9. That there shall be at least six vice-presidents, and that they shall be nominated and chosen in the same manner as specified above for the proposed council.

"10. That there shall be a treasurer.

"11. That there shall be three honorary secretaries.

"12. That an assistant-secretary be engaged, who shall act as librarian and curator.

"13. That the treasurer and secretaries shall be nominated by the provisional council, when formed.

"14. The above nominated office-bearers and council shall be submitted for election at a meeting of members of the united body, to be convened for that purpose, and scrutineers to be appointed at such meeting.

"15. One-third of the council shall retire at the end of each year, but such members of council shall not be eligible for re-election until a year has expired from the time of such retirement, and that no member shall remain on the council longer than three consecutive years.

"16. After discharging the liabilities and obligations of each society, the funds of each shall be merged into one fund.

   (Signed) JAMES ROBINSON.
        ARNOLD ROGERS.
        JOHN TOMES.
        SAMUEL CARTWRIGHT, Jun.
        THOMAS UNDERWOOD.
        ROBERT HEPBURN."

These propositions displayed abundant evidence of the deep interest in the future of the dental profession which the committee, both individually and collectively, felt. As the product of their joint and earnest efforts, it was most creditable to them all alike; and it was evident to those who knew the spirit and candour of the signataries that this document had cost them much in the direction of those sentiments which they held so tenaciously. There were the traces all through it of struggle. Had not the permanent benefit of the future dentist been the supreme idea in the minds of each and all concerned, no such conclusion could have been even hoped for, much less arrived at. Considering the amount and quality of conflicting opinion around them at that time, it was a matter of congratulation that so much forbearance and mutual conciliation had been manifested. The important consideration was, would these terms prove acceptable to the supporters of the two societies? So far as the Odontological Society was concerned, when the proper moment for their discussion came, they were duly submitted and approved. It remained, therefore, to be seen how they would be dealt with by the College of Dentists of England. Those whom the matter concerned had not long to wait in suspense. A meeting of the members of the college was announced to take place on the evening of January 8, 1858, for the purpose of considering the proposed plan of union. In the meantime, however, the Odontological Society had resolved to hold its first public dinner; which event was to take place on the 2d of that month, at the Freemasons' Tavern, Great Queen Street, London. To this festival Mr. Robinson, as president of the College of Dentists, had been invited; in itself an earnest of goodwill towards the institution he represented. In return Mr. Robinson very properly, and with a generous spirit, waived all other considerations, and accepted the proffered courtesy; believing that by so doing he would facilitate matters in many directions, and smooth the path towards a better understanding on all sides. By his influence he also obtained the support of the personal presence of several other members of the College of Dentists of England on the occasion. Mr. Arnold Rogers, in the absence of the president, occupied the chair, and was supported on the right by Mr. Robinson, and on the left by Mr. Jacob Bell, the latter gentleman being then the president of the Pharmaceutical Society. Many were the friendly expressions used, and great the cordiality experienced by gentlemen of both sides. Differences seemed to die a hasty and very natural death in the particular atmosphere of goodwill, and expectations of the best order appeared to grow and strengthen as by an instinct. In proposing the health of the president of the College of Dentists of England, Mr. Rogers made the following among other remarks, which will serve to throw a little light upon events which were in the immediate future:—

"I speak," said Mr. Rogers, "from behind the scenes; I have never had the pleasure of Mr. Robinson's acquaintance until, as one of the delegates, I met that gentleman upon this important business (the question of amalgamation). I shall never forget the cordiality of feeling displayed by the delegates of the College of Dentists, nor their heartiness in the cause of dental surgery, and their disposition to carry out every arrangement by which the profession might be benefited. When we came to compare notes, there was scarcely any difference between us; and I venture to say that if the delegates had the power granted to them, we should have settled the question there and then. We had eight hours most agreeable companionship. There was sometimes a little controversy, but it was all conducted in a most amicable disposition. I do not say there was any sacrifice of principle, for there was nothing to sacrifice; nor was there any compromise, for we were both pointing to the same object, and it would have puzzled the Lord Chancellor to have detected any real difference between us. . . . I consider that the circumstance of our having had two courses has been the happiest thing for the profession."

Mr. Robinson in reply said—

"With regard to myself and the gentlemen present, I assure you we never had any other wish than to raise the status of the profession. The best way to do that has been the subject of difference between us, but we certainly have broken the ice now, and I trust we shall all be able to unite and form ourselves into one strong and powerful body of dentists, equal to any other profession in the kingdom."

Although these were *post-prandial* observations, and as such may be accepted at only a certain value, yet subsequent events proved them to be very faithful representations of the sentiments held by an ever-increasing number of dental practitioners. Undoubtedly this gathering together, under pleasant social circumstances, of gentlemen who had held aloof from each other, and even had opposed each other, was no unimportant element in the direction of future union and progress. It seems strange that up to the year of grace 1858, a useful and honourable profession had been so uncared for and integrally separated as to permit two practitioners of position, like Mr. Rogers and Mr. Robinson, to be altogether unknown to one another in the manner Mr. Rogers thus stated. The occasion in question appeared to be a happy prognostic for the dentists of the United Kingdom, and the interest concerning the forthcoming meeting of the college members was heightened materially thereby. On the 8th of January the gathering at No. 5 Cavendish Square was duly held. Mr. Robinson, as president, was in the chair, and sixty-one members were present—a number which could hardly be said fully to represent the college on so important an occasion, as the names on the list at that time numbered, with the associates, somewhat over three hundred.

The president, in introducing the subject, announced that the propositions to be submitted were to be considered as a whole, and not to be taken *seriatim*. This constituted the first difficulty. It next transpired that the council of the college in their deliberative capacity were not unanimous upon the subject. This produced a feeling of uneasiness. There were, evidently, those present who would not allow the matter to pass without critical analysis. Such was the overwrought sentiment which existed, that a sense of jealousy was manifested in even the way in which the idea of amalgamation originated. "Who," it was demanded, "first made the proposition to unite the two bodies?" And here, it was apparent, lay the value and importance of Mr. Reid's procedure. This question having been satisfactorily answered by Mr. Underwood, the meeting went as far as receiving the propositions of the delegates. The real contest then began—Mr. Mackenzie, Mr. Lintott, Mr. Turner, Mr. Matthews, and Mr. Perkins making strong objections to the terms before them. The chief difficulty, at least with many, appeared to be in the forfeiture of the name. The College of Dentists of England was certainly a good and euphonious title, which had been determined upon after much discussion, and was admittedly most appropriate for an educational institution. No wonder that Mr. Rymer objected to the new scheme, considering the earnestness and sustained zeal he had exhibited in inaugurating, and so far helping to develop, his idea of what would meet the necessities of the profession. He firmly believed that there were within the dental ranks men competent to examine future dentists, and in every way capable of instructing them in the various departments of their profession. Besides this, he had been led to the conclusion that an independent existence was that which dentistry, as such, needed and demanded. Amongst others, therefore, Mr. Rymer, while desiring an amalgamation with the Odontological Society, felt that the terms proposed were incompatible with what he considered principle and honour. The meeting was a prolonged one, and after an animated discussion, the proposed terms of the delegates were put from the chair. The votes recorded were—For the amalgamation, 27; against it, 34—majority, 7.

The measure was accordingly lost. The result thus attained was productive of much feeling on all sides. The college delegates, Messrs. Robinson, Hepburn, and Underwood, construed it into an expression of want of confidence in them, and consequently resigned their official positions—the first as president, the two latter as members of council. Messrs. Rogers, Ghrimes, Fox, and the writer having supported the delegates at the meetings of council, and also at the general meeting, felt that the same course was alone open to them, and they also consequently vacated their official positions. With regard to those members of the governing body who had voted against the plan proposed, it may be asserted that much regret was experienced by them at the failure of this attempt at union; so much so, indeed, was this the case that they by no means abandoned the hope of succeeding through another attempt which they were prepared to make. Outside the college regret deepened into dissatisfaction, because it was generally thought that had the meeting in question been more numerously attended, the opposite result to that which had been arrived at would have been secured. With the Odontological Society there was the settled determination to do no more in the direction of uniting or attempting to unite with the College of Dentists. The council and members generally of that society had placed the measure in the hands of three gentlemen in whom they had unlimited confidence. Their proposals had been accepted by them, and when they were rejected by the College of Dentists in meeting assembled, they concluded that it was unnecessary to try further. This resolution was confirmed by their determination to hold no more correspondence with the Dental College on the subject. At the annual general meeting of the college, which was held January 21, 1858, the subject, as might be expected, was included in the report presented to the members for adoption. The chairman, Mr. P. Matthews, brought it forward, expressing his own regret, and that also of the council, that the proceedings on this important matter had terminated in the way then so well known. He also alluded to the great loss the college staff had sustained in the resignation of those gentlemen whose names have been already mentioned. Admitting that the meeting, whose decision had produced so much sensation throughout the profession, had been deprived of the opportunity of a full expression of opinion by the members generally, through the fact that no provision had been made in the laws for receiving votes by proxy, Mr. Matthews acknowledged the necessity of immediately attempting to remedy that palpable defect. There can be no doubt that the feeling of that meeting was that the amalgamation question was either not settled at all, or not properly settled. Mr. Rymer himself was under that impression, for he remarked that he should use his influence with the council to call another meeting to reconsider it.* Mr. S. Tibbs expressed his earnest desire that the gentlemen who had resigned, as a consequence of the rejection of the terms proposed, should be pressed to continue in office or withhold their resignations until the question had been submitted in such a manner as that town and country members might have the opportunity of recording their opinions. Mr. Tibbs was a vice-president of the college, and he believed that if this action were taken the decision of the former meeting would be reversed. In submitting his proposition to the meeting then assembled he met with a very cordial response, every hand being held up in token of acquiescence. Mr. Robinson, in concurring with the unanimous wish of those present, that he and others who had resigned should return to office, and speaking on behalf of those gentlemen who had resigned, said— " We now go on, then, upon these terms :—If we are beaten by proxy upon the amalgamation question, we consider ourselves open to take any course we please ; and if we should not be beaten, we shall join in any and all measures to advance the interests of the associated members and of the profession at large." This meeting ended by Mr. Matthews vacating the presidential chair in favour of Mr. Robinson, a vote of thanks being passed to the former gentleman for the efficient manner in which he had fulfilled the duties of his office, to Mr. Fox for his exertions as curator, and, finally, by the adoption of a resolution proposed by Mr. Rymer that the special meeting for the alteration of the bye-laws should be adjourned to a day not named. On the 8th of February 1858, the meeting here alluded to was held at the college rooms for the purpose of adding the following words, by way of amendment, to Law No. 13, viz. :—" Members of the college residing beyond twenty miles of Charing Cross shall be entitled to vote by

* Quarterly Journal of Dental Science, vol. ii. p. 95.

proxy in the election of council and officers, and all other questions of importance in general, and special general meetings." Mr. Robinson was in the chair. Mr. Matthews proposed the motion, and Mr. Underwood seconded it. Such, however, was the spirit of disagreement, even upon such a plain matter as this, that an amendment was proposed. The power to move an amendment was ruled against by the chairman, and after a considerable discussion on the original motion, the same was at length carried, with only one dissentient voice. Another and special meeting was held " to reconsider the terms of amalgamation proposed by the late delegates," which, through real or supposed technical difficulties touching the 13th law of the college, resulted in the dissolution of the meeting without any agreement being arrived at. This was on March 4th. It was speedily followed, March 27th, by a special general meeting of the college, " for the purpose of taking the sense of the members upon the course to be pursued in consequence of the rejection of the proposed terms of amalgamation." Mr. Robinson occupied the chair. Having explained that the then position of the council was considered to be anomalous, it had been determined to consult the members upon the position of the college. All the proxy papers which up to that time had been received were destroyed—a motion to that effect having passed the meeting. In consequence of the terms of amalgamation having been rejected, several of the original office-bearers declined being put in nomination for the new council. Mr. Mackenzie moved " that as the council has never been dissolved, it is still in active existence, and consequently cannot be in an anomalous position ; and that it be requested to call a general meeting to fill up the vacancies in its body occasioned by the resignation of some of its members." Mr. Underwood, with his usual clearness, stated that it was his decided opinion that the delegates were requested to return to office for the purpose of testing the feeling of the members at large upon the same terms which had been placed before the members on the 8th of January. This opinion, it is certain, was that of the delegates and those who supported them. However, Mr. Tibbs moved an amendment to the effect that a sub-committee of five should be appointed whose duty should be to endeavour to collect a council from amongst the members who would act with unanimity; which motion, having been duly seconded, was, after considerable discussion, carried. The gentlemen elected for this purpose were Messrs. Purland, Weiss, Bartlett, Imrie, junior, and Harding.

Apart from the feeling of disapprobation which was felt by many members of the college at the refusal to accept the terms of the joint-delegates, the college had to suffer the loss of its president, six vice-presidents, eleven members of council, its honorary corresponding secretary, and the curator and librarian. This may be considered the commencement of the throes of dissolution.

The president and council of the Odontological Society summoned a special general meeting of its members on the evening of the 19th of March 1858, to hear the report which the council had to make concerning its communications with the College of Surgeons on the subject of the introduction of a dental department into that body, and also what had been the results touching the proposed amalgamation of the society and the College of Dentists. The report presented the various facts with which it had had to deal in the order in which they had occurred. Hence we come to the statement of the well-known circumstance that eighteen gentlemen had, on 11th December 1855, sent in the celebrated memorial to the Royal College of Surgeons. That document has already been frequently alluded to; it is not, therefore, necessary to introduce it again here. It appeared that "no definite reply having been received to this memorial down to February 1857, and Mr. Headlam, M.P., having given notice that he would, during that session of Parliament, introduce a Bill for the regulation of the medical profession, it was thought desirable again to draw the attention of the college to that memorial, to solicit an answer, and to press upon their consideration the further suggestions contained in the following memorial :—

"*To the President, Vice-President, and Council of the Royal College of Surgeons of England.*

"LONDON, *February* 22, 1857.

"GENTLEMEN,—It will be recollected that a memorial was presented to your college in November 1855, in which the present state of the dental profession was set forth, with a statement of its educational requirements; and it was suggested for the consideration of the council, whether a department of dental surgery might not be instituted. The memorialists have not received an answer to that memorial, but they have heard incidentally that the charter held by the college does not empower the council to institute a separate department of dental surgery.

"Since the presentation of that memorial the Odontological Society has been formed, and the majority of the memorialists are members of its council. They collectively entertain the opinions expressed in the memorial, and beg to address you from their present position. The council of the Odontological Society, feeling strongly that dental surgery is, if legitimately pursued, strictly a branch of surgery, consider that the absence of an answer to the memorialists indicates that the subject of the memorial was favourably entertained by the president and council of the College of Surgeons, and that the legal difficulty has, for the present, interfered with the adoption of any definite line of action. They consider that the college presides over the subject of surgery, and regard an unsanctioned attempt to remove from its guardianship any department of surgery both as disrespectful to the college and injurious to the interests of the profession. If this interpretation of the silence on the part of your council be correct, they beg to suggest whether power may not be obtained, under the Medical Bill which is about to be brought before Parliament, which shall enable the college to establish a department of dental surgery, consisting conjointly of members of its council and of gentlemen engaged in dental practice. The excitement which at present prevails in the dental profession renders it necessary that some definite course should be at once adopted in respect to the education and recognition of dental practitioners. The council of the Odontological Society beg, therefore, to solicit the immediate consideration of the memorial, in order that they may be placed in a position to pursue such measures as may be deemed expedient.

    (Signed)   W. A. HARRISON, M.R.C.S.E.
JOHN H. PARKINSON.
ARNOLD ROGERS, F.R.C.S.E.
WILLIAM ROBERTSON.
THOMAS A. ROGERS, M.R.C.S.E.
JOHN TOMES, F.R.S.
H. J. BARRETT, M.R.C.S.E.
EDWIN SAUNDERS, F.R.C.S.E.
JAMES SALTER, M.B., M.R.C.S.E.
J. A. IBBETSON, M.R.C.S.E.
JOHN H. PARKINSON, Jun., M.R.C.S.E.
JAMES PARKINSON.
WILLIAM M. BIGG.
ALFRED CANTON, M.R.C.S.E.
HUBERT SHELLEY, M.B. Lond., M.R.C.S.E."

In the list of signataries to this address it will be noticed that the following, which were appended to the original memorial, do not appear, viz. :—Messrs. S. Cartwright, H. L. Featherstone, and J. L. Craigie ; while those of W. A. Harrison and William Robertson are new.

Within a month the college through their secretary replied to this as under :—

    "ROYAL COLLEGE OF SURGEONS OF ENGLAND,
                  March 13, 1857.

"SIR,—The memorial from the council of the Odontological Society of the 22d ult., together with a former memorial from certain practitioners of dental surgery, have been laid before the council of this college. I am desired to acquaint you that the reply to the memorial from the practitioners of dental surgery was delayed, pending the issue of the conferences between this college and the other medical corporations of the United Kingdom with reference to the legislative measure lately brought before Parliament. I am also desired to acquaint you that the legal advisers of the college are of opinion that the college cannot institute the proposed special examination in dental surgery without the authority of a supplemental charter, and that the council would not feel justified in applying to the Crown for such charter under their existing engagements with the other medical corporations above referred to ; but wishing the society every success in their laudable efforts to raise the character of their branch of the profession, would suggest that the society might petition Parliament to be placed, either independently or in connection with this college, under the supervision and authority of the general council proposed in the Bill of the medical corporations. At the same time the council entertain a strong opinion that the surgical qualification for the proposed examination of practitioners of dental surgery should be the same as that required for the membership of the college.— I am, sir, your very obedient servant,

"EDM. BELFOUR, *Secretary.*

"W. A. Harrison, Esq."

The petitioners had waited long—since December 1855—and patiently, and this answer arriving at last could not be said to carry much comfort with it. The explanation concerning the time which had elapsed was satisfactory enough, considering the importance of the subject which had absorbed it all; but the result of the council's deliberation upon the prayer of the petitioners was altogether unsatisfactory. Whatever the College of Surgeons thought its executive might desire to do for the dentists, the ability was wanting. An altered charter alone could effect the purpose proposed: this they did not feel disposed to ask for from the Crown— at any rate, not just then; and so the memorialists, if they still thought proper to pursue their course, might just as well do their own business by appearing as applicants, or rather suppliants, at the feet of Parliament. The final clause of Mr. Belfour's letter, even in the event of the memorialists obtaining the sanction of Parliament to be affiliated to the College of Surgeons, left matters pretty much *in statu quo ante.* It is not a matter of much surprise, then, to find the Odontological Society, through its council, taking up the pen to address the College of Surgeons once more. The society considered the college reply indefinite, and believing that there was some misunderstanding of their ideas upon the subject of what they proposed as qualifications for future dentists, a committee was appointed to address the college authorities again. The College of Dentists of England, and those who sympathised with it, were rejoiced beyond measure when the reply from Lincoln's Inn Fields reached the Odontological Society, and was made public through the "British Journal of Dental Science." The exultation which abounded was represented in the "Quarterly Journal of Dental Science" thus:—"In all the controversy that has taken place with respect to the dental movement, we have not read or heard of defence of the conduct of the eighteen, except from themselves. Even those who have most strongly opposed the establishment of the College of Dentists have admitted that these dozen and a half of gentlemen committed an act of unpardonable assumption. They would have had just as much right to speak for the surgeons of England as they had for the dentists; and we have too high an opinion of the distinguished men who sit on the council of the College of Surgeons to imagine for one moment that they would countenance such an imposition. They have stamped the arrogant pretension of the memorialists with the most withering brand they could affix to it, by not deigning a reply to their humble prayers; and the council of the college could have done nothing else, without being guilty of an assumption equally as unwarrantable as that of the petitioners; for by what right could the College of Surgeons deal with the whole body of dentists without the consent of the parties to be affected? When driven to it, the eighteen had to admit that they spoke only for themselves—that is, that they had no authority but their own, though they demanded from a body not entitled to grant it an act of professional legislation which was to affect every dentist in the kingdom. What would have been said of the College of Surgeons had it fiated such a proceeding as that? Why, that it and the eighteen were well matched, and that the sooner a reformation was introduced into its councils the better."

In the meantime, the Odontological Society appointed

a committee for the express purpose of addressing the College of Surgeons, in order to rectify any misapprehension concerning the views it held, and further to promote the all-important subject. The following memorial was accordingly drawn up, and presented to the college :—

" *To the President and Council of the Royal College of Surgeons of England.*

" ODONTOLOGICAL SOCIETY, *April* 4, 1857.

" GENTLEMEN,—The president and council of the Odontological Society beg to acknowledge a communication from the council of the Royal College of Surgeons in answer to two memorials addressed to the college on the subject of the dental profession. The memorialists beg also to state that they fully appreciate the consideration which has been given to the memorials, and the approval which the council has expressed in regard to the efforts they are making for the advancement of their branch of the profession. There are, however, certain points mooted, both in the memorials and in the reply to which the president and council of the Odontological Society respectfully request the further attention of the council of the college, and upon which they solicit a more explicit expression of its opinion. At the time the subject was considered by the college, a Medical Bill was before Parliament, and the council was pleased to suggest that the Odontological Society might petition Parliament to be placed under the general council proposed in the Bill, either independently or in connection with the college. But the Bill is now no longer before Parliament, the time of its introduction is indefinitely postponed, and its eventual introduction in the form recently proposed is, in the minds of many, a matter of great doubt. The council of the Odontological Society beg, therefore, to suggest, whether, under the new combination of circumstances, means for instituting a department of dental surgery, in the manner originally suggested by the memorialists, might not be taken, without immediate reference to a comprehensive Medical Bill ; and to ask, if such a step should at the present time be deemed inexpedient, whether the college, in any measure which may hereafter be brought before Parliament for the regulation of the medical profession, would induce, or render active assistance in inducing, the recognition of dental surgery as a department of the medical profession to be placed in connection with the College of Surgeons, somewhat in the manner proposed by the memorialists. In the communication referred to, the council expresses the following opinion :—'At the same time, the council entertain a strong opinion that the surgical qualification for the proposed examination of practitioners of dental surgery should be the same as that required for the membership of the college.' The president and council of the Odontological Society are fully prepared to show that the acquisition of a fair amount of proficiency in the requirements *peculiar* to dental practice necessitates close application on the part of the student over a period of little short of three years ; and are of opinion that any attempt to materially shorten that term would be attended with great disadvantage. If three years be added to the curriculum already enjoined by the college, the education of the dental surgeon becomes more extended, both as regards knowledge and the period of pupilage, and more expensive than that required of the surgeon. The memorialists do not suggest education and an examination *inferior* to that required of the medical practitioner ; but propose a certain difference in *kind* only—not a difference in *degree*—an education and an examination specially adapted to the requirements of the dental surgeon as distinguished from that fitted to the general surgeon. They would suggest a curriculum extending over four or five years, and embracing all the subjects necessary to a perfect qualification. Under existing circumstances, the dentist must pursue his special studies either after he has passed the college or before he enters upon the medical curriculum. Either course is attended with so much inconvenience, and so large an expenditure of time, and the college diploma, when obtained, is regarded as so imperfect an indication of the possessor's fitness for the peculiarities of dental practice, that out of 1500 individuals who follow this branch of the profession scarcely more than 30 have become members of the college. The president and council of the Odontological Society are of opinion, that if a suitable course of education were instituted, and an examining board established by the College of Surgeons, upon the plan indicated in the communication from the Odontological Society, very few dentists would in future enter upon practice without previously acquiring the proposed qualification ; but that, if the existing curriculum be insisted on, and a special one superadded, the dental pupil would feel that a higher qualification was required of him than of the surgeon, and in the absence of a legal prohibition would probably dispense with the proffered qualification, and enter upon practice, *as at present*, with such attainments as may have fallen within his reach. The favourable manner in which the suggestions advanced by the memorialists have been received by the council of the College of Surgeons has encouraged the council of the Odontological Society to solicit attention to the foregoing points in connection with a reconsideration of the preceding memorials. They feel that the more fully the subject is investigated, the more apparent will it become that the establishment of a department of dental surgery by the College of Surgeons upon the principle advanced by the memorialists, to meet the existing necessity, will not only prove advantageous to dental practitioners and the public, but to the medical schools and the profession at large. The anxiety for educational advancement among members of the dental profession evinced by the present agitation, renders it necessary that some measure should be taken for the recognition of this branch of the profession; and the president and council of the Odontological Society feel that the College of Surgeons is the proper source from whence these measures should emanate. They beg again, therefore, most respectfully to direct the attention of the council of the college to the subject, and to solicit a decided expression of its opinion upon the general points advanced in this and the former address.

  (Signed) W. A. HARRISON, M.R.C.S.E.
       ARNOLD ROGERS, F.R.C.S.E.
       JOHN H. PARKINSON.
       EDWIN SAUNDERS, F.R.C.S.E.
       JOHN H. PARKINSON, Jun., M.R.C.S.
       SAMUEL CARTWRIGHT, Jun., M.R.C.S.
       JOHN TOMES, F.R.S.
       JAMES PARKINSON.
       THOMAS A. ROGERS, M.R.C.S.E.
       HUBERT SHELLEY, M.B. Lond., M.R.C.S.E.
       WILLIAM M. BIGG.
       ALFRED CANTON, M.R.C.S.E.
       H. J. BARRETT, M.R.C.S.E.
       G. A. IBBETSON, M.R.C.S.E."

This document was valuable as explanatory, to a far greater degree, of the views and desires of the petitioners than those which had preceded it, and it must not be forgotten, in considering it, that it was not now the embodiment, to this point, of the sentiments of the eighteen gentlemen only who first memorialised the College of Surgeons. It was fairly to be understood as representing the feeling of the entire Odontological Society on the subject. This gave to it a very much greater importance, and although the continued petitioning from this quarter of the authorities in Lincoln's Inn Fields was still without the sanction of the profession at large, and also, that a portion, by no means an insignificant one, of the body of dental practitioners was distinctly opposed to the step thus taken, yet its increased representative quality could not be ignored or denied. In other words, there were very many more than eighteen members of the profession, and several of these men of the highest position as dentists, who not only had come to think, but were thus willing to act, with the original memorialists in asking for affiliation with the College of Surgeons. The council of the college doubtless recognised the augmentation of influence thus brought to bear: but whether it did so or not, there was no longer the disagreeable waiting for a reply as formerly. A pause of only four days sufficed to elicit the following answer :—

"ROYAL COLLEGE OF SURGEONS OF ENGLAND,
April 8, 1857.

" SIR,—I am desired to acknowledge the receipt of the memorial of the 4th instant, addressed to the council of this college by the president and council of the Odontological Society, acknowledging the receipt of the reply from the council of this college of the 13th ultimo to the former memorials from the Odontological Society, and suggesting—as the Medical Bill referred to in such letter of the 13th ultimo is no longer before Parliament, and its eventual reintroduction is, in the minds of many, a matter of great doubt—that the recognition of dental surgery as a department of the medical profession be placed in connection with this college. And I am desired in reply to the said memorial to state, that the council of this college have the strongest assurance that the Bill for the regulation of the medical profession will be introduced without delay on the reassembling of Parliament ; and that having entered into engagements with the other medical corporations in respect to the qualifications for obtaining a license to practise surgery, they are withheld, pending the fate of the said Bill, from entering into any negotiation, the object of which would be to admit members or associates of the college upon other conditions than those proposed by the Bill ; and that the council can therefore only repeat the recommendation offered to the Odontological Society in their reply of the 13th ultimo, that the society should petition Parliament, when reassembled, to be placed, either independently, or in connection with this college, under the supervision and authority of the general council proposed in the Bill of the medical corporations. I am, sir, your most obedient servant,

EDM. BELFOUR, *Secretary.*

"W. A. Harrison, Esq."

Although this response was not all that could be wished, still the Odontological Society could congratulate itself on the advance made, for such it really was; and so, having succeeded in gaining the attention and enlisting the sympathy of the College of Surgeons, it determined to leave nothing undone that could be accomplished; and, accordingly, believing that further explanation would make the future progress easier, it addressed another communication to the council. The following is a copy of the same:—

"ODONTOLOGICAL SOCIETY, *April* 30, 1857.

"GENTLEMEN,—We are desired by the president and council of the Odontological Society to acknowledge the receipt of the communication of the 8th instant from the council of the College of Surgeons in reply to the memorial presented by the Odontological Society on the 4th April, and to thank the council for the promptness of their reply. As it would appear from that reply that the council of the college feels some difficulty in entering at once upon the consideration of the establishment of a dental department, in consequence of its engagements with the other medical corporations in respect to the pending Medical Bill, we are desired to inquire whether the council of the Odontological Society may expect that measures will be taken for the institution of a department of dental surgery when the fate of the said Medical Bill has been determined? We are also desired to draw the attention of the council of the college to the fact, that the memorialists, in suggesting the establishment of a department of dental surgery, have contemplated, not that students who may pass such department shall be considered as *members* of the college, but as *licentiates of this department only,*—the terms of the reply of the 8th instant having led the council of the Odontological Society to suppose that this point has not been fully understood by the council of the College of Surgeons. And we are desired to state, that although the present position of the dental profession may not necessitate the immediate institution of an examining board, and a curriculum of education, yet that the feeling entertained by dental practitioners upon the subject is such as to require an assurance that this will be effected without any unnecessary delay. The president and council of the Odontological Society beg, therefore, to again call the attention of the council of the college to the points mooted in the memorial, and in the present communication.

    (Signed)   JOHN TOMES.
          SAMUEL CARTWRIGHT, Jun.
          THOMAS A. ROGERS.

"To the President and Council of the Royal College
  of Surgeons of England."

Gradually, then, the more detailed ideas of the petitioners were, as in this address, made plain to the College of Surgeons; and little by little the perseverance of the Odontologists was acknowledged by expressed hopes, assurances, and promises from the executive in Lincoln's Inn Fields. The willingness to enter into the consideration of the subject proposed to them was only equalled by the business-like promptitude of the replies sent. To those who know how difficult it is to gain the ear of corporations, as a rule, and with what wonderful facility and complacency the most important subjects are often quietly shelved, the result thus far secured will appear, as indeed it was, a very distinct success for the petitioners. There must have been an immense amount of energy displayed somewhere; and the author will have no difficulty in pointing to the spring and source of it in the proper place. Fifteen days more and the following reply came to hand :—

    "ROYAL COLLEGE OF SURGEONS OF ENGLAND,
        May 15, 1857.

"GENTLEMEN,—In reply to your communication of the 30th ult., I am directed by the president and council of this college to call your attention to the suggestion offered in their letter of the 13th of March last, of petitioning the House of Commons, or, at least, of putting yourselves into communication with the members of the House who have the charge of the Medical Bill. The council are of opinion that this mode of proceeding would be the most direct and effectual plan for promoting the object which the Odontological Society has in view. The council of this college, in sanctioning such application to the Legislature, cannot be unaware that they are encouraging the wish expressed by the Odontological Society of the connection of its members with the College of Surgeons; and the council beg to assure you that it is only in consequence of their present engagements with other medical corporations, and of the uncertainty in respect of the future powers of the college, pending the discussion of the Medical Bill, that they are now prevented from considering and duly weighing the conditions under which they would be disposed to accede to the proposal of instituting a new class of surgeon-dentists.—I have the honour to be, gentlemen, your very obedient servant, EDM. BELFOUR, *Secretary.*"

So far as this correspondence had gone, there was much to be gathered from it which would go to inspire with hope those who felt that association with the College of Surgeons would best promote the interests of the dental profession. Still this last letter left the work mainly in the hands of the Odontological Society. They were recommended to petition the House, or win over the members of Parliament connected with this Medical Bill to see with them in the matter. This involved an extra effort, and accordingly a deputation was selected and appointed to wait upon Mr. Headlam. Arrangements were made for an interview with that gentleman, and the same took place on the 2d of June. A technical difficulty, however, lay across the path. It appeared that at that particular stage of the Bill Mr. Headlam, being the proposer of the Bill, could not introduce a clause into the measure. He, however, not only did not object to a clause embodying the proposal of the Odontological Society to the College of Surgeons, as such, being inserted, but promised his support to it, if some independent member of the House could be obtained to propose it. This member was, therefore, to be sought and his acquiescence obtained, while the clause to be inserted must be drawn up, and that also with particular care. The council of the Odontological Society, therefore, put themselves into communication with the solicitor to the Royal College of Surgeons (Mr. Wilde), who drew up the following clause for the purpose in hand:—

"THE MEDICAL PROFESSION BILL NO. I.—*Clause proposed to be added after Clause* 38 : 'It shall, notwithstanding anything herein contained, be lawful for Her Majesty, by charter, to grant to the Royal College of Surgeons of England power to institute and hold examinations for the purpose of testing the fitness of persons to practise as dentists, who may be desirous of being so examined, and to grant certificates of such fitness.'"

The next step was to obtain the assistance of such a member of Parliament as had been indicated by Mr. Headlam. In reference to this, the late Mr. Arnold Rogers felt sure of the aid of Mr. Walpole, but, from causes beyond his control, that gentleman failed him. Mr. Tomes, however, with his usual caution and forecast, had reserved his action in the matter, and was prepared to ask Mr. A. Beresford Hope to introduce the clause, to which that gentleman courteously acceded.

The council of the College of Dentists, on the other hand, had not been idle. Their attention had, of course, been directed towards the Medical Bill, and Mr. Underwood, who from his first connection with the college had worked with great assiduity and zeal in its interests, called the notice of the members to what would be the effect of the measure on dentists without a medical qualification; hence the action taken by the executive of the Dental College, as already recorded. The decision on the part of the latter to reject the terms of amalgamation, and the resolution of the Odontological Society to entertain no further proposition concerning them, left the breach already existing between these two sections of the profession as wide, if not wider than ever. The result, as it touched the college party, was, that not long after the verdict had been given, a loss of about sixty members in all had to be sustained. The council of the college needed reconstruction, and eventually this was accomplished. Difficulty had been experienced by those to whom this duty had been assigned, especially in obtaining a gentleman to fill the presidential chair. The reason for the non-compliance with the sub-committee's request is given in the circular or report of their action in this matter. It is there stated that some gentlemen declined to be nominated unless previously assured that an amalgamation with the Odontological Society was certain. The names of these gentlemen whether proposed for the office of president or for seats at the council table are not given, but the fact is significant. When the meeting took place, May 21, 1858, the nomination papers appeared with a blank opposite the word "President," while twelve new names were printed as those of gentlemen designed for the council, together with one for the honorary corresponding secretary, and another for the librarian and curator. At that meeting between twenty and thirty only of the members attended. After a great deal of discussion, coupled with numerous protests from Mr. Fox, the house list, with Mr. Peter Matthews as president, was accepted by the meeting. One of the first acts of the new executive at No. 5 Cavendish Square was to issue a circular, signed by the honorary corresponding secretary, Mr. A. Hockley, and addressed to the members of the college. One of its statements was to the following effect, viz. :—" The bye-law requiring candidates for membership to undergo an examination prior to admission has not been submitted to a meeting of the body of members for sanction, and that the intention of applying for such sanction is not for the present entertained. All dentists practising as such exclusively and legitimately are therefore eligible for membership." It is needless to say that the abandonment, thus prefigured, of the examination test aroused many, and made them feel that the original ideas of the promoters of the college were being distinctly departed from. The author was therefore requested to prepare a counter circular, which is here appended, signed by fifteen London members and himself, as under :—

"38 EUSTON SQUARE, *July* 8, 1858.

" SIR,—A communication having been sent to each member of the College of Dentists of England, signed by Mr. Hockley, stating that the bye-law requiring examination as necessary for membership is not to be enforced, we consider that if this—the fundamental principle of that institution—be not acted upon, the college will sink into the position of a mere club, and fail to raise itself in the eyes either of the profession or the public. Should this be your opinion, we shall feel obliged by your signing the accompanying protest, and returning the same to the above address without delay.—We are, sir, yours, &c.,

"J. ROBINSON.   F. ROGERS.
C. CARTER.   C. ROGERS.
W. CRAMPTON.   A. J. ROBINSON.
C. S. FOX.   F. A. SASS.
S. GHRIMES.   W. D. SAUNDER.
R. HEPBURN.   J. L. STATHAM.
A. HILL.   T. UNDERWOOD.
J. W. MITCHELL.   B. WEST.

"I, the undersigned, hereby protest against the constitution and acts of the council of the College of Dentists of England, alleged to have been elected at a general meeting of members, held Friday, May 21, 1858, on the following ground, viz.—That by law No. 4 it is expressly declared 'that two-thirds of the new council shall consist of *members of the last year's council.*' Of the list of council as at present put forward, only eight were members of last year's council, and consequently a fundamental law of the college has been broken. And I further protest against all acts of the council as illegal, and demand that all moneys of the college expended by such council be refunded, each member of the council being personally liable for the same.

(Signed)   ———."

This document was portentous. According to its success might the college regard its future standing. It was promptly followed on the next day by one signed by Mr. Rymer, as honorary secretary to the council, in which he stated that there was inconsistency between the circular and the protest itself, and called upon the members "to determine whether lawful authority shall be supported, or whether faction shall be allowed to offer obstructions to all attempts at progress." The fact was, the amalgamation question had acted as a crucial test with a large number of those connected with the college. Many had felt that division and strife were intolerable, and looked eagerly forward to union, or at least combined action, throughout the dental ranks. With admirable tenacity Mr. Rymer held to the college scheme; but he could not help realising that a source of weakness had been originated by rejecting the delegates' proposals. The numbers on the council had been acquired, but it was evident to him and to others that the influence of those then occupying seats there was not of the order which those who had seceded exercised, both within and without the institution.

One week after Mr. Rymer's circular had been sent forth a meeting of the college was convened, July 16, 1858. Mr. P. Matthews presided, and several of the leading members appeared to protest against the then existing state of affairs. Mr. Underwood stated this, and declared that those gentlemen who objected to the action of the council, did so solely on the ground of its departure from the original and fundamental principles on which its existence was based. A copy of the protest which had been issued by the sixteen signataries, but now signed by sixty-eight members of the college, was handed to the chairman, with the demand that it should be entered upon the minutes of the college. Mr. Underwood then left the room, being followed by the major part of those present.

Whilst meeting followed meeting at Cavendish Square, the Odontological Society was turning its attention to two most important subjects. These were the formation of a dental school and a dental hospital. The society itself was to be viewed in the light of an advanced school. At its various meetings the members were to continue to unite for mutual edification by discussing such subjects as had been found worthy of combined thought. The dental school, or school of dental surgery, was to be so organised as that, by the delivery of lectures by members of the society, or by gentlemen in the profession of acknowledged ability, the students could be instructed in the various departments of their studies, so pre-eminently necessary to their being furnished and fitted for thorough scientific practice. Such an institution involved the necessity of an opportunity being given to the learners of seeing practically illustrated the theories taught them by their instructors. This could only be efficiently carried out at a special dental hospital. Although rich, even to profuseness, as the metropolis was at that time in the direction of charitable curative institutions, there was yet ample room for such an hospital among the rest. Its importance, even on public grounds, could not well be overrated, and on the score of professional educational needs it was unmistakable. The project, therefore, was most creditable to its proposers, and the results which have since been accomplished through its instrumentality are patent to all, and will be mentioned in the proper place. Although the originators of the College of Dentists subsequently asserted that it was their intention from the first to accomplish such a scheme, still to the Odontological Society must be accredited the praise of instituting the London School of Dental Surgery and the Dental Hospital of London. Before these important proceedings could take form there was much to be accomplished. The selection of an appropriate site constituted no mean difficulty; but this, with the other necessary preliminaries, was at length overcome. Mr. Harrison and Mr. R. Hepburn, with others, spent a good deal of their valuable time in endeavouring to secure a suitable house and premises for the hospital, and their labours eventuated in the possession of No. 32 Soho Square, upon lease for a term of years. Mr. Harrison acted as chairman of the committee of organisation.

On Wednesday, 6th October 1858, a meeting was summoned by the committee who had organised the institution, for the formal transfer to the committee of management which had been elected of the hospital itself and its future conduct, together with the duty of making the necessary arrangements for its public opening for the reception of patients. There were present on the occasion Messrs. A. Rogers, R. Hepburn, S. Ghrimes, J.

Tomes, W. A. N. Cattlin, W. A. Harrison, Dr. Babington, J. Parkinson, J. H. Parkinson, T. Dyer, S. Cartwright, jun., — Illingworth, J. Barrett, Campbell De Morgan, O. Clayton, Scott, W. M. Bigg, J. Hutchinson, E. Sercombe, and A. Hill. Mr. De Morgan was called to occupy the chair. Mr. Harrison, as chairman of the committee of organisation, explained the circumstances which led to the foundation of the hospital; and further, that that committee had organised the institution, taken the premises in Soho Square, had framed laws, obtained a highly influential list of vice-presidents, committee of management, trustees, treasurer, medical staff, and honorary secretary, for the future management of the institution, and had collected £192, 5s. 8d., with the promise of £63—total £255, 5s. 8d. Mr. Harrison announced that they were prepared to hand over the hospital to the care of the future committee of management so soon as that committee had legally elected from their own number a chairman and deputy-chairman for the year of office. Mr. De Morgan was then unanimously elected as chairman, and Dr. Babington as deputy-chairman, for the ensuing year. This having been effected, Mr. Harrison, in a formal address, transferred the hospital—the charge being duly accepted. The rent of the premises was stated to be £170 per annum, but tenants were ready to occupy a given portion at £70 per annum. Sub-committees were then appointed to proceed with the necessary details—viz., a furnishing committee, and also a publication committee for issuing prospectuses, &c.,—the writer being invited to act as honorary secretary. The event was one of the most auspicious kind, and all present felt that a distinct step towards the safe and efficient elevation of the profession had that day been taken. That the circumstance would be left unnoticed by the college party was not very likely. To show the difficulty which beset every effort at improvement in those days, it may be mentioned that the founding of this excellent institution was caustically animadverted upon by the opposite side in a notice which appeared in the college journal. Even the motives of the gentlemen connected with it were called in question, and the patrons' names being published evoked the ire of the writer. The notice of the opening of the Dental Hospital to the public was thus given in the "Quarterly Journal of Dental Science:"—

"On the 1st of November (1858) an institution under this title was opened in Soho Square. The hours for receiving patients is half-past eight to half-past nine every morning. We have heard nothing of the working of the charity, but one hour in the morning seems rather a short period for giving relief at an hospital. Great publicity is given to the institution, and the names of the dentists in connection with it are printed in large letters in the circular sent to the affluent soliciting contributions for the relief of the indigent."

Like all kindred efforts of benevolence, the Dental Hospital of London had to run the gauntlet of criticism, and endure the trial of opposing opinions. It was but an evidence of the ill grace of some of the profession that such remarks and insinuations should have ever appeared in print. Jealousy, however, is seldom seen in a reasonable mood, and is, perhaps, never philosophic. The attitude of the two societies towards each other from the time when the amalgamation question had been settled was that of determined opposition. Strong reaction had set in, especially with the College of Dentists, the executive and members of which together resolved to hold on their prescribed course on the original basis of independence. While the Medical Bills were before the late session of Parliament, the consideration of which had resulted in the passing of the Medical Act (1858), the college showed itself active on behalf of the profession at large, as has been mentioned already. From whatever cause, the results which were aimed at received attention, and were accomplished. The clause which would have operated prejudicially to the interests of dentists as a body was omitted, and the recognition of dentists as a professional class, entitling them legally to recover charges made by them as such, was allowed in the last clause of Mr. Cowper's Bill. Internally, the College of Dentists was reorganised, modifications and amendments of its laws being made from time to time. Distinct regulations concerning membership were made, and a curriculum adopted on the vote of town and country members, the latter recording their opinions by proxy. Instead of the transactions of the college being printed and distributed yearly, it was determined that after that year (1858) they should be forwarded to members and associates alike every three months. During the year the subject of painless dental operations, to be performed by means of electricity, was made known, and this idea was one which it was determined should be thoroughly tested by competent practitioners. A committee was formed from members of the college for this express purpose. The institution was to be one of a very practical nature, if it were possible to make it so, and most creditably and earnestly did the executive set itself to the accomplishment of this work. Lectures were delivered by eminent gentlemen, and papers of interest and merit were given by members of the college. Still the end that had been proposed by the Odontological Society—namely, the association of dentists, by examination, with the Royal College of Surgeons, rested heavily upon the efforts of the independent party, and was increasingly the *bête noire* of that time. The journals of either side discussed the subject constantly, and with an *animus* which was far from creditable. The "British Journal" was held up to scorn by the promoters of the college movement, while in return the action of the Dental College appeared to form a fit subject for ridicule or contempt by the Odontological Society's organ. Before discussing the subject of the college operations, and the intentions of its executive, it will be but just to record an important matter suggested by the late Mr. Bell, of Margaret Street, Cavendish Square,

At one of the college meetings, held August 25th in that year (1858), the following resolutions were proposed by him, and were carried unanimously, viz. :—

" 1. Candidates shall also be required to produce a certificate of having been articled to a dental practitioner for a period of not less than four years; such certificate to be delivered to the secretary of the college thirty days before the candidates shall be eligible for their dental examination.

" 2. Associates of the college enrolled, and pupils who shall have been articled to members of the college, previous to the foregoing resolutions coming into operation, shall be eligible for membership by passing a dental examination only.

" 3. Any member who shall maintain his membership for a period of three years after the ratification of these rules shall be entitled to the diploma of the college. And any person who may become a member previous to the foregoing regulations coming into force shall be entitled to the diploma of the college upon the expiration of the third year of his membership."

It was considered by many connected with the college, by Mr. Rymer in particular, that if the rules as then amended, and with these latter three included with them, could be strictly adhered to, there would remain nothing else to be acquired but a charter of incorporation to ensure for the undertaking complete success. What, then, they had to do was to steadily work forward in this direction, endeavouring to foster similar opinions among the outsiders, and affect to the utmost of their power the profession at large with the reasonableness of their ideas, taking for their motto, " Courage, perseverance, and hope." How far this could be considered justifiable was a matter of individual opinion, seeing that the Legislature had taken action in harmony with the petition of the memorialists to the Royal College of Surgeons. On the 6th of July, in a committee of the whole House, a clause was introduced into the Medical Practitioners Bill, by which the Royal College of Surgeons was empowered to institute examinations, and to grant certificates of fitness to practise dental surgery. The success of the Odontological Society's scheme was rendered all the more apparent from the fact that when, after due notice having been given, Mr. Beresford Hope proposed the insertion of the clause, the House adopted it without one dissentient voice. Over all the confusion and strife of party feeling which had characterised the year, this fact stood forth prominently as that which would most unmistakably affect the future of the dental profession. It was the most conspicuous event of the time, and it only remained to take the necessarily consequent steps thereupon, and await the manifestation of professional feeling on the subject, which time only could develop and declare.

CHAPTER VI.

The year 1859 opened with the introduction of a new dental journal, under the title of the "Dental Review." It was to take the place of the "Quarterly Journal of Dental Science," and would appear monthly. Its first editorial set forth its objects and intentions. It deplored the professional division which existed, and the writer's statements on this subject were—

"We join heartily in the regret, that from any cause whatever there should be any kind of discussion. We are for peace, and the law and practice of 'goodwill towards men.' Without cant, this is our creed. But while selecting this line of policy, while casting away from us all promptings to avenge even friends whom we have known to have been most cruelly and libellously pursued in the recent strifes, we should be wanting in firmness, as in rectitude, did we not support those broad principles of justice and equality, those catholic principles we may call them, without the acknowledgment of which no body of men can become efficient, not to say powerful."

With such a basis for future journalism to rest upon, the "Dental Review," whether knowingly or otherwise, had taken up a very difficult position indeed, considering the condition of things in the profession, if it was to carry out these principles in their integrity. Without referring to the reasons for discontinuing the "Quarterly," which had been from the first a staunch supporter of the college, for which object, indeed, it was originated, the "Review" could not hope to disguise the fact that it was to all intents and purposes the organ of the Dental College. How it was to steer a middle course under such circumstances seemed difficult to understand.

One month later, the opportunity of a test being applied offered itself, and the following remarks will speak for themselves. Commenting upon the fact that Mr. Matthews, then acting as president of the College of Dentists, had occasion to make certain statements at the annual general meeting of that institution in January of the above year, the editor remarks—

"These revelations must, indeed, have taken the meeting by surprise, for we venture to affirm that, disappointed as many of the pioneers in the dental reformatory movement must have been at the illiberal feeling which was manifested in certain quarters against the college, there were none who for a moment could have believed that a system would have been organised to undermine the foundations of the college worthy the darkest days of the Inquisition. Nor do we believe that *out* of the college would be found men with a spark of British feeling within their breasts who could look otherwise than with painful feelings upon the discreditable proceedings which have characterised the acts of some few—we trust and believe they are *but* few—whose feelings of virulence against the college have so far outrun all discretion as to lead them to employ the basest means to endeavour to throw discredit upon the fair fame of a body of their fellow-practitioners."

The "Dental Review" was evidently occupying the position of a distinct party supporter already, a step by no means unnatural, and most easily accounted for. The truth concerning that journal was simply that it would do, in its own style of course, exactly what its predecessor had done—viz., advocate energetically the college cause. How this was to be accomplished, and yet the ground of "peace and goodwill" to be held while the Odontological Society was determined to pursue its course, that being such an one as would, if successfully maintained, completely supplant the college by supplying the means for professional education and examination in a totally different direction, it was difficult to divine. It was evident to all concerned that the two societies would continue to try their strength against each other, and that neither side would lack a journal to support its views, or register its action. The truth of this is apparent from the tone of the leading article in the "British Journal." In that for January 1859, the editor, in alluding to the College of Dentists, and referring to the secession which it had suffered, says—

"Differences which had existed for some time between several of the leading men were in the first instance effectually terminated, and a party which at one time threatened to create a schism in the profession virtually ceased to exist, save in the shape of repeated advertisements in the daily papers. Who they now are, and what are their numbers, no one knows—we suspect not even their secretary. As a public party, therefore, we say they have ceased to exist; and as a petty club, holding together for self-glorification, their influence is no longer to be feared. They do but serve the useful purpose of a safety valve, through which may escape the vapourings of individuals who would be neither congenial associates in a professional society, nor themselves feel at ease therein, even if they had been admitted on the mistaken plea of liberality."

While the Odontological Society was more "in evidence" than it ever had been, and had taken up important ground as towards the profession, it is also true that the College of Dentists of England had not diverged from its original idea of becoming a means for the independent existence of the profession, and certainly was very far from being without influence, or ceasing to be, altogether. Regardless of the loss that had been sustained by the college party, it had held, during the year 1858, no less than twenty-nine meetings of council, besides its ordinary business and monthly meetings, and had arranged for regular lectures throughout the then current year also. Mr. P. Matthews, who up to the annual general meeting of the college had acted as president, on that occasion resigned his office. Under very disadvantageous circumstances he had conducted the affairs of the institution most creditably, and always with business-like method.

So far as the numerical strength of the college was concerned, there was less for him to do, the list of members having sunk to about one-half, or less than 150. But touching the circumstances surrounding the institution and arising within it, there had been hitherto no such difficult passages to pilot it through as fell to Mr. Matthew's lot to deal with. The fact of the Odontological Society's gradually augmenting strength, and growth in numbers and influence, was not to be overlooked as that which would have a very decided tendency to dispirit and dishearten him as a leader in an opposite cause. Nevertheless, like his colleague Mr. Rymer, he had strong faith in the ultimate success of the scheme, and most earnestly laboured to effect it. Although declining for the future to act as president, he did not withhold his services, or rather the continuance of them, as chairman at any meeting where they might be of avail. As a firm friend to the movement organised by Mr. Rymer, he had few as his equal, and, it may be safely said, none as his superior.

With regard to the Odontological Society, its principal action may be recorded as having been in the direction of promoting the establishment of the Dental Hospital of London. This had been accomplished by the joint efforts of gentlemen both within and without the society. In fact, several practitioners, who but a short time since were active and influential members of the College of Dentists, had co-operated with the Odontological Society in founding the hospital in question, and several of them were elected to the staff. Mr. Fox and Mr. Ghrimes had seats at the committee of management, Mr. James Robinson was one of the trustees, Mr. R. Hepburn, Mr. C. Rogers, and Mr. Underwood were to act as dental surgeons, and the writer held the post of honorary secretary. The power given by the Legislature to the Royal College of Surgeons to constitute a dental department in connection with their body had not yet been acted upon, and the Odontological Society felt that it was necessary to take such steps as would facilitate such a measure, by preparing a curriculum most likely to be accepted by the authorities in Lincoln's Inn Fields. To this end a committee was appointed "to draw out a scheme for the education of future dentists." This committee was presided over by (the late) Mr. Harrison as chairman. The following extracts from the report presented to the society early in the year 1859 will explain the action taken in the matter, and the principles which had been kept in operation throughout the committee's labours. The report says—

"It will be remembered that, in the memorials addressed to the council of the College of Surgeons, the council of the Odontological Society has stated that it sought to establish for the dentist a qualification different somewhat in *kind*, but not inferior in *degree*, to that at present required by that college from its members.

"This point your committee has kept in view, and it will be seen that, although in the curriculum proposed for the consideration of the council, certain courses of lectures required by the college from its members are omitted, other lectures have been added, which, in an educational point of view, will be found equal to those for which they have been substituted.

"Your committee has felt that, in proposing a course of education for those who may now enter the dental profession, it must also be guided by the two following considerations: First, that the curriculum must be such as would be received by the College of Surgeons, should that college form a dental department; and, second, that it must be such as would be received by an 'independent dental institution,' should it ultimately be found necessary to form such an institution."

These remarks make it evident that, although the first and principal difficulty had been overcome, there had been no positive assurance yet given that the council of the College of Surgeons would accept the power, and act upon it in the direction the memorialists so much desired. The determination to provide means whereby a full and sufficient professional education for the future dentist should be secured was a strong one; and there is no question or doubt whatever that the Odontological Society was firmly resolved to achieve this as the consummation of their efforts, first through the College of Surgeons, and then, if that could not be done, through an independent institute. The care and foresight of the committee is amply demonstrated in the following extract from the report :—

"Your committee is of opinion that it is necessary that the council should feel fully assured that the foregoing conditions are fulfilled in the subjoined scheme before it is adopted ; for inasmuch as the proposed school is to be brought into existence *before* the establishment of an examining body, it will be apparent that it will be absolutely necessary that the dental pupil, on commencing his studies, shall be fully satisfied that the curriculum to which he is conforming will be received by *any* recognised examining board which may be hereafter instituted.

"Your committee has not lost sight of the fact, that there are many students at present engaged in their pupilage who may hereafter desire to avail themselves of a recognised qualification ; and that it would be unreasonable to expect them to recommence their education, in order to conform to a curriculum established subsequent to the date at which they entered upon their professional studies.

"To meet these exceptional cases, your committee would recommend that any examining board which may hereafter be formed should be invested with a discretional power to admit for examination those who may have commenced their professional education prior to the establishment of a dental school."

Then followed the proposed curriculum, as under :—

LECTURES AND HOSPITAL PRACTICE TO BE ATTENDED AT THE EXISTING SCHOOLS AND HOSPITALS.

Courses of Lectures.

Two on Anatomy, with dissections (one being special).
Two on Physiology and Pathology.
One on Practice of Physic.
One on Practice of Surgery.
One on Materia Medica.
One on Chemistry.
One on Practical Chemistry.

Hospital Attendance.

Twelve months' surgical practice.
Six months' medical practice, with attendance upon clinical lectures.
Lectures and hospital practice to be attended at the Special Dental School.

Courses of Lectures.

Two on Dental Anatomy and Physiology (human and comparative).
Two on Dental Surgery.
Two on Mechanical Dentistry.
One on Metallurgy.

Dental Hospital Attendance.

Two years' attendance at a recognised dental hospital, or at the dental department of a recognised general hospital.

Candidates for examination to be required to bring proof of being twenty-one years of age, and of having been engaged at least four years in the acquirement of professional knowledge, and of having devoted a period of not less than three years in acquiring a practical familiarity with the details of mechanical dentistry under the instruction of a recognised practitioner.

The report concluded by expressing the opinion of the committee on the necessity of establishing a special dental hospital, together with the method of its organisation. As, however, this had already been accomplished—and, in fact, this very report was read at the society's rooms in the Dental Hospital, where it had taken up its abode *en permanence*—the matter needs not to be repeated. The president, the late Mr. J. Parkinson, announced on the occasion in question, that the council of the society approved and adopted this report. He also stated that between its commencement and its acceptance by the council of the society, the council of the Royal College of Surgeons had signified its assent to the proposal of the memorialists, and that a copy of the report had been forwarded to the authorities at Lincoln's Inn Fields, but up to that time no official answer had been received. Looking, then, at the condition of things as they existed in the early part of 1859, it cannot be denied that the position taken by the Odontological Society was much strengthened. They had been successful in two important directions, the first being the power which had been granted to the College of Surgeons to alter their charter so as to include dentists in their ranks, and the next the acceptance of the proposal of the memorialists that a dental department should be established. Added to this, the curriculum thus suggested by the committee of the society was under consideration, with every prospect of its being accepted by the college executive.

As may be supposed, the scheme of the Odontological Society thus arranged for met with criticism, especially by the opposite party, principally on account of the expenses it would involve. The ideas on professional education and examination, as stated in the "Dental Review," may be given in the words of one of its editorials thus—

"We affirm, as a principle, that if the dental body is to be advanced at all, the question of qualification must rest solely on examination, and that the idea of a coercive curriculum must be cast to the winds, as opposed alike to the spirit of the age and to common sense."

And again—

"We urge the profession to allow no apedom of a medical curriculum—of a curriculum coercive in its pretensions, and signifying nothing in its results—to be thrown in the way of improvement. The dentists, as an organising body, are in the first stages of life; and if, as a body, they would progress into manhood, they must pick up the modern in principle, and, of all things, eschew those old academic garments which, glittering feebly with tarnished embroidery, are as much out of character with the time as stage-coaches and hour-glass timekeepers."

It may be fairly asked, in face of such observations, what method did the College of Dentists itself recommend? The answer to this was given in the same article. The writer says—

"We would certainly advocate, as heartily as could be wished, the establishment of one, if not two, well-arranged dental schools, in which first-class instruction should be supplied at a moderate cost, in anatomy, physiology, elements of chemistry, and natural philosophy, dental surgery, pathology, and dental practice; and, in a word, every subject which shall tend to make the dentist an accomplished man, and to aid him in preparing for his examinational test. For all the rest we would trust a sound and practical examination, and would base qualification on this alone, leaving it with the candidate to gain the required information by reading a printed lecture, or hearing a written lecture, according as his own taste and opportunities may lead him on his way."

It was very much doubted at the time when these remarks were made public whether the opposition to the Odontological Society's method was the sole reason of a counter method. There still continued so much violent party spirit, that the fact of a plan emanating from that body at all was amply sufficient to call forth a different scheme, and bring the support of many to it. From whatever cause it arose, the College of Dentists objected not only to what had been done, and what was proposed to be further done, by the Odontologists, but gave, as above, an outline of what they considered better and more applicable to the necessities and interests of the junior members of the profession. It was while commenting upon the action taken by their opponents that the College of Dentists began to feel that there was a certain incongruity in their then position, as altered by the amended rules passed at the meeting in the August of the last year, contrasted with the programme which they were preparing touching ulterior steps. The "Dental Review" goes on to say—

"Tied recently from circumstances, by an absurd law also, to the College of Surgeons, the College of Dentists has sold its birthright for a mess of pottage, which its enemies have feasted on. If the college would stir and re-live, it must perforce reclaim its birthright; it must return to its original laws and its original independence; it must aim again at gathering all into one commonwealth, and at instituting an examinational test for membership, which shall be the primary step towards legal incorporation."

What remained, therefore, to be accomplished was the obtaining a charter; the appointment of a board of examiners from amongst themselves; the establishment of the rule that candidates for the membership of the college should not be expected to pass any particular curriculum, and that the reward of those deemed efficient before the court of examiners should be the college diploma. The first step to be taken was the rescinding of the laws so lately passed, and by which it was considered the principle of independence had been injured, if not actually lost. On the 22d of February in the year 1859 a requisition signed by ten members of the college was forwarded to the council, requesting that an early meeting of the members should be convened " for the purpose of taking into consideration the present position of the college, and to determine what course shall be pursued with regard to its future management." A meeting was accordingly called by the council for the 16th of March. It was numerously attended, and Mr. Matthews occupied the chair. The fact was elicited during the discussion which ensued, after the first proposition had been submitted, that a sense of despondency had been experienced by some of the members, and that the subject of dissolving the college had been mentioned at the council meetings. It appeared, however, that 170 members still existed, and, moreover, that a considerable balance was yet in the hands of the treasurer. Fresh courage instilled itself into those present, perhaps, from the numbers attending; and after the old ground of " independence " had been gone over, and it was found that, through some informality in the notice summoning the meeting, the proposition before them—which was to call upon the council to frame bye-laws by which the original principles of the college should be carried out, and which also included the making provision for granting diplomas without examination to members of the profession now in practice, with sundry other details—could not be carried, another resolution was submitted instead. The following is a copy :—

" Resolved :—That this meeting being now in possession of all the facts relating to the present position of the college, and feeling that the college, by departing from its original objects and intentions, has been deprived of much of its usefulness to the dental body at large, is of opinion that the regulations passed September

22, 1858, should be rescinded, and that a special meeting of the members be called by the council to consider such question."

This resolution was adopted. Another resolution was also submitted and likewise adopted. It was to the following effect :—

"That, for the information of the members of the dental profession, the council of this college be desired to communicate with the College of Surgeons, to know their intentions with respect to granting dental certificates ; and that, should the College of Surgeons give no satisfactory reply within one month, this college pledges itself to consider the question answered in the negative."

Although this meeting may be considered a rallying point in the history of the Dental College, it could not be concealed from the ordinary observer that it was from a very palpable and painful condition of weakness that it had rallied. The chief and leader of the movement admitted very frankly what had been his own experience. He had been "deeply depressed," and very naturally so too ; for there had appeared many vacant places in the original list of members, and, coupled with this, a noticeable inertness and want of support had been manifested. So much so, indeed, was this the case, that from Mr. Rymer himself had emanated a resolution in council having for its ultimate object the power and the opportunity to dissolve the college. When one so full of determination and uncomplaining energy as Mr. Rymer had shown himself to be felt constrained to take such a step, there can be no doubt whatever of a prime necessity being in existence. For two years and a half, with a devotion which was simply admirable, he had laboured strenuously for the attainment of what he conscientiously believed to be the means of securing the permanent benefit of the profession. When others flagged or failed in their faith of success, he resolutely proceeded in the cause, permitting nothing to daunt him. Surely there had been enough to dishearten the bravest, yet he held on perseveringly ; so that if, under the then circumstances, his heart failed him temporarily as he looked around him, there was no reason for surprise; the real matter for astonishment rested in the fact that he had never once evinced anything like discouragement before.

About a month later another meeting was called, which resulted in the amendment of the college laws in accordance with the views then entertained by its members.* The varying events in the profession were not only watched with interest both by dentists and the medical profession generally in England, but attracted no small amount of notice of dental practitioners in America and elsewhere. Commenting upon the condition of things at this time, the "New York Dental Journal" remarked, after reviewing the steps which had hitherto been taken to ensure dental reform in this country:—

"Thus grew up the '*Odontological Society*' and the '*College of Dentists;*' and the difference between them seems to have been just this: The Odontological Society, very properly relying little upon their own unaided efforts for stability, feeling that a spinal difficulty was rapidly becoming chronic, and that they were indeed weak, proposed to combine with the College of Surgeons, and obtain their diplomas in the old manner. The College of Dentists, on the other hand, wished to throw aside all connection with that body, and, obtaining a charter, educate their own men for their own profession, and in their own way—thinking a dentist could but obtain his education from dentists, and not from surgeons. Fortunately for the progress of the profession in England, there were found men who were unwilling to sacrifice their independence and prospect of proper education and future success to the childish scruples of a few old fogies. They saw that a profession including so many members as our own, a science in which something new is daily being discovered, surely were entitled to their own teachers as well as their own exponents. Thus the Dental College came to be established; and it is with pleasure that we are able to record its complete success thus far. Lectures are being read by the best men in England; professorships are being established; and there is little doubt but the COLLEGE OF DENTISTS will yet become as successful, as creditable, and as honoured an institution as the LONDON COLLEGE OF SURGEONS."

---

* See Appendix.

Such a notice as the above, coupled with others of similar import, may have served, and very probably did, to stimulate the hopes and efforts of the college party. It is certain that, from some cause or other, the determination to proceed with the institution on its original basis was formed. On the occasion of receiving the report of the committee on "Electricity as an Anæsthetic in Dental Operations,"*—a committee whose appointment reflected credit on the College of Dentists—Mr. Matthews took the opportunity to observe, "We have many eminent physicians who have sent in their adhesion to us, offering their services to forward our views in every respect; and a great number of members of the College of Surgeons of England have assisted us, and are glad to find that we are going on well. This gives us encouragement to do our utmost night and day to carry on the College of Dentists of England." On the 24th of June 1859, George Waite, Esq., M.R.C.S., and a member of the Dental College, was by the council elected to the office of president. In this month it was announced that the Metropolitan School of Dental Science had been fully organised, under the immediate auspices of the college, although practically distinct and separate from it. The court of examiners, also, was about this time constituted, some of whom, the profession was informed, were members of the College of Dentists, others fellows or members of the College of Surgeons, but unconnected then with any dental association, and others independent dentists unconnected with the College of Surgeons. The charter by which the institution alone could be consolidated and enabled to claim respect for its proposed certificates or diplomas was, however, still unpossessed, and to some the difficulties in the way of its obtainment appeared both numerous and formidable.

In the meantime the Odontological Society had been hard at work. Since its inauguration the Dental Hospital

---

* For entire report see "Dental Review," vol. i. p. 438.

of London had been working so as to fully justify the highest anticipations of its founders. Their object was to ascertain the practical value to the profession of such an institution—the importance to the public being perceptible from the first—before further action in the direction of providing a proper school in connection with it. In the interval between the opening of the Dental Hospital and the middle of the year 1859, the council of the Royal College of Surgeons having obtained a charter,* as has been already stated, took the initiative, and insisted that a curriculum should be drawn up, which was to be submitted for their approval, and steps taken to organise a school of dental surgery, by which a practical effect should be given to the legislative enactments that had been passed. The first requirement was at length met by the now well-known curriculum being formulated.† At the same time the London School of Dental Surgery became a fact, and the education of the student in dentistry was provided for in the fullest manner, with the ultimate object of the licentiateship of the Royal College of Surgeons of England being the coveted prize of all who should pass the examining board of the latter institution.

To revert again to the College of Dentists. The announcement was made in the August number of the "Dental Review," that what it had in its last issue predicted concerning the appointment of a board of examiners was fulfilled, and that the following gentlemen had been called to the office aforesaid:—

> Mr. James Harley, M.C.D.E.
> Mr. Robert T. Hulme, M.R.C.S., F.L.S., M.C.D.E.
> Mr. Peter Matthews, M.C.D.E.
> Mr. B. W. Richardson, M.D., L.R.C.P.
> Mr. James Robinson, D.D.S., M.C.D.E.
> Mr. Alexander Stewart, F.R.C.S.E.

---

* This had not yet received the Royal assent.
† See Appendix.

Mr. Somerset Tibbs, M.C.D.E.
Mr. George Waite, M.R.C.S., M.C.D.E.
Mr. T. Spencer Wells, F.R.C.S.

These gentlemen met to decide upon the requirements which they deemed necessary from all candidates for examination at their hands, July 26, 1859, and the decision was for the following subjects:—

1. Anatomy of the Head and Neck.
2. Structure of the Teeth.
3. Elements of Surgical Pathology
4. Injuries of the Teeth and Jaws.
5. Diseases connected with Dentition.
6. Operative and Mechanical Dentistry in all departments.
7. Pathology of the Teeth.

Gentlemen successfully passing an examination on these subjects would be thereby entitled to the use of the letters M.C.D.E., indicating thereby that they were members of the College of Dentists of England. It was further announced that the examinations would be essentially of a practical character, and would be held quarterly. The condition of the College of Dentists at this time may be best described by a quotation from an editorial in the "Dental Review." The writer asked—

"Does the college want more to give it strength? A little more. It wants law. Give it incorporation, and its stability is complete. Towards this the members must advance, they must neither hesitate, nor pause, nor tire, till this great object is attained—*their charter*. . . . But the charter is, after all, the true compact. The dentists of England must have a charter."

This was easy enough to write, and looked well enough when written, but the question was, Were the essentials in hand which would justify a hope of the attainment of this desideratum? The important fact appeared to be overlooked or forgotten, that a certain amount of influence, arising from the professional and acknowledged position of those who asked for a charter of incorporation, would be absolutely necessary in pressing such a claim or demand. This the institution in question did not possess. The secession from its ranks of several gentlemen, who would have contributed largely to the success of the scheme, had they remained in connection with it, naturally left it so much the weaker in this matter. The seriousness of their resignations told more against the project than the mere loss of numbers to the body at large. Whatever was the estimate of the step thus taken in the minds of the college executive and the members generally, the opposite party very naturally counted the secession in itself a direct gain to them, and a double gain when several of the seceders went over to them. It was not merely like so many guns captured from the enemy, but those very guns turned against the artillery of the opposing side. To put a good face on adverse circumstances was, perhaps, creditable and politic too; but that did not necessarily neutralise the effect of palpable weakness. The idea which obtained with many at the then position of things was, that the two societies had no need to combine. It was set forth that the Odontological Society was a great good in its own specific department. As an organisation for the elaboration and perfecting of the scientific portion of dentistry, a large and free course was open to it. On the other hand, the College of Dentists of England had its own distinct sphere of operation in the direction of educational and dental politics. Numbers of gentlemen held these views, and felt that such a division would prove of the greatest practical value. Whatever was the opinion upon this point of those outside the Dental College, the executive there determined to hold on its way towards the desired goal, and set itself to bring to perfection its own internal arrangements for that purpose. It was announced that three courses of collegiate lectures were to be delivered during the coming winter. Professor Erichsen had been engaged to deliver the first course on a surgical subject. Mr. Hulme would take the second course, his subject was to be the development of the teeth; and

Dr. Richardson was appointed to give the third course, on subjects relating to special pathology and the history of dental tissues. Four conversaziones were also to be held at the college, while the examiners would be prepared to fill their office with regard to the students desirous of passing their ordeal. The 5th day of October was fixed for the opening of the Metropolitan School of Dental Science, and six courses of lectures were to be given—viz., on "Physiology, or the Laws of Life;" on "Elements of Surgery;" on "Dental Surgery;" on "Dental Mechanics;" on "Chemistry and Metallurgy;" and on "Comparative Anatomy." The students had the promise of three medals, as prizes to the successful competitors, the council having resolved to offer these as a stimulant to earnestness and exertion. However the college, as an independent institution, had been opposed by those holding contrary views, it would be idle, and unjust as well, to ignore the benefit which, as an educational centre, it was desirous of conferring upon the younger men of that day. Its most determined adversaries could not overlook the fact that advantages in this direction were palpable enough, although the attempt to compete with the Royal College of Surgeons they felt assured would end in ignoble failure.

One or two events of importance occurred towards the close of this year which deserve record. The first was the circumstance of action taken by the newly-constituted Medical Registration Association concerning the use of the words "surgeon-dentist" by those practitioners who were entirely unconnected with the Royal College of Surgeons. The vigilance committee of the association had successfully prosecuted one individual using the prefix "surgeon," and then gave notice to Mr. Brookes, a dentist practising at Banbury, that it was their intention to adopt the same course with him if he did not abandon the use of the same word within a reasonable period after the letter they addressed to him. This led, of course, to a reply from Mr. Brookes, who was a member of the College of Dentists, and also to a communication from Mr. Rymer, as honorary secretary to the council of the College of Dentists, in which the proposed action of the association was argued against, deprecated, and a desire expressed for a speedy solution of the question at issue. In order to this, Mr. Rymer, who had hitherto styled himself "surgeon-dentist," expressed his willingness to be proceeded against. A lengthy correspondence ensued between the honorary secretary of the Medical Registration Association, Dr Ladd, and Mr. Rymer in his official capacity. The College of Dentists was up in arms on the subject, and issued an address to the entire dental profession, of which the following is a copy :—

"*Address to the Dental Profession.*

"The council of the College of Dentists of England deem it but right to acquaint the profession generally—whether members of the college or otherwise—with certain proceedings arising out of a recent attempt to tamper with a most important provision contained in the new Medical Act, which, had it proved successful, must have worked with the most reprehensible injustice on the great body of dental practitioners. The Act referred to concludes with a clause in which it is enacted that *nothing* therein contained 'shall extend, or be construed to extend, to prejudice or in *any way* to affect, the lawful occupation, trade, or business of chemists and druggists and dentists.' In the session of Parliament just closed a Bill was introduced into the House of Commons, entitled 'The Medical Act Amendment Bill.' This Bill, as *originally introduced*, would not have called for any remonstrance on the part of dental practitioners; but on the evening of Tuesday, July 26th, Lord R. Cecil gave notice of the following motion :—' That the words, "or licentiate in dental surgery" shall be added after the words "licentiate in midwifery" to the qualifications described in the fourth head of schedule (A) of the said first recited Act.' The subject of this motion was immediately brought before the notice of the council of the College of Dentists; and as it was apparent that if the clause should be carried in the Legislature, a privilege would be granted to a small party of dentists, to the detriment of the general body of existing practitioners; and, moreover, as the Medical Act itself clearly expresses that dentists (*i.e.*, as a body) shall not in *any way* be affected by it, the council resolved to take immediate steps to frustrate a movement evidently intended to be carried surreptitiously, and which could only be regarded as the more unprecedented because a privileged exclusiveness was sought to be conferred on a *non-existent* class of practitioners. It was never for a moment believed that Lord Robert Cecil was the originator of the motion of which he had given notice; and the council having communicated officially with his Lordship, ascertained that he had not been candidly informed as to the real feeling and position of the profession; that the motion had been drawn up by Mr. Tomes; and that Lord Robert Cecil would not have taken any steps in the matter had he been told plainly, as he ought to have been, that the motion was one upon which the dentists would be very far from unanimous. That any individual should presume to influence legislation for the benefit of a certain few, and to the detriment of the general body, otherwise than in an open and straightforward manner, is a proceeding of which the profession will be able to form a just opinion. The council at once resolved to present a petition to the House of Commons, of which the following is a copy :—

" '*To the Honourable the Commons of the United Kingdom of Great Britain and Ireland, in Parliament assembled.*

" 'The humble petition of the president, vice-president, examiners, and council of the College of Dentists in council assembled,

" '*Showeth,*

" 'That your petitioners humbly beg to represent to your Honourable House the great injustice which would be done to the general body of dentists of this country in case any amendment to the Medical Act (1858) be passed which would have the effect of allowing an *existent* or *non-existent* class of practitioners, to be called " Licentiates in Dentistry," or by any other partial title, to have their names entered on the medical register. The Medical Act, in the last clause, clearly expresses that nothing in the Act contained shall extend, or be construed to extend, to prejudice or in *any way to affect* the lawful occupation, trade, or business of chemists, and druggists, and *dentists*. Your petitioners humbly submit that if a class of men (existent or non-existent) are to be allowed to register under the Medical Act, that Act will be rendered anomalous, inasmuch as dentists in practice will be prejudiced and materially affected by any measure which does not confer privileges on *the entire body of practising dentists*. That the College of Dentists of England having been established by the dentists of England in open meeting, the officers and council elected by the members deem it their duty humbly to inform your Honourable House that it is intended to apply for a charter of incorporation for the college forthwith, and that it is the opinion of the council that any partial grant of privilege, such as to licentiates in dentistry, would act alike to the prejudice of the profession and the public.

"' Your petitioners, therefore, trust that no legislation will take place in reference to the question during the present session of Parliament, and humbly pray your Honourable House to reject any measures which may tend to prejudice the general body of British dentists.

'"And your petitioners will ever pray,' &c.

[This petition was, of course, signed by the entire executive and staff of the college.]

"This petition was placed in the hands of Mr. Brady, M.P., for presentation, who kindly promised to give it his support. In opposing this attack on the rights of dentists, the council have desired to act in a spirit of entire liberality, not only striving to protect their own members, but all those who practise dental surgery, and who are recognised *as entitled* to protection in the Medical Act. The absolute necessity for professional organisation, such as is afforded by the College of Dentists of England, can no longer be questioned, when, but for such organisation, independent dentists might at this moment be suffering, without redress, from the spirit of exclusiveness existing in a mere mistaken but persevering individual or party. Thus, whilst the college is engaged in the great work of providing efficient instruction and in regulating examination, the general interests of the entire body are not neglected. That there is need for vigilance on the part of dentists, independently of such *secret* proceedings as the one just exposed, recent prosecutions would appear to indicate. The title 'surgeon-dentist' *has been* objected to as illegal; although the right to assume it was never questioned before the passing of the Act, and the last clause, already quoted, is specially intended to prevent dentists from being deprived of *any* privilege they were in possession of. If the title 'surgeon-dentist' be objected to, it is time to be prepared for protection from any attempt on dentists' rights under the 32d clause, which enacts that none but registered persons shall recover charges for (amongst other things) the performance *of any operation* of a surgical nature. Now, the council of the College of Dentists has no doubt that the last clause of the Medical Act will avail to protect fully the rights of dental practitioners, but not without a strong organisation of the members to resist attempts that are made, and may in future be made, on their privileges. It is also to be borne in mind that, if Lord Robert Cecil's clause had been carried through Parliament, none but a 'licentiate' in dentistry could have been entered on the register; it is time, therefore, to organise, in order to resist attacks which evidently threaten those practitioners in dentistry whose rights are protected by the Medical Act of 1858. In order to give greater efficiency to the authority of the College of Dentists, it is intended to apply for a royal charter of incorporation, and it is requested that every practising dentist who thinks a charter desirable will append his name to the petition (a copy of which is enclosed), and return it to the secretaries with as little delay as possible.

"Signed on behalf, and by order of, the council,

"GEORGE WAITE, *President.*
SAMUEL LEE RYMER, } *Hon.-Secretaries.*
ANTHONY HOCKLEY,

"*August* 30, 1859."

It was evident to all outsiders, and to the Odontological Society especially, that the College of Dentists were not only on the alert to discover any attempt to infringe upon what they considered the rights of the general practitioner, but resolute to put forth all their power to nullify all action by their opponents in such a direction. Their promptitude thus displayed had a double effect. It was the throwing of the *ægis* of their protection over their own members, and was a plausible bid for an increase in the numerical strength of their own body. In due time a memorial or petition for a charter of incorporation for the Dental College was forwarded to the Queen's most Excellent Majesty in council, signed (*pro forma*) by six members of the college,[*] the result of which had, of course, to be patiently waited for. According to previous announcement, the Metropolitan School of Dental Science was opened on the day named, October 5, Dr. B. Richardson delivering the inaugural address. This gentleman had fully espoused the college views concerning the needs of the dental profession, and, from his point of vision, forcibly advocated them in a very able and full lecture. Many gentlemen of note were present on the occasion; and this new feature of the college enterprise was one which gave the greatest satisfaction to all concerned. The

* See Appendix.

event itself was commemorated in the evening of the same day by a dinner at the Freemasons' Tavern, when sixty gentlemen sat down together—the company including the lecturers, students, and friends of the school. The session was thus inaugurated under very promising circumstances; and it was evident that, whatever might be the fate of the college itself or the school, that a very important channel of instruction to dental students was opened for their special advantage. It was subsequently stated that the lecturers would not have to deliver their respective addresses to empty benches, twenty-five young men having entered the school as students. These were further stimulated to honest exertion in their studies by the offer from Mr. James Robinson of a ten-guinea prize, to be given for the best thesis on a subject to be determined by the council. This prize, with Mr. Robinson's usual liberality, was to be given in perpetuity. With such gentlemen as had consented to lecture at the Metropolitan School of Dental Science, the college was justified in feeling the highest satisfaction. On the following day, October 6, Mr. G. Waite, who had been elected president of the college, delivered his inaugural address, which was well received; and the action of the College of Dentists at that time was favourably noticed by the "Medical Times and Gazette," and by several of the daily journals. The "Dental Review" also went the length of asserting that new members and associates were coming in, and old members, who, in the late unhappy disturbances, retired for a time from the contest, were returning in full friendliness and good-will. So far as the College of Dentists was concerned, the year had furnished it with much work and more experience; and this eventful period of its existence came to a close with an amount of reanimation among its members which was prophetic of sustained life, if not of increased vigour for the future. Among its last acts in 1859 was the preparation of a somewhat elaborate diploma, which, under certain regulations, it would be prepared to issue to its members, it having, as an institution, been in existence the self-prescribed time prior to issuing such a distinction—viz., three years.

From the opposite side, too, the outlook was clear and also encouraging. The "British Journal" was enabled to state, before the year 1859 had anything like terminated, that the Odontological Society had steadily increased in numbers—in November of that year the list included nearly 150 names; the Dental Hospital of London was in full work; the London School of Dental Surgery was organised and in excellent operation; a library and museum was rapidly forming; and, last of all, in September the announcement was made that the dental charter was complete, it having received the royal sign manual. A board of examiners was, therefore, provided at the Royal College of Surgeons, and arrangements were being made for the consequent granting of dental diplomas by that body. It was not a difficult question to decide who were the victors. Seeing that the Odontological Society had added many, and in some cases influential, names to their list of members; that the course of events had brought about the acceptance by the college authorities at Lincoln's Inn Fields, and also by the Legislature, of the proposals they had made for the education and examination of future dentists, and that the institution of the Dental Hospital and its dental school had both been projected, and were thus far a success, there remained very little more to be done to constitute for that society a complete triumph. The dentists at Cavendish Square could not help realising the important advantage their opponents had gained. The hope they once fairly entertained of obtaining a charter for their college was dimmed, if not eclipsed, by the fact that a connection with the College of Surgeons for dentists, advocated by the original memorialists, pressed by the Odontological Society, and recommended by the Medical Registration

Association as the representative of the medical societies throughout the country, had taken definite form, and had passed into law by the act of the Legislature itself. Nevertheless, the general acceptance of this new state of things by the body of dentists at large was still wanting. The Odontological Society believed that in due time that would not be withheld; but the Dental College thought otherwise, and its members determining to set in themselves the example of unflinching opposition, resolved to leave nothing undone which could be done by them for proving that large numbers of town and country dentists sided with them in condemning affiliation with the Royal College of Surgeons as a blunder. Amid the expressions which took the printed and public form of editorials and general correspondence in the two opposing journals—the one side breathing taunts or exultations, and the other, stern, uncompromising defiance—the year 1859 died out.

CHAPTER VII.

The year 1860 opened under circumstances which fostered the highest expectations of that portion of the profession who either from the first, or gradually, and afterwards, approved of a connection with the Royal College of Surgeons. Those thus desirous of a closer intimacy with the medical body were looking eagerly forward to the time when the steps that had been taken to promote this end should be developed in a practical result. The authorities at Lincoln's Inn Fields, being empowered to act as the original memorialists suggested, having deliberated upon the entire scheme, resolved that, for facilitating the possession of the new degree of Licentiate in Dental Surgery by students in the provinces, certain provincial schools should be recognised as well as those in the metropolis. The board of examiners at the Royal College of Surgeons had been instituted, and at the proper time these gentlemen were prepared to fulfil their office. Their names, it need scarcely be added, inspired the highest respect. They were Mr. W. Lawrence, Mr. Joseph Green, Mr. J. M. Arnott, Mr. T. Bell, Mr. J. Tomes, and Mr. A. Rogers. In the meantime the College of Dentists had been deciding to issue a diploma in connection with that body, so that the profession had laid before it the two documents from which it might choose. From this point of view the contest looked very unequal. The weight of authority and dignity so evidently preponderated in the direction of the Royal College of Surgeons, that it was to be expected the majority of those desiring to possess a qualification to practise dentistry, which would be of real worth, would naturally find their opinions gravitating towards their old-established and widely-acknowledged institution. It would be untrue, however, to ignore the feeling which existed in the minds of many, that the independent principle had sufficient force and merit in it to influence a considerable number. At any rate the College of Dentists, through the executive, determined to bring the matter to an issue as speedily as might be. However, before any examination had taken place at the Royal College of Surgeons, or the diploma of the Dental College had taken visible form, it was agreed upon by those who leaned towards the former method of obtaining a certified status that a public protest against the College of Dentists and its proceedings generally should be issued. In the month of February therefore the following document appeared :—

"A certain number of dentists having associated themselves under the assumed title of 'The College of Dentists of England,' and having signified their intention of issuing diplomas of fitness to practise dental surgery to those who may consent to such regulations as they shall propose, we, the undersigned practitioners in dental surgery, deem it to be our duty publicly to protest against the proceedings of this so-called College of Dentists of England, as being wholly unsanctioned by law, unwarranted by precedent or professional usage, and opposed to the opinion and feeling of the great majority of the leading practitioners in dental surgery. And we more especially protest against the issuing of diplomas without legal authority, believing that such diplomas are calculated to mislead the public, by whom they may be mistaken for the legally authorised dental diplomas to be granted by the Royal College of Surgeons of England, through its dental department, consisting of surgeons and dentists in equal numbers, and organised in accordance with the provisions of a special charter granted to that body by Her Majesty in September last, in conformity with the Medical Act."

This was a veritable throwing down of the glove and entering the lists for a trial of strength. The challenge thus given had no sooner seen the light than the opposing party determined to answer it with all possible boldness. Accordingly, immediately afterwards, the College of Dentists issued the annexed "Counter-Protest":—

"We, the undersigned, being members or associates of the College of Dentists of England, and others engaged in the practice of dentistry, in reply to a Protest, published in the 'Times' of February 28th, 1860, do hereby enter the following counter-protest:—1st. That the College of Dentists of England was founded at a public meeting specially convened, in the year 1856, for the purpose of bringing about an honourable organisation of the dental profession. 2d. That as the college at its commencement had educational objects in view, extending to dentists throughout the kingdom, the title of 'College of Dentists' was agreed upon as the most expressive of such objects. 3d. That in taking this step no legal right whatever was infringed, there being no other institution of the same kind in the United Kingdom or its dependencies. 4th. That many of the names affixed to the protest against the College of Dentists are those of gentlemen who assisted in the establishment of the college, were once members of it, and assented to its name. 5th. That the College of Dentists is striving to advance the interests of the dental profession, and at the same time to secure for the public a properly-qualified class of practitioners—(1) By providing first-class lectures in the higher branches of science, delivered by men of scientific rank and reputation. (2) By establishing a school of dental surgery, for the teaching of anatomy, physiology, surgery, dental surgery, chemistry, dental mechanics, and comparative anatomy to students in dentistry, the chairs at which school are filled by able and practical teachers, and the usefulness and necessity of which educational establishment is fully proved by the excellence of the attendance. (3) By founding prizes for competition on subjects pertaining to the advancement of the science and art of dentistry. (4) By founding a museum and library. (5) By instituting a board of examiners for ascertaining that none but gentlemen, duly qualified by their knowledge and skill, be admitted to the privileges of membership. 6th. That the College of Dentists took up the subject of an examination for its membership before the certificate to be issued by the College of Surgeons was even planned, and that the suggestion that an attempt is being made by the College of Dentists to confuse the one examinational certificate with the other is an entire and wicked fabrication. 7th. That, on the contrary, the College of Dentists wishes its certificate to stand out as an independent and honourable distinction, indicating the one principle, that the organisation and status of the dental profession can be better provided for by an institution of its own than by its becoming an appendage to the College of Surgeons, contrary, as it is believed, to the wishes of the members of that corporation. 8th. That in the attempt to establish their policy the members of the College of Dentists have tried to act in the open character of Englishmen, and only desire to be allowed to carry out the principles they advocate in a straightforward and generous spirit.—Dated Feb. 29, 1860."

The rapidity with which the counter-protest was made to follow the protest was an evidence of the activity and decision of the College of Dentists. Both documents were largely signed, although exception was taken to the names of many which were affixed to the instrument emanating from Cavendish Square. What the public thought of either the one or the other it would be difficult to say, but there is no doubt that the 4th clause of the counter-protest told against it in the minds of many practitioners. It was evident that if many who had been associated with the Dental College were now leagued against it, there must have been serious reasons for such a decided step being taken by those so placed and so acting. In the March number of the "British Journal of Dental Science" the clauses were dissected *seriatim*, their various points of weakness exposed, and their logic disputed. The great thing to be done was to have an examination held by the board of examiners at Lincoln's Inn Fields. This would practically test the estimation in which the certificate to be given by the College of Surgeons was held. Fortunately for the memorialists and their now numerous and influential colleagues, this ordeal was soon to be arranged. It was announced that on the 13th day of March the examiners would meet for the above purpose, and a considerable number of names of gentlemen were accordingly sent in as candidates for examination —so many, indeed, that it was impossible in the allotted time to dispose of them all, and consequently a second examination was determined upon, to be held on the following day. The granting of these certificates by the authorities in Lincoln's Inn Fields was not without marked results so far as many medical practitioners were concerned. In commenting upon the subject, the "Lancet" of March 10th, 1860, had the following remarks:—

"It had been thought that these college dental diplomas are likely to be mistaken for college surgical diplomas, and that quacks, availing themselves of this opportunity to register, will also use it for surgical practice. We do not think the argument worth much in either case. If there be a chance of mistake, this will involve a little care on the part of those interested in preventing them. It is sufficiently obvious that the diplomas of a self-constituted college, without any charter or other recognised legal standing, will labour under a great disadvantage as compared with those of the Royal College of Surgeons. Any attempt at simulation would so degrade the College of Dentists as to produce its immediate dissolution. We cannot but retain the opinion which we have formerly expressed, that the dental profession has everything to gain by attaching itself to the College of Surgeons. Due precautions being taken, both bodies of practitioners will profit by the connection."

This was in accordance with the views held from the first by this the principal medical journal. The Odontological Society, in its unremitting efforts to bring about a distinct and decided connection between dental practitioners worthy of the name and the medical profession, had all along received support from the "Lancet." However, all the medical journals did not take the same view of the subject, and the College of Dentists felt that while that was so, they had an extra stimulus to persevere. The "Medical Times and Gazette," under date February 25th, spoke out as follows:—

"These dental licentiates, like the licentiates in midwifery, will call themselves surgeons, and are not likely to confine their practice to their specialty. Instead of a high order of dentists, we shall have a low class of surgeons thrust upon us. This, however, is a trivial mistake compared with the blunder the council has made in granting their diplomas to men who have not complied with the educational regulations of the college. We all feel that the council has done us an injustice. We all feel that we have been wronged."

The "Medical Circular," of February 29th, complained in a similar manner thus—

"The progress of specialties in the College of Surgeons is going on unchecked. This honoured institution is becoming the head and home of all the half-educated pretenders who have hitherto been considered the reproach to the profession Dentistry is to be legally recognised as a distinct branch of surgical science, with its special diploma and privileges. The Queen has granted a charter to the college, enabling it to carry out the provisions of the Medical Act ; and a board of examiners, consisting of three members of the council and three dentists, has been established. There can be no doubt that if the dentists avail themselves to any extent of this offer, and connect themselves parasitically with the college, it will be with the intention of practising as surgeons under the *ægis* of the college diploma. Every petty town in the country will have its certificated dentist poaching upon the practice of the fully-qualified man. . . . We regard the special diploma as bad in principle and ruinous in policy, except to those gentlemen, perhaps, who are benefited by the fees."

Both these journals continued to be exceedingly irate at the action of the College of Surgeons, and gave expression again to their indignation. The "Medical Times and Gazette," in its issue March 10, again reverted to the subject, and, among other things, said—

"The council of the College of Surgeons, acting on the 48th clause of the present Act, without any reference to the wishes of the profession it ought to represent, is about to admit to its body not only men who have passed a special examination, but men who assume a retrospective qualification by virtue of having operated on teeth, and worked at the mysteries of gold-plate, bone, or vulcanite. We may thus expect, granting that this folly is not stopped by the firm and manly voice of the profession, to see introduced among us a number of persons who, claiming relationship with a surgical corporation, will pass themselves on the public as surgeons, and being neither surgeons nor dentists, will pretend to be everything. That such a suicidal course can be allowed to pass without remonstrance is impossible. . . . Let it be strongly proclaimed that we want no certificated specialists, and won't have them, and no power whatever can sustain them in honour. We make this remark with the best feeling to the members of the dental profession. In their own sphere we can work with them as brethren, consult with them as equals, but they must keep to their own sphere—not intrude upon ours."

This outburst of fretful jealousy and unjust insinuation serves to show to some extent the difficulties in the way of dental reform and progress. The "British Medical Journal" of March 10th, after a long denunciation of the action of the College of Surgeons, concludes its remarks by direct reference to the College of Dentists and its plan thus—

"Taking things as they are, there are a large number of dentists; and of these there is a powerful section aiming to maintain a college of their own and claiming their own independence. These men, we learn, have spurned the temptation offered by the College of Surgeons; they disdain to creep into the medical profession surreptitiously and disgracefully. They are determined to prove that the worth of their profession is not to be increased by their buying the privilege of becoming appendages of a body in which they would be regarded as intruders, but that it is to be maintained and augmented only by independence, industry, and conscientiousness. The medical profession will do well to act in concert with these men in resisting the disgraceful acts of the College of Surgeons."

Referring to the same subject, the "Medical Circular," in its number for March 21st, remarks that—

"The confidence that now prevails between the surgeon and the dentist would be severed; the former would regard the latter with jealousy, and would refrain from sending him patients. The result would be that the dentist would be worse off in consequence of his connection with the college than he is now apart from it. A considerable number of them would, doubtless, invade the practice of the surgeon; but the remainder would scarcely know how to live, and would be driven to connect the drug trade with their other business. The necessities of the profession would lead to the creation of a new order of dentists disassociated with the college, and these only would receive patronage and support. Let the dentists carefully consider their position before they embrace the council of the College of Surgeons' proposition."

Although somewhat amusing from the present point of view as such sentiments, and so expressed, must be to the dental reader, at the time they were ushered into the light of day they had a very different effect indeed. It need hardly be said that the doleful predictions thus uttered have not been fulfilled, nor has the surgeons' province been at all invaded. The "Dental Review" did not keep silence. It said—

"The College of Surgeons may assume authority; it cannot change a sentiment, nor blend into one two professions which are by natural circumstances and boundaries entirely separated; still less can it do so by virtue of a mere scrap of paper which gives no legal right, and which does not affiliate in any one particular the men who possess it with the institution that sold it— which, in short, neither makes a dentist nor a surgeon; and, without making surgery dignified, makes dentistry a vassalage."

While the heat of contending parties was becoming palpably stronger, the three days appointed for examination—viz., the 13th, 14th, and 20th of March 1860—saw no less than forty-three gentlemen, most of whom were distinguished members of the profession, submit to the ordeal, and receive the dental diploma. Whatever, therefore, might have been the opinion of other dentists, or medical practitioners generally or in particular, there could be no doubt about the estimate formed of the licentiateship in dental surgery by those who thus submitted voluntarily to be tested upon their qualifications to practise their special profession. So long as the scheme propounded by the original founders of the Odontological Society was in nucleus, or even approaching completeness, there was a fair opportunity for discussing its merits and opposing its advance; but when it had become *un fait accompli*, opposition appeared useless. However, this was not the idea of the College of Dentists' party; and whether the executive said as much among themselves, or secretly thought so, there can be no doubt that from that moment the doom of "independency" was proclaimed. The council of the College of Dentists had appealed to the medical profession on the subject of dentistry being a separate and distinct profession from surgery, and had received some

3000 names of gentlemen acquiescing in that view. One of the most energetic workers in connection with the Dental College, Mr. Peter Matthews, its former president and treasurer, in the month of April, having previously retired from the college, presented himself at Lincoln's Inn Fields, and received the new diploma. The list of such recipients continued to increase, until in June, just three months after the first examination had taken place, the number of licentiates in dental surgery was no less than eighty-eight. This list, alphabetically arranged, was somewhat triumphantly published in the June issue of the "British Journal of Dental Science." In the meantime the supporters of the Dental Hospital of London, with others, had formulated the London School of Dental Surgery, which on the last day of April in that year was consummated. On that occasion, and amid much hearty applause, Mr. Samuel Cartwright, jun., delivered a most excellent inaugural address. This took place at the Dental Hospital, where a goodly company of influential and representative gentlemen was assembled. Consolidation of what had been already accomplished by the instrumentality of the Odontological Society was now the principal aim of that party. In the meantime, the College of Dentists had set the engraver to work, and secured an ornamental diploma, which it was proposed to confer upon its members, not simply on account of their membership, but also as a guarantee of the holder's fitness to practise dentistry. The document was somewhat showy, bearing at the top the college arms and inscription; beneath which was the following statement:—

"By virtue of the powers vested in us by the council of this college, we, the court of examiners, have diligently examined ————, and have found him competent to exercise the art and science of a DENTAL SURGEON. We have, therefore, this day admitted him a member of this college."

This was followed by the signatures of the president, examiners, secretary, and registrar, concluding with the date. There can be no question as to the real motives of the projectors of this diploma. They were doubtless most anxious to do all they could towards affording the public a guarantee which should ensure against incompetency. They felt, and without question, the disastrous results of charlatanism, and earnestly desired to check, if not suppress it. Their examination was to be real and not fictitious, while the issue of a diploma would go far to meet the universal longings to possess an authoritative acknowledgment of the holder's capacity. But beyond this it is morally certain that the granting of diplomas by the College of Dentists was meant as an overt competitive act with the College of Surgeons. Two certificates were in the field, and it remained for the profession to elect which it should obtain. The "Dental Review" left nothing unsaid to promote the acceptance of the instrument emanating from Cavendish Square, nor was the "British Journal of Dental Science" silent upon the all-absorbing subject. The College of Dentists must be credited with exemplary diligence in seeking to improve its position. The prizes had been distributed by the Metropolitan School of Dental Science, at a most enthusiastic meeting. The lectures in connection with the college were being delivered before numerous auditors. To the already well-filled list of objects for the museum specimens of interest and value were being added, and more promised. The formation of a good library was under consideration, and about this time, June 1860, the council were proposing to seek for more accommodation in larger premises than those then occupied. The large measure of success which had been obtained by the opposing party, instead of quenching zeal and obliterating hope, seemed but to add fresh vigour to those connected with the College of Dentists, and stimulate the executive to further effort on its behalf. It may be, perhaps, safely asserted that at no previous period had there been more unflinching resolution manifested by the upholders of "independency" than at this time. They were determined to develop all their resources, and show an uncompromising front to the foe. One of the characteristics of the College of Dentists' diploma was, that all submitting to examination in order to obtain it were not bound by the ordinary curriculum. Using the phraseology of the editor of the "Dental Review," the following is a description of the liberty here alluded to:

"We ask you not whether you come from east or west; whether you are self-taught or master-taught; whether you have studied twenty years or twenty months; whether you have worked in winter or summer; bring with you a good character, and prove demonstrably that you possess the standard of knowledge which we consider requisite, and your membership with us is secure."

This principle had considerable fascination, doubtless, for some, especially for such as could, perhaps, with difficulty afford to meet the expenses of the recognised medical schools; and the conclusion arrived at in the minds of many was that under such a method the examination proposed would be less stringent or severe than that imposed at Lincoln's Inn Fields. Whatever motive actuated the gentlemen proposing to submit to either of the two examinations, the value of a certificate emanating from a chartered body like the Royal College of Surgeons was undeniably greater than that issued by an unchartered institution, as the College of Dentists continued to be. This would have been still true, even had the Dental College a majority of the well-known and most influential practitioners to support it, which, indeed, it had not. However much the licentiateship in dental surgery might be ridiculed by those who said they saw in it nothing of worth to the possessor or to the profession, such a document carried with it a legal recognition of the holder's fitness to practise, and in no other direction could such an acknowledgment be found. For the dentists of this country to have won for themselves such a position, and in so short a time, reflected the highest praise not only upon those who had originally proposed it, but also upon every one who had been instrumental in supporting the enterprise from its commencement to its close. In four short years the profession had arisen and shaken itself from the dust and disgrace of former times, and by dint of sheer hard work had secured for itself a legal standing; and it may be fairly assumed that a corresponding social improvement was thereby attained. If the national instinct in the direction of liberty had been aroused, as it certainly had, yet it would be futile to deny that another instinct equally strong had not been dormant—namely, that which not only looks towards but leans upon law and order. In the certificate of the Royal College of Surgeons this instinct was met; and while no immunity from distasteful services in the community was granted, such as the full membership secured to medical practitioners, yet the acknowledgment of dentists from a legal point of view was a distinct and most important step in advance. Ardent spirits are always to be found in every reform movement; but the history of all such revolutions teaches us that they are not the safest guides. Unless the florid imaginations and full demands of men of this temperament are gratified there is sure to be a manifestation of discontent on their part. Even those who had thus laboured and won the new position would have preferred something more than the certificate allotted to them. But, although not absolutely content, they were well pleased with what had been accomplished. In all legislation and new enactments not only is the justness of the law to be considered, but also the appropriateness of the time, and the fitness to receive, and willingness to accept and obey on the part of those legislated for. It is very certain that the propounders of the "licentiateship" scheme felt they had done that which would best suit the needs of the dental profession, and were content to wait until time had done its allotted work in proving the soundness of their views. They were rewarded before the year 1860 came to its close by seeing more than a hundred members of the profession holding the new dental degree. The Dental Hospital of London had been doing quiet but efficient work, the patients being more double in number than those of the preceding year.* The London School of Dental Surgery was giving signs of real vitality, and the Odontological Society was more than ever *en evidence,* both from a practical and scientific point of view. The effect of all this both upon the College of Dentists and the outsiders in the profession may be readily imagined. Whether Mr. Rymer and his friends considered it politic to openly admit defeat, there can be but little doubt as to what both he and they must have felt at the distinct success, or rather series of successes, which had been achieved by the opposing ranks. They could, nevertheless, look back upon their efforts as the year closed with honest pride. The second session of the Metropolitan School of Dental Science was opened in the month of October, and an interesting and instructive address delivered by Mr. T. Hulme, M.R.C.S.* A conversazione followed on the 30th of the same month. The president of the college (Mr. Waite) gave his address and reviewed the progress of the institution, alluding to the lectures which had been given to the members of the college by Professor Erichsen, Dr. Richardson, and Mr. Hulme on the important subjects of "Diseases of the Maxillary Bones," "Anæsthetics," and the "Anatomy and Development of the Teeth" respectively. Mr. James Robinson, in conjunction with Mr. Tibbs (of Cheltenham), vice-presidents of the college, desiring to stimulate the students to real industry, had offered a prize of thirty guineas for the best essay on "Caries of the Teeth." So far from acknowledging defeat, the executive had been searching for a separate building in which the college might be installed; but not being able to succeed in that

* In the month of May this hospital and school were recognised by the Royal College of Surgeons.

direction, they contented themselves by securing a renewal of the lease of the rooms at No. 5 Cavendish Square, together with increased accommodation for the larger attendance of members and others who they fully expected would support their cause. Those who had been looking forward with eager anticipation to unity of action between the two contending parties, were disappointed on reading the last words which the editor of the "Dental Review" published towards the end of that year on that subject. The writer remarked—

"The College of Dentists of England, now consolidated, enters on this new session with better days before it than it has yet seen. In its attempts at reform it has accepted the broadest policy. It stakes its position, not on an obedience to existent prejudices, nor on personal compromises, but on the faith of an introduction into its future life of young, unbiassed, working intellect—of intellect represented by men who, trained in independence, lured by scholarly friendships into unity, educated by early learning into strength, and sustained in principle by association, will identify the institution that has reared them with their own lives, improve it by their labours, and consolidate it the more."

The friends of "independence" were thus filled with courageous hope, if not sanguine expectation, concerning the ultimate success of their project, and their faith not only in the soundness of their principles, but in the applicability of them, and their acceptance by a large number of the up-coming generation of dentists, must have been unusually strong, especially with such a fact as the 13th day of March in that year had placed on permanent record. Mr. Robinson had for some time past changed his views concerning the Odontological Society, and the side of the profession it represented, and had accordingly espoused once more the college cause. He had been elected to the treasurership, and determined to advance the interests of the institution as much as he possibly could. Originally one of the trustees of the Dental Hospital of London he became dissatisfied with that charity, and resigned his office. His private reason, subsequently made known to the author, was his personal dislike to be associated with one of the gentlemen on the staff; but the true motive lay in the direction of his strong desire to inaugurate a similar hospital to be identified with the College of Dentists of England. The struggle between the two sections of the profession was destined to be prolonged, and the "British Journal of Dental Science" accepted this as the then situation, and in the leading article in its first number for the following year, 1861, after comparing the relative positions and prospects of either side, said, in concluding, "We look upon the 'College of Dentists' as a positive evil, calculated to mislead the public, and to encourage a low tone of professional conduct among dental practitioners." Although it might have been inferred from the opening remarks of the editor of the "Dental Review" that a more peaceful era had dawned, many felt that such, indeed, was not the case. The latter journal remarked, "With the new year we come before our readers full of expectation, not unalloyed with anxieties. We buried with the last volume all feeling of rivalry, political and general." What the feelings of the large mass of dentists occupying neutral ground may have been, it is not easy to declare. Perhaps it would be nearest to truth to say that they were content to wait still longer, and watch the course events might take as the relative strength and efficiency of the combatants to represent them were manifested. In the hope of displaying these qualities the college party firmly believed in the prospect of success. If the assertion that its strength was gradually augmenting, the numbers of its supporters were increasing, the certificate or diploma of membership was publicly recognised, and the possession of that document a thorough guarantee of the holder's fitness to practise or to fill public appointments, could be received as a reliable statement, its efforts in its own chosen direction were justifiable enough. The clouds overspreading the sky of the profession were murky and threatening, nevertheless, and there were not wanting those who apprehended stormy days in the immediate future. Although continued conflict was in one sense much to be deplored, yet there can be no doubt that the complete trial of the merits of the respective methods of reform had in it enough of advantage to permit its continuance unchecked. An angry tone of feeling between the editors of the two dental journals displayed itself in the early part of this year on the subject of advertising, as it was hinted, if not positively asserted, took place among the members of the College of Dentists. Threats were made by the conductors of the "Dental Review" to arrest what the editor called "libellous and scurrilous attacks." A correspondence accordingly ensued between these two literary champions which ended in nothing, or, at least, nothing that could be called satisfactory, as is usual in similar cases, as a rule. What was far more interesting and suggestive withal was the commemorative dinner of the establishment of the dental licentiate degree. This event took place at the Albion Tavern, London, on the 13th of March—the late Mr. Arnold Rogers being chairman. As the first anniversary dinner of those concerned it proved a signal success, and words of encouragement, direction, and hope for the future were freely given by the speakers on the occasion. Gentlemen from Scotland, Ireland, and distant parts of England were present, and the social ties of the profession certainly were made all the firmer, while the reminder thus given to those who still stood aloof of what had been already accomplished for the benefit of all, had in it the element of utility. The list of names of gentlemen who had taken this degree was gradually becoming larger, and it was an act of policy thus to meet and let their brethren be made aware of the fact. On the other side the college party felt constrained to rejoice that two of their members (the late Mr. Cox Smith, of Chatham, and Mr. Tweed, of London) had been appointed to public posts—the former to Fort Pitt Establishment, and the latter to the Essex and Colchester Hospital On the occasion of the distribution of prizes in connection with the Metropolitan School of Dental Science in April of this year, statements were made as to the progress already made, and that which was intended for the furtherance of education which could not but be indicative of a certain amount of success. Among other matters which the Faculty of Lecturers had to report, it appeared that several gentlemen already in practice had entered at the school with the express intention of making themselves qualified to pass the examination necessary to obtain the diploma of membership of the College of Dentists. A course of lectures on Practical Chemistry was about to be commenced under the superintendence of Dr. Bernays, and notice was also given of the intention to institute a dental hospital or infirmary in direct connection with the college and school. It was evident that the Metropolitan School of Dental Science was doing a healthy work for the students there. The various prizes distributed on that occasion had been obtained by the prizemen after substantial and continuous effort, and were contested for by keen and anxious minds. Whatever some may have thought as to the value of the licentiate's degree, it was plain to all that the College of Dentists still had an earnest following.

About the middle of this year the "Lancet," which had all along supported the views held by the Odontological Society, published a trenchant article concerning the College of Dentists, commenting upon its *raison d'être*, comparing it to the "Morisonian Institute" or "College of Health," and complaining of the conduct of some of its members in the direction of unprofessional conduct by means of advertisements, and setting forth the necessity "for the interests of the licentiates in Dental Surgery now affiliated to our body," ... "to all who value their social and intellectual status, that they should not be supposed to be represented professionally by a body which can consent to practices so undignified, or allow its name to be paraded as a sanction to proceedings so entirely opposed to the canons of professional conduct." The fact is, the Odontological Society had determined to keep a strict watch over the College of Dentists and the conduct of its members. There was no disguise as to its resolution to take advantage of anything and everything which could be fairly brought against it. The rival bodies were in real earnest in opposing each other, and whenever the medical press could be helpful to the course which each proposed, that help was eagerly sought for. When the article in question appeared, it created a profound sensation among the executive of the College of Dentists, and the "Dental Review" in alluding to it admitted that "a more serious attack against our independent institution was, perhaps, never before made." The result was, that Mr. Waite, the president, published a long, temperate, and expostulatory reply. He admitted that, notwithstanding certain stringent rules, "It has happened, in a few instances, that certain persons who have taken up our membership have proceeded in a way the council entirely condemns." He also asserted the *tu quoque* concerning certain of the dental licentiates, and put in evidence of the council's action in such matters, that that year two names had been struck off the college list and three others refused admission on account of their perpetrating the offence complained of. Mr. Waite gave the number of those associated with the college at that time as 160, and summarised the proceedings of the body in the following remarks:—" Thus we have, in the five years of our existence, had delivered eleven distinct courses of lectures from men who, by position and practical knowledge, were best fitted for the task. We have inaugurated a school for systematic instruction in dentistry and the collateral sciences for our junior brethren. We have published four yearly volumes of 'Transactions,' which have been largely reprinted and circulated both in this country and in America. We have opened a reading-room, library, and museum. We have appointed committees to investigate special scientific questions. We have instituted liberal prizes for the promotion of dental science, and we have provided during the session for monthly discussions and readings. Finally, to give our membership more value, we have lately originated a system of admission of members by examination, the examining board having been selected with all the judgment we could bestow upon the selection." Mr. Waite concluded his reply by stating the fact that 3000 members of the medical profession gave them their countenance and encouraged them to proceed. It was evident that the College of Dentists had not been idle, but on the contrary had, with all the influence it possessed, pushed forward after its own method the movement of reform on the basis of education. It must be admitted, however, that that influence was limited; and its limitation was the more apparent by the contrast of the names of its supporters with those who were upholding the opposite scheme. While the majority of the recognised leaders in the dental ranks were to be found identified with the working out of the means for securing the licentiateship of the Royal College of Surgeons, it was manifest to every impartial observer that the executive of the Dental College had really but small hope of eventual and permanent success. The question of how to deal with advertisers, and how an arrest of their unprofessional habits could best be effected, was once more brought into prominence. Unfortunately, that question had to deal with something deeper down than mere habit or practice. The cause of advertising lay in the instincts and proclivities of the men who indulged in it; and no law, however far-reaching in its effects, or wise in its conception, can ever be depended upon to eradicate such an evil as all good men then deprecated and still deplore. The process of moral purification must of necessity be slow; and it was, perhaps, from an over-anxiety on the part of the higher-minded and zealous supporters of those things, which such felt were necessary to consolidate the good already done, and become the means of achieving still more good in the future, that these offences against professional conduct assumed such ugly proportions in their eyes. The spirit evinced by both sections of the dental body was of that type which would not permit of any outrage of acknowledged canons without extracting from it material for political capital or party purposes. It was a time of trying of strength. But wherever offenders were to be found, there was cause for congratulation in the fact that they were noted and denounced. The above letter in the "Lancet" created a feeling of great irritation among the College of Dentists' party, and the advice given by the "Dental Review" was to give every opposition its counter, and remain firm in the principle of independence. On the other hand, the editor of the "British Journal of Dental Science," after commenting upon and criticising Mr. Waite's letter, concluded his article by saying—"All will agree with us that it is deeply to be lamented that a profession highly useful to the public, and honourable to its representatives, should be subjected to the degradation which is entailed in the publication of falsehoods by a body of men pretending to represent the dentists of England." So far as the candidates for the licentiate's degree were concerned, their number was gradually on the increase. Up to the end of July in this year (1861) one hundred and thirty-one had obtained that distinction, and of that number twelve out of the seventeen dentists appointed to the Metropolitan Hospitals possessed it. The medical profession was evidently interested in the progress of events. The "Lancet" adverted to the subject again, and Mr. Waite again replied. Comments appeared in the dental journals supporting either side, and there were not wanting contributors to the discussion, which was conducted in a far from amicable spirit. Such was the *animus* evoked, that the "Dental Review" in one of its articles had the following statement, which was put forth as very like a threat:—"A correspondent, writing to us on the advertising question, suggests that we print a carefully-compiled and authenticated list of every advertisement that has been put forth by every living dentist. The list certainly would be a startling fact; and if we do publish it, will indicate that many who, under the treacherous protection of time, are bold in condemnation of the modern advertiser, were better employed in performing a wholesome penance in liquidation of past delinquencies." Such words were not without their significance "to all whom they might concern," and doubtless produced a certain amount of fear and trembling in more directions than the humbler paths of professional life and their occupants. The question or rather subject of advertising raised a considerable amount of discussion, apart from what was made public. So far as the "Dental Review" was concerned—and its utterances may be taken as reflecting the sentiments of the College of Dentists—its conclusions were that in the then condition of the profession "the admission of a truthful advertisement must be allowed." Here, as in so many other particulars, the opposition of ideas to those held by the Odontological Society was apparent. The latter association condemned entirely public announcements under all circumstances. It laid down a sharp line of demarcation, and those who passed over to the side which permitted the use of advertisements of any sort were considered by it to have renounced their claim to be quoted as professional gentlemen, and had voluntarily sunk themselves to the lower level of tradesmen. This year was characterised mainly by the determination of both sections of the profession to advance in their chosen paths. The Odontological Society held its regular meetings with increasing interest and scientific utility. The licentiateship was steadily sought after, and the number of those who obtained it became greater at each examination of the board. The Dental College carried on its usual meetings, and the Metropolitan School of Dental Science was stirring itself, and exhibiting increased activity, while there were the social features of conversaziones and dinners, intermingled with the more prosaic demands of study and application. The one notable fact of the year, however, for the college party was the inauguration, on the 11th of November, of the National Dental Hospital. This event took place on the premises, No. 149 Great Portland Street, Dr. Brady, M.P., being called upon to preside. Such an institution had been suggested by Dr. Alfred Carpenter, of Croydon, some four years previously, but the National Dental Hospital was, doubtless, due to the untiring energy and determination of the late Mr. James Robinson. The Metropolitan School of Dental Science was not itself sufficient to carry out the requirements of the College of Dentists without such a sphere of demonstrative and practical utility as a dental hospital could alone supply; and as the one had been established, and was in working order, it was expedient that the complementary hospital should be brought into existence. The Dental Hospital of London was in full work, 7000 cases having been admitted in the course of the year; and the London School of Dental Surgery was proving a thorough success also. Each side congratulated itself upon its career, and was determined to pursue its course with unabated vigour. Conflict, it was evident, was not yet to cease, and the hopes of union, and consequent peace between opposing parties, were still faint and dim.

With the commencement of the following year (1862) came a matter which served to divert the thoughts of the profession from the harassment and fret of political subjects. This was the appearance of Mr. Makins' work on metallurgy. To have secured the services and co-operation of such an authority on the above subject in connection with the London School of Dental Surgery was an achievement of which the promoters of that enterprise might well be proud. As lecturer on this important branch of study, Mr. Makins was creating a deep interest in it among the students there, which was very gratifying. But the issue of the "Manual of Metallurgy" was a distinct gain to the entire profession. The author of that work had not only directed his attention to the consideration of the precious metals, but also to such others as were necessarily used by dentists in their laboratories and operative practice. This contribution to the gradually accumulating literature of the profession was as timely and welcome as it was practical and to the point. It certainly served then, and, indeed, still continues to do so, as a stimulus to study in that important department of knowledge. The work was very favourably reviewed, and occupies the place of a book of reference on all the subjects of which it treats. So far as the College of Dentists was concerned, there was every evidence that its executive intended to continue the efforts which it had been making. A change occurred in the staff of lecturers at the Metropolitan School of Dental Science. Mr. Perkins, who had been hitherto, with the occasional assistance of Mr. A. Hockley, lecturing on dental mechanics, was compelled through failing health to resign his post. Mr. Hockley was called to succeed him, and delivered his introductory lecture in November 1861, and continued his course in the following year. This extra duty must have proved a considerable tax upon his time and energy, seeing that he held the office of honorary secretary, in conjunction with Mr. Rymer, to the College of Dentists. When the author vacated that office, Mr. Hockley succeeded him, and bestowed both time and labour in the most commendable way in the sphere to which he had been called by his brother practitioners. Mr. Purland, who had been acting as librarian and curator to the college, also retired in the early part of the year, and was succeeded by Mr. R. T. Hulme. These changes were to be expected, occurring as such things do in all societies; but a vacancy in the college staff occurred shortly after for which no one could be said to have been prepared. This arose from the sudden death of Mr. James Robinson, the treasurer of that institution. The melancholy event took place on the 4th March 1862, and created a shock and surprise throughout the profession generally. A further allusion will be found in this work touching this sad circumstance. The opponents of the college were steadily at work, watching and waiting the course of events, and using all the available means at their disposal to keep the merits of their method constantly before the profession. The large mass of neutrals did not appear likely to become less by the adoption of the plans and principles of either of the contending sides. In fact, the apathy exhibited by this class of practitioners was very tedious to deal with by collegians and odontologists alike. After more than five years of strife and struggle, the expectation that the profession, more or less as a whole, would elect its leaders for the future was not at all an unreasonable one. Those, however, who had been waiting for such a decision to be made were not destined to see their hopes gratified.

The depression experienced by those who were so energetically endeavouring to confer what they fully believed would be lasting benefits upon those who would succeed them was none the less because it was not very frequently alluded to. The disinterestedness which many of the more prominent members of the profession on either side were showing was manifest from the fact that, in several instances, there were no members of their families destined to enter the dental ranks. It becomes very certain, therefore, as a conclusion in all reflective and impartial minds, that what was being done was only possible to men of indomitable perseverance and unfaltering faith. When the 13th of March came round, the licentiates in dental surgery again met at the Albion Tavern to commemorate the granting of the degree. On that occasion Mr. Thomas Bell occupied the chair, and was supported by Messrs. Laurence and Arnott of the Royal College of Surgeons. Whatever the indifference of the bulk of dental practitioners to the movement progressing in their midst, this gathering proved itself a means of increasing the determination on the part of those who had been thus far successful to persevere in the direction they had been pursuing. It must have been a great reward to all who had so unremittingly worked to secure affiliation with the Royal College of Surgeons for the dental profession to hear from such an authority as (the late) Mr. Lawrence such words as these: "We are, indeed, as our chairman has said, *all one body*—associated in the accomplishment of a common end; and let me say, that it is simply impossible for one branch of the profession to be elevated, without that elevation redounding to the credit of the general body." And also, "I can say, however, for the council of the College of Surgeons, that we feel a deep interest in the welfare of the dental profession; and are ready to promote its welfare in every way in our power." Mr. Lawrence had warmly expressed the ideas, the fulfilment of which were thus being celebrated, and his powerful influence, in conjunction with Mr. Arnott and Mr. Green, had materially smoothed the way for the acceptance of the memorialists' views by the executive at Lincoln's Inn Fields. Another gratifying proof of the estimation in which true service to the cause of professional advance was held appeared in the determination to present Mr. Tomes with a testimonial to that effect. For years past Mr. Tomes had been labouring for the general good; and not only by his personal presence and counsel at the several meetings which had been held, but also by his valuable contributions to dental and scientific literature, had shown himtelf to be a real friend to the profession. The idea of a "Tomes' Testimonial" once mentioned, it speedily took form, and reached maturity. Mr. S. Cartwright, jun., kindly consented to act as chairman of the Testimonial Fund Committee, and used all his influence to secure the best possible results. Mr. T. A. Rogers acted as treasurer, and in the course of a very short time found out that his office was not a sinecure. Subscriptions, limited to one guinea, were freely given, coupled with the kindest expressions towards the, to-be, recipient. All preliminary arrangements having been completed, July 16th was fixed as the day for the presentation to take place. This, moreover, was made the occasion of a public dinner by the subscribers, which was held at the Freemasons' Tavern, London. Mr. Samuel Cartwright, jun., presided; Mr. A. Rogers being vice-chairman. A very large number of the subscribers came together, and Mr. Cartwright, after highly eulogising the efforts Mr. Tomes had so continuously made for the true advance of the dental profession, presented the testimonial in graceful terms to him. The gift took the form of an elegant tea and coffee service, on a doublestage centrepiece—the whole forming a beautiful design, in sterling silver, mounted on a stand. A silver shield bore the following inscription:—

Presented to

J. TOMES, Esq., F.R.S.,

BY SEVERAL OF HIS BROTHER PRACTITIONERS, IN ACKNOWLEDGMENT OF THE MANY VALUABLE SERVICES HE HAS RENDERED TO HIS PROFESSION, JULY 16, 1862.

The gift was accepted and acknowledged by Mr. Tomes in appropriate terms; and the occasion was one of great pleasure to all concerned, and helped in no small degree to cement newly-made friendships, and was not without its effect in the direction of strengthening that cause with which he had so prominently identified himself.

The International Exhibition of this year had, as a matter of course, drawn several foreign dentists to this country; and this circumstance was utilised by the College of Dentists of England, it being in the opinion of that body a fitting opportunity for offering some sort of hospitality to their foreign brethren—some token both of courtesy and goodwill. It would have been well had there been a general combination for such a purpose; but from some cause or other, or, perhaps, from many causes, the profession was not in a condition thus unanimously to concur. On the 23d of July a dinner in honour of the foreign dentists then in England was given by the Dental College at the Freemasons' Tavern, London, which was attended by several practitioners from Germany, America, &c., together with not a few members of the medical profession of this country. The chair was taken on the occasion by Mr. Waite, president of the college, and many fraternal and friendly sentiments were expressed. Drs. Parmly, Abbott, Steinberger, with Mr. Hulme, Dr. Richardson, Mr. Rymer, and others, were among the speakers.

The unhappy American war then raging precluded many eminent dentists from visiting London; but the College of Dentists, it may be supposed, felt that such an act of hospitality as that just related would also stand somewhat in the light of an appreciating acknowledgment of the recognition which had been bestowed from time to time upon the promoters of "independence" by their Transatlantic brethren. If there could have been large numbers of American practitioners present on the occasion, it would have been still more pleasant to have welcomed them as guests; as it was, there could have been no other feeling than that of gratification in meeting those who had come around the hospitable board thus spread by the executive of the

Dental College. There appeared, quite up to the end of this year, the same determination on the part of the two opposing sections of the profession to relinquish nothing in their several attempts at supremacy. It is true, nevertheless, that the minds of many of the best men were truly weary of continued strife; and it was to them at least a great relief to hear, as it was asserted some did hear, a faint whisper of peace.

CHAPTER VIII.

THE prognostics in which the more hopeful members of the profession had ventured, at the close of 1862, to indulge concerning the blending of the two sections hitherto so diametrically opposed to each other, gave evidence of their correctness in the opening of the year 1863. Although not publicly known, preparations had already been commenced, with the object of bringing about the fusion. Mr. Rymer had felt that the successful institution of the licentiateship at the Royal College of Surgeons had destroyed all reasonable expectation of establishing permanently the movement which he had organised. He had arrived at this conclusion only after having tested to its full extent the probability of success attending his efforts, and those of his fellow-labourers in the college cause. He had striven heartily, and in the most unselfish and disinterested manner, to accomplish what he sincerely believed would best meet the requirements, and advance the interests of the dental profession. His hope was strong in the good results to be obtained through the National Dental Hospital and the Metropolitan School of Dental Science, both of which had been the outgrowth of the College of Dentists. By the abandonment of the latter institution, however, he saw that these two channels of benefit would not necessarily be closed. The expectation of obtaining a charter for the Dental College was evidently a vain one, in the face of the fact that the Royal College of Surgeons had been empowered to admit dentists to examination and association there. To continue the College of Dentists as a mere opposing institution he considered both unnecessary and unworthy, while to resign connection with it, and, as he justly calculated, with such a step to draw with him all high-minded and true-spirited men associated with it and himself, would only be to leave it open to unscrupulous persons, and thus really to inaugurate a new danger and difficulty. There remained, therefore, nothing for him to do but to consent to amalgamation with the Odontological Society, endeavouring to secure the co-operation of as many of his colleagues as possible, and with them to obtain honourable terms of capitulation. To this end propositions were made and submitted to the Odontological Society.

Mr. Rymer had consulted with Mr. Vasey, an influential member of the Odontological Society, and had ascertained through him that Mr. Tomes was willing to confer with him (Mr. Rymer) on the subject. It was considered necessary, that, as the former terms of amalgamation had been rejected by the College of Dentists, this body should make the new proposals. A council meeting at the college was then called, the subject discussed, and a resolution unanimously passed, wherein the desirability of union was expressed. This was forwarded to the council of the Odontological Society, who approved it, and appointed a sub-committee—Messrs. A. Rogers, S. Cartwright, and J. Tomes—to meet a similar sub-committee from the other side. The College of Dentists deputed Messrs. Imrie, Hulme, Weiss, and Rymer to represent it. These gentlemen met at the house of Mr. A. Rogers, December 22, 1862, and the result of this was the following proposal:—

" Resolved :

" 1. That the title 'The Odontological Society of London,' be abandoned, in favour of the title 'The Odontological Society of Great Britain,' for the purpose of embodying the members of the College of Dentists of England, under the latter title, with the members of the Odontological Society.

"2. That the byelaws of the Odontological Society relating to the election of members, namely, laws 5, 6, and 7, be suspended; and the members of the College of Dentists who are such according to the strict interpretation of the laws of that body, be embodied as members of the Odontological Society of Great Britain.

"3. That the interpretation of the laws of the College of Dentists respecting the use of professional advertisements shall be interpreted as excluding those members who use any other advertisements than a simple announcement of change of residence.

"4. That the members of the College of Dentists who are embodied in the Odontological Society of Great Britain during the suspension of the laws of the Odontological Society, viz., 5, 6, and 7, respecting the election of members, shall not be required to pay an entrance fee.

"5. That on the embodiment of the members of the College of Dentists with the members of the Odontological Society, under the title of the Odontological Society of Great Britain, three ordinary members of council, and one town and one country vice-president, be added to the present council of the Odontological Society from the council of the College of Dentists; but that at the expiration of three years from the date of such addition the members of the council shall revert to the number which at present constitutes the council of the Odontological Society.

"6. That after the embodiment of the members of the College of Dentists, the suspension of the laws respecting the admission of members shall cease; and that the laws by which the Odontological Society is now governed shall govern the Odontological Society of Great Britain, except as respects the temporary increase in the number of office-bearers.

"7. That the property of the College of Dentists and of the Odontological Society shall become the property of the Odontological Society of Great Britain.

"8. That the members of the joint-committee of the Odontological Society and the College of Dentists hereby subscribe their names to the spirit of the subjoined resolutions.

S. CARTWRIGHT, jun.
WILLIAM IMRIE.
JOHN TOMES.
FELIX WEISS.
ALFRED CANTON.
ROBERT THOMAS HULME.
ARNOLD ROGERS.
SAMUEL LEE RYMER."

The College of Dentists having, upon consideration, nominated four gentlemen instead of three, the Odontological Society added the name of Mr. Canton, to preserve equality of numbers.

Allusion to these resolutions was made in the report presented by the council of the College of Dentists at the annual general meeting of that body, held January 22, 1863, and in the course of the evening Mr. Rymer was called upon by the chairman, Mr. Perkins, who presided in the absence of the president, to introduce the subject to those present. Having done so in a few explanatory remarks, Mr. Rymer read the whole of the resolutions, forming, as they did, the report of the sub-committee appointed to negotiate the terms of union between the two bodies. Some discussion followed on the name proposed; but when the proposition for the terms arrived at to be accepted was put, the meeting unanimously adopted it. On March 2d, a special general meeting of the Odontological Society was held for the purpose of taking into consideration the foregoing terms of amalgamation—Mr. S. Cartwright, jun., the president, in the chair. Mr. Cartwright introduced the subject by detailing the steps which had been taken to secure the formation of the joint sub-committees appointed to consider the method by which the union of the rival bodies could be effected, and spoke in cordial terms of the enterprise, the adoption of which had already passed the council of the society. In an able speech Mr. Harrison moved the following resolution: "That this meeting fully approves of the amalgamation of the Odontological Society of London and the College of Dentists of England on the terms agreed to by the sub-committees of their respective councils, and cordially agrees to accept the union upon those terms on the formal dissolution of the latter body." Mr. James Parkinson, in a few remarks, expressed his entire confidence in the result that had been arrived at by the sub-committee, and warmly seconded Mr. Harrison's resolution. The sub-

ject being then open to discussion, several pertinent and important questions were asked by gentlemen present, and satisfactory replies given from the chair. The general tone of the meeting was distinctly that of approval, but one gentleman—Mr. Napier—rose and expressed his disapproval of the project. He was, however, fully answered by Mr. Cattlin, Mr. Bigg, and especially so by Mr. Harrison; and when the motion was put from the chair, Mr. Napier was left, as Mr. Tomes subsequently remarked, "in a glorious minority of *one*." After this decision there remained only one other resolution to be adopted to conclude the entire business of this most important meeting. In moving that resolution, which was to the following effect, viz.: "That it be left to the council of this society to carry out the arrangements for completing the union of the two bodies on the terms proposed, in such a way as may seem best," Mr. Tomes gave expression to these, among other remarks, which are of interest as evidences of his mind then, and may be useful to remember under the present circumstances of the profession as well:—
"When a body of men are willing to abandon their own special views in favour of a common cause, and have acted in the spirit in which the College of Dentists have acted on the present occasion, it is not for us to scrutinise the past too closely; but it is for us to receive them with liberality, placing implicit confidence in the future. If in adopting a liberal course we can embrace a number of men who have been in the habit of advertising, and thereby induce them to abandon this unprofessional practice, it will be to the general advantage of the profession. Before taking my seat I must protest against the general accusation of inferiority preferred against the members of our profession. There are many practitioners unknown to us who hold as high a position in town and country as those who frequent this room. We are too apt to class those we do not know with the inferior men with whom we happen to

be brought into contact—a tendency calculated to produce mischief, and one we shall do well to abandon." It need scarcely be added that such sentiments, and expressed by such an indefatigable worker in the elevation of the dental profession as Mr. Tomes has ever proved to be, were received with loud cheers. On the 20th of March, a special general meeting of the College of Dentists was convened, to take the necessary steps for securing the names of gentlemen as office-bearers, to represent the body in that capacity in connection with the Odontological Society, and for the formal dissolution of the College. Mr. William Imrie, president, was in the chair. The result of the ballot showed that Mr. William Perkins, Mr. William Imrie, and Mr. Somerset Tibbs had been elected vice-presidents, and Mr. R. T. Hulme, Mr. H. T. Kempton, and Mr. S. L. Rymer members of council. The votes for the dissolution of the college were—by members present, 38; by proxies, 47—total 85. Two votes against the dissolution were registered, with one neutral. Thus, then, after nearly seven years of existence and severe struggle, the College of Dentists of England ceased to be. Its efforts for what its promoters sincerely considered the general good had been unremitting. As an enterprise it had developed many excellent qualities in its advocates and supporters. Through its instrumentality agencies had been set in motion which could not fail to be beneficial to those who had been associated with it, and there can be no doubt that the final act was one of deep regret to many concerned. The idea of an independent institution had been fairly put before the profession by Mr. Rymer, accepted by a large number of the practitioners, both in London and the provinces, in public meeting assembled, and with large expenditure of time, money, energy, and perseverance it had been advocated. This attempt had received both internal and external support from the medical profession to a considerable extent; nor did it lack encouragement from the Transatlantic brethren. It failed, however, simply because it was surpassed. The Odontological Society's scheme outrivalled it, and when it thus expired, it was but the inevitable result of conflict with a superior force. The amalgamation of the two bodies took place at a meeting of the Odontological Society, held May 4th (1863), when the official list of members, presented by the council of the late College of Dentists, was formally read. One hundred and eleven ordinary members, and three honorary members, constituted the addition thus made to the Odontological Society of Great Britain. Mr. Arnold Rogers, with his usual courtesy, said many kind and encouraging words on the occasion, and Mr. Rymer, with modesty and good taste, replied on behalf of those with whom he had been so long and intimately acquainted. This event was a happy inauguration of an entirely new era. It was not only the formal cessation of hostilities between parties who never should have been in opposition, but also the blending of hitherto hostile forces in a common pact for the common good. The feeling of relief throughout the entire profession was manifest enough. There may have been, and doubtless were, lingering in the minds of some, doubts as to what would be the outcome of this amalgamation. No movement of any importance is ever made without its due proportion of doubts and fears. There are always to be found men ready to magnify evils and difficulties, but who are either without the power or will, or both, perhaps, to rectify or remove them. Purists, too, are not absent at such times, men who would have an all but Utopian condition of things, and from their own fancied exaltation talk words into an atmosphere too highly rarified for ordinary individuals to breathe. While such members of the profession as Mr. Arnold Rogers, Mr. Cartwright, and Mr. Tomes were evidently inspired with a well-founded hope in the matter, there was not much room for despair among others who were less informed.

Whatever faults the Odontological Society may have had to find with any of its members, it is but just to those who came into its ranks from the College of Dentists to say, that they have not thus unenviably distinguished themselves. The effort which Mr. Rymer had made to advance the interests of his fellow-practitioners, though thus ultimately ineffectual, had been both sincere and thoroughly disinterested. It was determined, therefore, by those with whom he had laboured, that some mark of their appreciation of his work should be offered him, and, with him, to Mr. Hockley also, who had been so indefatigable in the office of honorary secretary to the College of Dentists. A "Rymer and Hockley Testimonial Fund" was opened, Mr. R. Hulme acting as honorary secretary and treasurer. This fund was very cordially subscribed to; and on the evening of May 11th (1863), after the meeting of the Metropolitan School of Dental Science for the distribution of prizes, a large number of gentlemen, most of whom had been connected in the past with the late College of Dentists, adjourned to St. James' Hall for the purpose of presenting the above-named gentlemen with tangible proofs of their respect and esteem. Mr. Purland occupied the chair, and in an appropriate address recounted some of the circumstances which had characterised the efforts which had been made, and after eulogising the untiring energy which had been displayed by both Mr. Rymer and Mr. Hockley, presented the testimonials to them. The various objects, which had been chosen by the recipients themselves, bore the following inscriptions:—
"Presented to Samuel Lee Rymer, Esq., May 11, 1863, by members of the College of Dentists of England, as a token of respect, and in acknowledgment of his services to the dental profession. College of Dentists of England, founded by Samuel Lee Rymer, Esq., December 16, 1856, united to the Odontological Society of Great Britain, May 4, 1863." "Presented to Anthony Hockley, Esq., May 11, 1863, by members of the Col-

lege of Dentists of England, as a mark of respect, and in acknowledgment of his services as honorary secretary. College of Dentists of England, founded December 16, 1856, united to the Odontological Society of Great Britain, May 4, 1863."

These presents were, of course, appropriately acknowledged by the gentlemen in question, and such offerings proved the high estimation in which genuine disinterested effort was held by all concerned. In fact, the circumstance of the college scheme having failed was at such a moment lost sight of in the remembrance of the sustained perseverance which had been shown to make it succeed if possible. Whatever political opinion might be held by other members of the profession, it was pleasing to know that years of real labour had thus met with a practical recognition. The amalgamation of the two bodies having taken effect, it was determined that for the future the Metropolitan School of Dental Science should be carried on at the National Dental Hospital. Mr. H. T. Kempton continued to hold the office of secretary to the school, a position which he had assiduously filled from its formation. One of the strongest evidences of the complete fusion of the two societies was given by several gentlemen, formerly members of the College of Dentists, presenting themselves for examination with a view to taking the licentiateship degree at the Royal College of Surgeons. During the months of June and July in this year (1863) some twenty practitioners received the certificate. Such a step on their part was worthy of all commendation. They thus not only took a recognised position, but also afforded the assurance of real union with their former opponents. When the College of Surgeons accepted the proposal to grant certificates of proficiency to practise, one of the stipulations was that the certificate would be available to all who had been in practice up to the year 1859 without their passing through the prescribed curriculum. In September, therefore, of this year (1863) this term of grace would expire. The "British Journal of Dental Science" called attention to this important fact, and the "Dental Review" in a very sensible article echoed it. From this time onwards the rivalry of opposing factions ceased, because there existed no need for conflict. What remained to be accomplished, therefore, could be defined in one comprehensive word—"development." To effect this was certainly worthy of quite as much energy as had before been displayed in another direction. The activities of life in all its departments are, perhaps, less perceptible in times of peace than in those of war, but the result of well-directed action, such as was then necessary, was as honourable as any laurels hastily snatched in the heat of conflict. It was anticipated by some that the leaders in the past movements would suffer from the inevitable reaction which would ensue. The faith of others in the leading men of the profession was strong enough to allow them to look for continued effort in the direction of real progress. One mark of advance was perceptible in the establishment of a Dental Students' Society in connection with the Dental Hospital of London. This society owed its origin to Mr. W. Hele, then a student at the above institution. It was to be a sort of junior Odontological Society, where papers on the principles and practice of dental surgery could be read and discussed, under the presidency of one of the members of the medical staff. An opportunity would be thus given for the students to accumulate interesting facts as they occurred to them in their daily practice, and lay them before their *confrères* as occasion offered. Another, and a by no means unworthy result, would be open to them, namely, that of marshalling their ideas in their minds, and then giving expression to them in correct language. There are many influential men who, for want of early training in the art of public speaking, although intellectually furnished, are of little or no use to others, seeing they are not capable of expressing themselves in such a way as to place their stores of information at the service of those who would gladly and respectfully listen to them. It was a good omen to see the embryo dentists thus assembled, willing to have their opinions submitted to, and discussed, changed, or even exploded by, each other. This society has continued, with some exceptions, to exist to the present time. The anniversary dinner of the dental licentiates continued to be held, and, as a means of strengthening old ties and forming new ones, it was useful enough. That it should be used for another purpose was suggested in the "British Journal of Dental Science" for March 1864. In the number of those who had taken the licentiateship degree were to be found, here and there, those who could not refrain from advertising, and made the degree itself contribute to their design in this direction. This unpleasant fact was, although vexatious to real reformers, perhaps to be anticipated. In all departments of professional life individuals of this type are to be found, men who worship personal advance so ardently as to obliterate all other and nobler sentiments. To such the power of asserting their connection with a recognised and acknowledged body ever proves too strong a temptation to be resisted for long together. That all such delinquents should be made to understand that they had thus forfeited all claim to fellowship with those upon whose honourable position and practices they sought to draw was correct enough, and the "British Journal" proposed that they should be quietly excluded from any and all participation in the amenities and reciprocities of these annual gatherings. It does not appear, however, that, while they lasted, this suggestion was distinctly acted upon. Nothing is at all likely to correct and eradicate the obnoxious system of advertising but a higher and proper admission of what a profession demands by those whose proclivities at present lean so strongly towards public announcements. While the world outside condescends to patronise advertisers so much as it does, the unprofessional practitioner finds too readily a reason for displaying his "quasi" attainments to allow such a wide field to remain uncultivated. Restrictive laws are all but useless, owing to the difficulty of their effective operation, and there remain, therefore, but education and example on which the true practitioner may hope to rely. A further step in the prohibitory direction was the ballot-box at the Odontological Society, and this suggestive and practical little instrument has been freely exercised. A feeling began to manifest itself among the licentiates generally that their position should be more distinctly acknowledged as members of a branch of the medical profession. This they considered would, in some degree, be effected by their being permitted the use of the library and museum, and also being allowed to attend the various lectures delivered at the Royal College of Surgeons. At the anniversary dinner of the licentiates this subject was formally alluded to in an excellent speech delivered by Mr. Harrison. Mr. William Lawrence, F.R.S., was chairman on the occasion, and some of the remarks of such a high authority are worthy of record, and might be remembered with great advantage now. Having sketched the rise and progress of the dental reform movement, and eulogising the efforts which had been made, Mr. Lawrence proceeded to say, "Among those who sit at this table are many members of the college, and some among them have attained the higher grade of fellowship. This is all plain and easy, without reference to the course of education and examination proposed for the future. It is open to any one who is not inclined to submit to that rigid examination to come as the former members of the dental body have done, and to become members like other surgeons. The difference between those gentlemen who mean in future to practise as dentists with the licence of the college and members possessing the diploma, is not that the dental surgeons will be less informed than the members, but, if that curriculum is to be thoroughly carried out, they will be better informed. That curriculum lays down a surgical and anatomical examination nearly equal to that of members of the college, and in addition it prescribes a long course of special education which does not belong to the practice of surgery. Well, if they undergo that examination, why are they not to be members of the College of Surgeons in the same way as those of their brethren who have undergone the usual examination for the membership? That is a question I cannot answer. I don't see any reason why they should not, but I speak for myself. My opinion is, that they will be absolutely better informed. I think the course taken by the body of dentists in endeavouring to improve their education, and thus to render their body more worthy of the public confidence, and more capable of giving efficient assistance to those who seek their aid, does them the highest credit. I have watched with great interest the whole course of these proceedings, from the first application to the college to the present time. I have always sympathised with the efforts those gentlemen were making, and I have had great pleasure in seeing their success, so far as it has gone up to the present time." In his concluding speech Mr. Lawrence further said, "I think a person who is decently acquainted with reading, writing, and arithmetic, if he gets thoroughly acquainted with his own profession, will become a very useful member of society, though he does not know Latin or Greek, nor the elements of mathematics. Some of the most distinguished members of all the branches of our profession are totally ignorant of these, but yet they are good men, and capital practitioners." Whether the desire of the licentiates in dental surgery to have their names placed on the register was reasonable or absurd need not be entered into. It was not, from the easily-excited jealousy of the full members of the College of Surgeons, in any way likely of being accomplished. The "Medical Times and Gazette" took the subject up, and mildly censured Mr. Lawrence for what he had advanced, especially the concluding remarks of that gentleman, above quoted. Although the most eminent surgeons admitted that the curriculum for securing the licentiateship was full and sufficient for the holder of it to consider himself incorporated into the medical body, the above journal, echoing the sentiments of many medical practitioners, pronounced the stern verdict, "Outside still." Mr. Harrison addressed a letter in reply to the editor of the "Medical Times and Gazette's" remarks, but this was not published in that journal. It was very evident that Mr. Lawrence's observations were taken hold of as a pretext for opposition to any hope the licentiates in dental surgery were indulging of finding a place for their names on the register. The editor could not for a moment reasonably conclude that Mr. Lawrence advocated scanty education in any member of the medical body. The fiat was that unless those whose determination it was to practise as dental surgeons, and dental surgeons only, would submit to an expenditure of time, money, and energy in the acquisition of knowledge of subjects utterly useless to them, they must not presume to hope for a position which would entitle them to protection. There can be no difficulty in concluding from what feeling such sentiments sprung. The idea that licentiates once registered would be likely to practise general surgery under the shadow of such a privilege was akin to that which a little time before found expression in the notion that if admitted to a connection with the College of Surgeons, by examinations for the licentiateship degree, the holders of it would assume themselves to be equal with general practitioners. Such fears were alike fallacious and absurd. It needed not Mr. Harrison's letter to prove that dentists had in their own clearly defined practice more than enough to fully absorb all their time and attention.

While there have been and still are instances, enough and to spare, of surgeons dabbling in dentistry, it would be difficult to produce a single case of a fully-qualified dentist acting the part of a medical man. There was, perhaps, at this time too much desire on the part of the dental practitioners to push their position, while on the other side, viz., that of the medical profession, there was not lacking a strong feeling of mistrust as to what, and how far, such action might lead. Such a condition of things was by no means unnatural, and it needed a considerable amount of tuition to convince the more zealous dentists of the undesirability of precipitating matters too hastily. Time would have to elapse before the important advantages which had been gained by the dental body would be heard of and appreciated by the general public, or cordially acknowledged by the medical profession at large. In one direction it was legitimate to look for recognition—that was in the appointment of dental officers to the general hospitals, as vacancies occurred. To this the editor of the "British Journal of Dental Science" properly called attention. Towards the close of this year the subject of extending the term of grace by the Royal College of Surgeons in connection with the licentiateship degree was mooted. The idea of opening the college doors again to those members of the dental profession who, when the original time had elapsed, were still without the degree, was pretty general. It was certain that there yet remained many practitioners who, from their acknowledged position and acquirements, ought to have had their names enrolled on the list of licentiates, but had not done so. There were reasons strong enough in the minds of such for their abstention hitherto, and those reasons were adduced and discussed. It was, nevertheless, evident that the number of properly-certified men should be increased as much as possible. The advocacy of their cause was commenced in the "British Journal of Dental Science," and espoused particularly by Mr. Vasey, who has on all occasions shown a warm and liberal feeling towards all honourable dental practitioners. In a letter to the Journal Mr. Vasey said, "My own opinion is, that any respectable member of the profession who was of age and in practice at the time the charter was obtained, should have the privilege of offering himself for examination at any time without going through the curriculum. Examples in favour of this could be easily given. I cannot but think that the council of the college, if memorialised, would grant the privilege. If those gentlemen interested in gaining such privilege for the profession will forward their names and addresses, I shall willingly undertake to have a memorial properly presented, provided the signatures obtained are sufficiently numerous to warrant our soliciting the attention of the council." There were opponents to this scheme, of course. With much reason it was said, that those who had shown so much langour and indifference to the progress of the profession as to neglect the opportunity when offered to them, ought not thus easily to reap the advantages which others had won after so much patient sowing and unwearied exertion. There were certainly two aspects of the question, and the result of its promulgation will be seen further on.

During this year the death of Mr. Samuel Cartwright, F.R.S., occurred, and although for some time entirely retired from practice, the news of his decease was received with pain by the profession at large. He had been one of its brightest ornaments, and in himself had exemplified to what a pinnacle of prosperity large gifts and high qualities, when properly and steadily employed, could raise the possessor.

Early in the year 1865 an important step was taken in the direction of presenting a memorial from the licentiates in dental surgery to the council of Medical Education and Registration, with a view to obtaining the privilege of enrolment on the register. This instrument contained so full and explicit a statement of the facts concerning the position and claims of the licentiates that it is here given in full. It was signed first by the three (then) examiners on the dental board—Mr. Thomas Bell, Mr. J. Tomes, and Mr. Cartwright, which signatures were followed by twenty-five other licentiates, who were also members or otherwise connected with the College of Surgeons.

" *To the General Council of Medical Education and Registration of the United Kingdom.*

"We, the undersigned Licentiates of Dental Surgery of the Royal College of Surgeons of England (a degree founded by the college on section 48 of the present Medical Act), although entitled to register under that Act in virtue of our other professional qualifications, considering it to be desirable, and believing it to be only just, that those persons who have taken this degree should be allowed the privilege of registering as 'Licentiates in Dental Surgery,' under the proposed amended Medical Act, beg respectfully to bring this our view of the subject under the consideration of your honourable board. We are aware that the following objections have been raised to this privilege being allowed to the possessors of this degree—First, that if the privilege were granted to persons who have taken this degree only, they would, under the 34th clause of the present Medical Act, be considered in law as 'duly qualified practitioners,' and might, if so disposed, practise legally any or all branches of the medical profession without having received a full medical education, and thereby interfere with the interests of the fully-qualified medical man. Second, that to grant this privilege to them would be to infringe upon and injure the existing rights of those persons at present practising dental surgery who do not possess this degree, by giving the new Act a retrospective character. And third, that it is open to those persons practising dental surgery, who desire to possess the privilege of registering under any Medical Act, to take the degree of 'Member' of the College of Surgeons, as well as that of 'Licentiate in Dental Surgery,' and to register under the former title.

"To the first of these objections we respectfully submit, that the very slight additions we have suggested to the wording of the 31st and 34th clauses of the present Medical Act would, if adopted, make it clear, beyond the possibility of a doubt, that the possessors of this degree only, if registered as 'Licentiates in Dental Surgery,' *could not* legally practise any other branch of medicine or surgery; and, therefore, that the incorporation of these, or similar words, into any amended Medical Act, would fully meet and do away with this objection. To the second objection we also respectfully submit, that the few words proposed to be added to clause 55 of the present Medical Act *completely protect* all the existing rights of those persons at present practising dental surgery who do not possess this degree, as also the prospective rights of those at present preparing to practise dental surgery who have it in their power to take this degree, and so meet and do away with this objection. And to the third objection we respectfully submit—First, that the argument on which it rests is founded upon an imperfect knowledge of the amount of 'special study' required to form the duly-qualified dental surgeon, as we think will be apparent to your honourable board by a reference to the accompanying curriculum of education required by the College of Surgeons for the degree of Licentiate in Dental Surgery. Next, that to expect the full course of education required for the 'Membership' of the college to be added by the dental surgeon to the curriculum required for his special diploma, in order to give him the power of registering under such Act, would be to exact a more extended and more expensive professional education, both in respect to time and money, from the dental than from the general surgeon—a requirement which we respectfully submit would be both unnecessary and unjust. And, lastly, that to be registered as a 'Fellow' or 'Member' of the college only, does not, *in itself*, afford any proof that persons so registered are duly qualified to practise the specialty of dental surgery, as we think will also be apparent to your honourable board after referring to the curriculum above named. Entertaining these views, we think it right to bring them under the attention of your honourable board, and we pray that you will take them into your favourable consideration."

At a meeting of the board, held at the Royal College of Physicians April 7th, this memorial was introduced by Dr. Storrar in a temperate speech, which he concluded by submitting the following motion, namely—"That the memorial of the Licentiates in Dental Surgery of the Royal College of Surgeons be referred to the committee on the amendment of the Medical Acts." The motion was duly seconded by Mr. Hargrave, then discussed, and finally carried. At a subsequent meeting of the board, held April 13th, Dr. Andrew Wood objected to the petition of the memorialists, principally on the ground that all persons on the register should be fully qualified, and that the introduction of specialists would create confusion in the public mind, and be a serious blot on the Medical Act. He advised that the Licentiates in Dental Surgery should apply for an Act of Parliament for themselves, and keep a separate register. It was evident, from the consideration of the subject by the amendment committee and the board itself, that the prayer of the memorialists could not be assented to. This, indeed, was the result. A correspondence ensued in the columns of the "Lancet," the editor of which journal, however, was favourable to a dental register being added to the medical register, though distinct from it. A hastily summoned meeting of dental licentiates was convened on the 24th of April, and presided over by Mr. Harrison, when the position of affairs was discussed, the resolution of which was, that it was undesirable to press the matter further at present, the meeting agreeing to content themselves with endeavouring to obtain the introduction of a clause into the new Medical Bill exempting licentiates in dental surgery from serving on juries, &c. A standing committee was then chosen, consisting of Messrs. Harrison, Cartwright, Tomes, Underwood, Rymer, and T. Rogers, whose duty it would be to take such action as was deemed advisable by them for obtaining the above-stated privileges. It must be acknowledged that there were reasonable difficulties in the way of licentiates registering, however much the possessors of that degree felt the justice of their claims. As professional men they could not but experience annoyance at their liability at any time to be called from their practices, perhaps in the height of the season, to attend for days in succession at the courts of law. The friends of education and advance were destined to meet with checks and obstacles more or less irritating. One of these was manifested in the fact that no place was found for a list of the gentlemen who had taken the new degree in the "Medical Directory." From whatever circumstance this arose, it produced in the minds of many the feeling that, wherever and whenever possible, they would be made to realise their inferiority to full members of the College of Surgeons. The mistake, however, was not allowed to remain long unrectified. The author undertook to compile and publish a "Dental Licentiates' Directory and Local List." This was speedily done, and certainly answered the end in view, as, since then, an alphabetical list of their names has regularly appeared in the "Medical Directory." To revert to the proposal made by the editor of the "British Journal of Dental Science," in connection with Mr. Vasey, that the

College of Surgeons' portals should be again opened, under circumstances already detailed, it was somewhat dispiriting to find that those for whose especial benefit the idea had been ventilated responded but very languidly to it. Like other matters, it appeared to require time.

The consolidation of the profession and its general advance were evident facts, however. The Odontological Society continued its useful scientific career and increased its list of members steadily. The number of practitioners holding the licentiate's degree was nearly three hundred, while the Metropolitan Dental Hospitals, as well as the dispensaries and similar institutions in the provinces, were producing good fruits as the reward of those disinterestedly connected and working in and with them. The following year, 1866, was one of comparative quietude. The introduction by Dr. Richardson of his new method of producing local anæsthesia by means of the ether spray created much interest in the profession. The proposed alteration of the Odontological Society's bye-laws caused some amount of disturbance among its members; and Mr. Waite's proposal to form provincial branches of the above Society met with an apparently general approval. The characteristics of the year 1867 were not either stirring or numerous. Its principal features were the animated discussion that arose from the resolution of the Odontological Society to adopt the title of "Fellow;" the inauguration of the Odonto-Chirurgical Society of Edinburgh, of which an account is given in another part of this work; the very pleasant circumstance of the presentation of a testimonial to Mr. Arnold Rogers; and finally, the creation of a "defence fund" on behalf of Mr. Statham, a dental practitioner who had to answer in a court of law to a gross charge of having forcibly extracted several teeth from a patient's mouth against that individual's consent while under the influence of chloroform. The action against Mr. Statham ignobly failed; and in order to indemnify him in the matter of costs (some

£700), his professional brethren, together with many and influential medical men, subscribed to this fund. The circumstance is worthy of notice, not only on the ground of the evidence it manifested of the principle of combination—once, and not long ago, a thing altogether impossible among dentists—but also as the proof of the amicable spirit of the medical profession towards dental practitioners.

The importance of such an institution as the Dental Hospital of London was proved by the fact that, on the occasion of the annual general meeting of the governors of the Charity in January of the year 1868, the medical committee's report stated that no less a number than 17,300 operations had been performed during the past year. The increase in the number of students attending was marked, and in such progress that the friends of reform and education found ample material for encouragement. The National Dental Hospital, too, was doing its part both as a Metropolitan Charity and a school for the instruction of dentists. Nitrous oxide as an anæsthetic was introduced to the notice of the profession in the early part of this year. Its resuscitation—Sir Humphrey Davy having more than half a century previously proclaimed its merits as an agent for obtunding sensibility—was due to Mr. Horace Wells, of America, that gentleman having proved its specific action in 1844. Dr. Colton, in 1863, brought it prominently before his professional brethren; it was subsequently taken up by Dr. Evans, of Paris, who added some improvements to the apparatus necessary to its exhibition, and then came to England, generously giving a handsome sum to be applied in further investigating its merits under the supervision of the anæsthetists to the Dental Hospital of London, Messrs. Potter and Clover. A committee of investigation was appointed by the Odontological Society, and thus a full and fair opportunity was given for ascertaining to what extent it could be admitted to the *répertoire* of the dentist in this country.

The year 1869 was a quiet season in the profession. The important investigation of the merits of protoxide of nitrogen as an anæsthetic was proceeding under the auspices of a select committee, appointed for that purpose, in connection with the Dental Hospital of London and the Odontological Society.

In due time the preliminary report was given, and printed in the "Transactions" of the Odontological Society, as follows:—

"Your committee, in proceeding to carry out the inquiry intrusted to them, were of opinion that the subject presented itself for consideration under the following heads:—

" 1. To ascertain how far this agent was an efficient anæsthetic.

" 2. If so, whether it was as safe, or a safer anæsthetic than those in general use.

" 3. What were its special advantages and disadvantages as compared with other anæsthetics.

" 4. To ascertain, if possible, how far it produced its anæsthetic effect, with a view to devise the best probable remedy, or remedies, for any alarming or dangerous symptoms that might arise during its exhibition.

" 5. To ascertain the best, most convenient, and cheapest method of procuring the gas in a pure state.

" 6. The safest and most convenient method of administering the gas.

" 7. Whether there were any special conditions of the system, any given age, &c., which would contra-indicate its use; and,

"Lastly, To collect and tabulate as many cases and facts as possible, so as to arrive at as full conclusions on these various points as could be arrived at within the time allotted to themselves, before making their first report.

" Pursuing this plan as fully as circumstances permitted, your committee first instituted a number of experiments on the lower animals (including dogs, cats, rabbits, guinea-pigs, mice, and birds), from which they at once ascertained—

" 1. That the pure gas, so administered as to preclude the inhaling of any atmospheric air with it, *was* a powerful anæsthetic, more rapid in its action, although more evanescent in its effects, than chloroform and the other anæsthetics then in general use;

" 2. That if its administration were pushed beyond a certain point, it was capable of producing death; but,

" 3. That even when death appeared most imminent from its use, allowing the animal to breathe fresh air, in most cases, brought it rapidly round.

" With this information, obtained from their experiments on the lower animals, your committee proceeded to avail themselves, cautiously, of the opportunities afforded them at the Dental Hospital of London and other hospitals, and of such opportunities as they respectively had in private practice, to carry on their observations of the effects of the gas, when exhibited to the human being, *pari passu* with further experiments and observations on the lower animals; and although they are not yet prepared to offer to the members of the Odontological Society, and the committee of management of the Dental Hospital of London, definite opinions as to the effect of this agent, under *all* the heads of investigation which they have just enumerated, they beg now to offer to both those bodies, in this as a preliminary report, certain facts connected with the exhibition of this agent (the result of their observations *thus far*), which they think will prove interesting and advantageous to the profession in a practical point of view, as forming some guide for its safe exhibition, and for determining the class of cases for which they think it peculiarly suited. Your committee have arrived at the conclusion from their various observations of the effects of this gas when exhibited to the human being, and especially from their experiments with it upon the lower animals, that, properly administered, it is at least as safe, and for short operations as efficient, an anæsthetic as any other now in use; but that, while it possesses certain advantages over these other anæsthetics for such operations, it labours also under certain disadvantages, when compared with them, for the longer operations in surgery; and also under some other special disadvantages which they subjoin. The following are what they consider to be its comparative advantages and disadvantages:—

"ADVANTAGES.

"1. The rapidity of its action in producing anæsthesia; the average time required for this being (see Table I. of this report) from 63 to 81 seconds, according to the age and sex of the patient.

"2. The rapidity with which patients recover from its effects as an anæsthetic; the time required for this being, according to the same table, from 100 to 120 seconds.*

"3. It is more agreeable to most patients, being when pure quite tasteless.

"4. It is less irritating to the air passages; coughing or struggling for free respiration being rarely witnessed after its use, except in cases of very nervous persons.

"5. The comparative freedom from nausea and vomiting after its use; the average number of cases where actual vomiting has occurred being under one per cent.

"6. The absence, as a general rule (after the recovery of complete consciousness), of giddiness, headache, and many other unpleasant effects, which are well known to follow the use of chloroform, and other anæsthetics.

* Patients generally recover *so completely*, as well as quickly, as to be able to walk, speak correctly, and write with a steady hand within four minutes from the commencement of the inhalation.

"DISADVANTAGES.

"1. Its unsuitableness for long operations, owing to the shortness of its anæsthetic effects.

"2. Its unsuitableness (or, at any rate, ineligibility) for operations followed by much smarting and pain, for the same reason.

"3. Where very delicate operations have to be performed, the inconvenience to the operator from the muscular twitchings which often occur from its use.

"4. It is more troublesome to administer, and requires more complicated and cumbrous apparatus for that purpose than other anæsthetics do.

"5. It is more inconvenient and troublesome to transport than the other anæsthetics in use.

"6. It is more expensive, and more difficult to procure in a pure and efficient state for use at all times, if wanted on an emergency.*

"The grounds on which your committee have arrived at these conclusions, so far as regards the effects of this agent, are founded on the tabulated results of 1380 cases in which its administration has been carefully watched and noted down by the different members, both in public and private practice; and on the tabulated results, also, of 1051 cases reported to them by practitioners of reliable authority who have used it in London and the provinces; and they offer these opinions, therefore, with considerable confidence so far as conclusions can be arrived at from this comparatively limited number of cases. With regard to the manner in which this gas produces its anæsthetic effect, this is a physiological problem on which your committee do not feel themselves yet in a position to give any positive opinion. But the result of their experiments on the lower animals would lead them to recommend the

---

* The committee are of opinion that these latter objections will probably be met and overcome after a short time, should this agent come largely into use.

following course to be adopted in case any alarming symptoms should arise during its administration :—

"TREATMENT UNDER ALARMING SYMPTOMS.

"1st. The immediate withdrawal of the gas, and the access of fresh air.

"2d. If this is not at once followed by respiratory movements, resort to artificial respiration in the usual way.

"With respect to the best method of procuring a perfectly pure gas, your committee, having had the valuable assistance of Messrs. John Bell & Co. in aiding them to arrive at a conclusion on this point, would recommend the following."

(Here the committee give full and detailed instructions for the manufacture of the gas, and the reader is referred to the Odontological Society's transactions, *in loco*, for the same, as also for the mode of administration, which likewise engaged their attention, and is alluded to in the concluding part of their next observations.)

"With regard to the best apparatus for administering the gas, your committee feel that there will be, as there now is, a difference of opinion on this point; but after having seen several tried, would recommend that introduced by Mr. Clover, which is a slight modification of his well-known apparatus for administering chloroform. Whatever may be the apparatus used, however, they beg to impress upon the administrator that it is absolutely necessary, for the production of the perfect anæsthetic effect of the gas, that it should be so constructed as entirely to prevent the inhalation of any atmospheric air during its administration. With respect to the best and safest mode of exhibiting this gas—the apparatus being chosen—your committee would recommend the following plan (some parts of the directions in which, it will be observed, apply particularly to Mr.

Clover's apparatus); and they would especially draw the attention of the profession to the symptoms to be expected during its administration—to be watched—and, when alarming, to be guarded against—which are therein enumerated."

(Here follow the committee's instructions on this head.)

"As regards the question, 'Whether there are any special conditions of the system, any given age, temperament, constitutional derangement, &c., which contra-indicate the use of this gas,' your committee have to state that, so far as their present experience goes, they have met with nothing to absolutely contra-indicate its use—having administered it to both sexes, at all ages, from one to sixty-six years, to patients of all temperaments, to women in different stages of pregnancy and suckling, to persons acknowledged to be the subjects of asthma, epilepsy, &c., and to persons labouring under many other constitutional derangements, without any ill effects following; but they would, nevertheless, recommend great caution in its administration to persons suffering, or presumed to be suffering, from organic diseases of the brain, heart, arteries, lungs, &c., and to persons of very plethoric habit and short neck, such as would be considered especially likely to be injured by venous congestion about the head, even where no organic disease was supposed to exist. They throw out this precautionary advice, not because they have as yet seen any untoward symptoms arise in such cases (although they have exhibited the gas in several such), but because they are of opinion that it would be in such cases, if in any, that untoward symptoms would be likely to arise from its exhibition. Lastly, with reference to the various heads under which your committee have considered this subject, they would direct the attention of the society to the following tabulated results of their combined observations, as being interesting in themselves, and of some practical importance in guiding the profession in the administration of this gas.

Table I.

Average Time required to produce Anæsthesia.	Average Duration of Anæsthesia.	Average Time from commencement of administration to recovery.
Males . . 81 Seconds.	24 Seconds.	115 Seconds.
Females . . 76 ,,	28 ,,	120 ,,
Children of 15 years and under . 63 ,,	22 ,,	100 ,,

"From this table it will be seen that children are the most readily affected by the gas, that they remain for the shortest time under its influence, and that they recover the most quickly from its effects; whilst females, although more quickly influenced than men, remain longer in a state of anæsthesia, and take more time to recover from the effects of the gas. The time required for producing anæsthesia, its duration, and the time required for recovery, in each class of cases, on an average, will also at once be seen from it.

Table II.

Ages of the Patients to whom the gas was administered.	Males.	Females.
Under 10 years of age	4	10
Between 10 and 20	124	169
,, 20 ,, 30	144	225
,, 30 ,, 40	47	48
,, 40 ,, 50	17	17
,, 50 ,, 60	4	2
,, 60 ,, 70	2	1

    Males 342
    Females 472

    Total 814

Being the number, sexes, and ages, of the cases from which Table I. is formed.

"In drawing up this report, your committee have purposely avoided, thus far, making special reference to the very large number of cases stated to have been treated under the action of this gas in America (now said to amount to upwards of 200,000), with the occurrence of but one death, and that in a patient who was suffering from extensive disease of both lungs; and they have also purposely avoided referring to a large number of cases which have been treated under its action on the continent of Europe. This was because they had no *special data* connected with these cases on which they could form particular calculations, or from which they could draw special inference or inferences; unless it were one—but that an important one—viz., that this gas must, with this large mass of evidence in its favour, be regarded as a very safe anæsthetic.

"They cannot, however, close their report without drawing the attention of the profession to the very favourable statements regarding its efficiency and safety as an anæsthetic which have been received from both these sources. Your committee think it right, also, to record here their great and special obligations to Dr. G. Q. Colton, of New York (to whom is due the merit of having reintroduced this gas into use in America, and who must undoubtedly be considered to have had the largest experience of its use of any man living), for much valuable information communicated to them by him during two visits he paid to London last summer, when on both occasions he administered this gas frequently at the Dental Hospital of London, and freely and willingly communicated to your committee and the medical officers of that institution the results of his large experience of its use. In conclusion, your committee beg to state that they have added, as an appendix to this report, the result of their observations in certain peculiar cases in which this agent has been administered, and also of peculiar effects produced by it in other cases (put together without any special arrangement), considering that these details would prove both interesting and instructive to the profession at large; and they venture to express their hope that, in bringing the results of their experiments and observations on this subject, thus far, before the members of the Odontological Society and the committee of management of the Dental Hospital of London in the manner they have now done, they will be considered to have laid before both these bodies some valuable as well as interesting information, which will meet the requirements of the profession pending the prosecution of further experiments and observations which they purpose making on this subject, and hope to lay before them at some future time.

(Signed) " W. A. HARRISON, *Chairman.*"

Considering the important position which protoxide of nitrogen has subsequently taken in connection with the operative department of dental surgery, too much stress cannot well be laid upon the benefits which this committee conferred upon the entire profession by their careful investigation of the whole subject. It was especially to be commended that the Odontological Society, acting in concert with the Dental Hospital of London through the managing committee of that institution, determined to accept this new agent only after careful and comprehensive investigation by gentlemen on whom the most complete reliance could be placed, as members of the dental profession in this country. To have data of their own on which they could form an independent judgment was clearly a step in the right direction. The very flattering accounts which had been received from America and elsewhere they were happy to accept; but it was deemed far more expedient to make full trial of the gas under a select committee of their own members, ere they endorsed unreservedly all the statements which had been made by others in its favour. The result, so far as the committee had then gone, was of the most assuring character, and certainly prepared the profession generally for its free adoption. It was, in fact, a distinct step in advance, and contributed plainly to professional progress. The thanks of all are due to those gentlemen who, under Mr. Harrison's leadership, devoted so much time and attention to the subject placed before them. The knowledge thus obtained concerning the gas produced the disposition on the part of many to further investigate it, and improve if possible the apparatus for its exhibition. The apathy of the undiplomaed practitioners in the matter of petitioning to have the Royal College of Surgeons opened to them was very significant. Mr. Fox, as the editor of the " British Journal of Dental Science," alluded to it again and again, but nothing seemed to stir these gentlemen to action. Mr. Fox, in the journal for May 1870, addressed a leading article directly to the interested parties, offering a donation towards a general expense fund on proper and fully-stated conditions, concluding with the following proposition:—" Let us, then, have sent to us first of all the names of a sufficient number of gentlemen who will at the same time promise, as our correspondents have done, to subscribe a certain sum each. From among these a *small* committee should be appointed. To this end we would suggest the following plan : as soon as not less than fifty gentlemen have sent us their names as willing to co-operate in this movement, we will publish the list, and we will then ask each of these gentlemen to send us privately the names of seven gentlemen whom they would vote for to act as a committee, with power to add to their numbers. On receipt of these votes we will—if our friends see fit to allow us to take upon ourselves these preliminary steps —make it our business to obtain the permission of the seven gentlemen who have most votes to publish their names as ' *The Committee.*' Failing the consent of any of them, we should substitute the names of those who stood next in point of number of votes. The duties of this committee will be clear and simple: they must first appoint some gentleman as treasurer, well known in the profession; then draw up a memorial to the Royal College of Surgeons of England; compile a carefully-revised list of every dentist in the United Kingdom—and to this end we can offer them material assistance, having been for some time preparing such a list; forward a copy of the memorial, with a circular requesting his signature to it, to every respectable practitioner, and take measures for its proper presentation and support." This plan was feasible enough, and was one of the many evidences of the desire Mr. Fox has often displayed to help, in his measure, his brother practitioners. This called forth some correspondence in the journal, and secured some contributors. The idea of "registration" appeared to be the paramount measure in the minds of some; but the expectation of its accomplishment could not be seriously entertained while the number of licentiates was no greater than it was at that time; and the difficulty of names being obtained, whereby it might be hoped to be augmented, was painfully *en evidence*—to say nothing of the opposition it was so likely to receive at the hands of the medical profession. The only grain of hope which could be imparted was given in a letter from Mr. Harrison, who, as chairman of the Committee of observation, as it might be called, stated that the committee had placed itself in communication with the promoter of the Amended Medical Act Bill, Lord de Grey and Ripon, and that from the reception his Lordship had given to the views set forth in the committee's plans, there was every prospect of the interests of the dental profession being secured in the proposed alterations under the new Act. In the direction of investigation, especially with regard to nitrous oxide gas, the profession was not idle. A carefully-prepared statement of the process and results of its use in a certain number of cases of extraction was issued by Mr. M. Harding, then dental house-surgeon to the Dental Hospital of London. It was a matter of surprise to many at this time that Dr. Richardson should inveigh against this new agent in all but unmeasured terms. This, however, was the case. In an article which that gentleman wrote for the "Popular Science Review," he stated that "although it produces insensibility, it causes at the same time darkening of the arterial blood, painful, rapid breathing, a countenance terrible to behold, and imminent approach to death."[*] In the meantime this eminent investigator had discovered "methylic ether," a paper on which he read in the month of March before the Medical Society of London. It was evident that, if not absorbed in politics, the dental profession would have no cause to be idle in matters which touched its interests in the closest manner. In order that the nitrous oxide gas should be fully tested, Mr. Fox suggested in his journal the formation of a special fund to meet the expenses consequent upon its frequent use. This was in a measure responded to, several gentlemen contributing to the fund. Although Mr. Fox had been unremitting in his exertions to press forward "the dental diploma question," and had published a pamphlet on the subject, it was not until the month of September in this year that he was able to print the list of the supporters of this movement, together with their subscriptions, these latter amounting to the sum of £85, odd. In the meantime, however, the "Lancet" had advocated the cause, and this afforded no small encouragement. In the following month the announcement was made that a committee had been chosen, consisting of Mr. James Parkinson as treasurer, Mr. Oakley Coles, honorary secretary, with Mr. E. Sercombe as chairman, acting in concert with Messrs. S. L. Rymer, Joseph Steele, J. Dennant, J. Haslam, W. J. Newman, and J. Scully. The object of this committee was, as stated in the "British Journal of Dental Science," "to place the pro-

[*] British Journal of Dental Science, vol. xiii. p. 239.

fession in the same relation to the Royal College of Surgeons that it held in the year 1863, with regard to those whose professional education commenced prior to September 1859." Added to this, however, was the compilation of a Dental Directory, to effect which the committee had asked the services of Messrs. Gregson, Kempton, and Fox. Ten years had now elapsed since the first granting of the Dental Licentiate's degree, and it was satisfactory to find that at the close of 1870 three hundred practitioners had passed the ordeal of examination at Lincoln's Inn Fields. The profession itself was in steady progress, unmarred by bickerings and strife. The various institutions in the metropolis and the provinces alike seemed to have settled down to real, persistent work. The Odontological Society was growing in numbers and usefulness, its "Transactions" being first carefully compiled, then excellently printed and published for the information of those who were interested in the scientific aspect of their profession. Mr. Joseph Fletcher bestowed much time in the preparation of these "Transactions" for the press, and the result of his labours was seen in yearly volumes whose appearance, as well as contents, did credit to him and the society with which he was connected.

Bichloride of methylene was to receive attention as an anæsthetic, its merits being tested by the side of methylic ether and nitrous oxide. The subject formed material for writers such as Messrs. J. A. Salter, Spence Bate, A. Coleman, H. L. Jacob; while Messrs. Clover and Braine—authorities of eminence in anæsthetics generally—did not withhold their testimony. These two gentlemen advocated the use of gas, as preferable to other similar agents, in the operation of tooth extraction. Mr. Clover indeed said, as the result of his experience up to that time, that he considered in 98 per cent. of cases of tooth extraction nitrous oxide was the most suitable. This was after having administered the gas to no less than 3014 cases. Mr. Braine's experience led him to differ from Dr. Richardson, Mr. Salter, Mr. Rendle, Mr. Spence Bate, and others. His testimony was in favour of the gas, and both at the Odontological Society, and through the medium of the medical press, he very plainly stated his preference, and gave forcible reasons for it. During the year 1871 the controversy in the matter of anæsthetics was the most noticeable feature of the day. It was pleasant to observe that men were not satisfied with the dictum of some one else, but resorted to experiments and tests themselves. While there were leading men to whom the uninitiated would of course look, and to whose opinion they would unhesitatingly bow, nevertheless many determined to learn by the safer, if sometimes mortifying method of failure, which agent they personally could employ with the greatest amount of benefit to their patients. Verily art and science flourish in times of peace, and when such a year as this is compared with a period of convulsion and war, such as the profession had known not very long before, the satisfaction in contemplating the happily-changed circumstances was extreme. When men lay aside the sword for the pen, and squabbling egotism for general edification, the benefit is simply incalculable. To take up the records of this year and quietly to peruse them, yields ample encouragement to every wellwisher of the dental profession. The laboratory appeared to be in active operation, from what was stated orally, or by means of the journal; the surgery was the centre for continued and vigilant observation of dental affections, their cause and cure. Chemistry was being unfolded and developed by keen eyes and careful hands, and made to minister to the necessities of humanity, when most urgent; while instruction at the hospitals and schools was being imparted and received, and the general advance in education and professional acquirements secured through the various agencies, which, in themselves, furnished the best and most available assurance of improvement. The process by which it was hoped that the list of licentiates should be augmented was at work, the committee appointed for the purpose meeting and diligently transacting the necessary business, hoping to be able to compile a perfect list of every class of dental practitioners, so that the true condition of the profession might be ascertained. That the interest attaching to this object, which had for its ulterior result the opening of the college doors again, had been aroused was certain, and the proof of that lay in the fact that £106 were then in the hands of Mr. Parkinson, the treasurer. The Dental Hospital of London had been working in so thoroughly efficient a manner that its exchequer suffered, and to an extent that made it necessary to take means for its replenishment. To this end a public dinner was organised, and eventuated in some £500 being subscribed, and this was done amongst the freest acknowledgments of the usefulness of the institution both as a charity and school of instruction. In mechanical dentistry the profession received an addition under the name of "celluloid base," a composition of solid collodion, and proposed to be fitted to the model by means of pressure, after having been subjected to the action of oil heated to a temperature of 300 degrees. This preparation promised to revolutionise the profession, and it was supposed would supersede vulcanite. The idea was of American origin. In alluding to America, it must not be omitted that this year a recognition of the claims that the late Mr. Horace Wells had upon the medical and dental professions, by his introduction of the valuable anæsthetic, nitrous oxide, was thought proper. The idea originated with Mr. Fox, who had had an interview with Dr. Colton, when that gentleman was in this country, and from whom he learned that the circumstances of the widow loudly called for amelioration. Accordingly an influential meeting assembled at the house of Mr. Clover, F.R.C.S., to consider what it would be desirable to do in order to express sympathy with the family of the late gentleman. Mr. Clover presided. The meeting may be thus summarised. Mr. Erichsen eloquently advocated the cause of Mrs. Horace Wells, and moved the following resolution, which was seconded by Mr. Woodhouse Braine, and carried unanimously, viz. :—" That in the opinion of this meeting it is desirable that subscriptions should be raised for the widow of the late Horace Wells of Hailford, Connecticut, United States, in consideration of the services rendered to humanity by her late husband in the realisation of the idea of Sir Humphrey Davy, and consequent introduction of nitrous oxide as an anæsthetic."

The second resolution, which was moved by Mr. W. A. Harrison, seconded by Mr. Turner, and carried unanimously, was " that this meeting resolve itself into a committee, with power to add to its numbers, for the purpose of carrying out the first resolution." Mr. Erichsen was requested to act as chairman of the committee, Messrs. Clover and Braine as treasurers, and Messrs. Fox and Sercombe as honorary secretaries.

However much some practitioners of this country have thought proper to think lightly and speak disparagingly of their brethren across the Atlantic, and however that evidence of narrow-minded partiality may have been returned with interest from those on the other side, it was very pleasant to notice this effort to acknowledge painstaking investigation which had resulted in a universal benefit to mankind, although the searcher and practical donor of the blessing had not only been unrewarded, but eclipsed by the introduction of chloroform—cowed and so disheartened as to seek a vain refuge in death. To see such a work of practical charity in full exercise was a fitting close to the year.

Allusion has been made in this work to the feeling that was manifest in the direction of obtaining the privilege of admission to the museum and library, and to the lectures delivered at the college. The opening of the year 1872 was marked by the concession of these things by the college authorities, a decision arrived at in the closing part of the former year. The willingness to accede to a reasonable request made in an appropriate manner was exemplified in the following notice:—" At the ordinary meeting of the council, on the 14th December, the following resolutions agreed to by the board of examiners in dental surgery, on the 2d of November 1871, for the consideration of the council, were adopted:—

" I. That it be recommended to the council that paragraph 10 of the regulations relating to the diploma in dental surgery be altered, as follows:—

" 10. Of having attended at a recognised dental hospital, or in the dental department of a recognised general hospital, the practice of dental surgery during the period of *two years* (instead of during *two winter and two summer sessions*).

" II. That it be reported to the council that, in the opinion of this board, it is desirable that the diploma in dental surgery should bear the college arms, and that the diploma should be so altered in form as to admit of its being signed by the president of the college as well as by the examiners.

" III. And that it be recommended to the council that a ticket of admission to the museum, to the library, and to the college lectures be presented to each candidate on his obtaining the diploma in dental surgery."

Not only were these alterations and consequent concessions to be accepted thankfully by all the students seeking to obtain the degree of the college in their specialty, but the phraseology employed was noticeable and worthy of remembrance by the whole profession. The degree itself, as the result of long, arduous, and difficult effort by the most eminent and disinterested practitioners, had been subjected to a very large amount of ridicule, and even contempt, by many both in the profession and outside of it too. It was asserted that, after all, it was but a "certificate," and conveyed no privilege to its possessor. That it was but the evidence that dental surgery had become a sort of appendage to general surgery, and nothing of advantage could accrue to the licentiate who had become a voluntary vassal of the great corporate body of Lincoln's Inn Fields. Throughout this important notice, however, the degree was spoken of as a "diploma," and a diploma only. The word "certificate" does not once appear. And this, doubtless, was not the result of mere chance in the choice of expressions. The licentiates in dental surgery had therein the direct proof that whoever might choose to undervalue or misrepresent the document which proved a thorough fitness to practise, the College of Surgeons deliberately affixed to it a certain recognised value and stamp. Whatever others might, therefore, say as to the pre-eminence that full membership bestowed, the council of the College of Surgeons thereby distinctly admitted that this diploma was the distinguishing mark of proficiency in those who held it to practise the art and science of dental surgery. It did not come too soon. The toil which it had demanded to secure it, as well as the capacities of those who had submitted to the ordeal of examination, deserved this distinct acknowledgment of its value by those highest in authority and best capable of judging. One good result of this edict was to be hoped for in its stimulating every licentiate to uphold the dignity of the diploma by his unswerving obedience to the canons of true professional conduct. It could not be said truthfully that those who had worked so indefatigably to obtain the benefits of a higher status for the dental profession were slumbering, or at ease, for not only were there true friends in the dental body still, but friends who had influence, and generously used it for their fellow-practitioners' benefit. The governors of the Dental Hospital, at their annual general meeting in January of this year, heard the report read by the excellent honorary secretary, Mr. Coleman, in which it appeared that no less a number than 19,702 cases had been registered during the year which then terminated, out of which 1879 operations had been performed by the assistance of nitrous oxide gas. Beginning, as this now necessary charity had, with some 200 or 300 operations in its first year, 1859, the number now reached most amply certified its abundant usefulness. On the occasion in question, Mr. E. Saunders, who had for some time past entertained the idea, suggested the desirability of the removal of the hospital to a position in London where better light could be obtained, and fuller scope given to its ever-busy staff. He had already been seeking, and hinted that in all probability had found, a better site for the charity. Mr. Thomas Hyde Hills, who on that occasion acted as chairman of the meeting, and has ever been a true and benevolent friend to it and the dental profession, concurred in Mr. Saunders' views, and promised a donation to the £2000 which would be necessary to carry out the contemplated removal. The proposal very soon acquired the evidences of ultimate success, and in the March following £700 had been already subscribed. It is but just that the fact should be stated of Mr. Saunders' liberality in this matter. Out of the £700 thus obtained, this gentleman had given the handsome sum of £500. During the next two months £200 more had been either received or promised, so that the list was being rapidly augmented. Mr. Saunders worked very heartily in this matter, using not only his purse but his personal influence, and pen also, in order that his idea might be carried out to a successful issue. The natural result was, that subscriptions, of a less amount than that contributed by a few of the wealthier members of the profession, were systematically received and duly announced. The managing committee of the Dental Hospital of London thoroughly discussed the project, and took the opinion of the medical staff upon the desirability of the proposed removal. The manner in which the entire subject was presented to the medical committee at first made it difficult for that body to deal with it. It appeared that if an adverse vote were given by the medical officers, the whole onus and responsibility of failure would rest upon them. Several of their number, not seeing the absolute necessity of a change of locality in the clear light in which Mr. Saunders and his supporters had viewed it, resented this as an unjust conclusion. The consideration of the subject was fully entered into by them, and while all claimed an equal interest in and desire for the present and future prosperity of the institution to which they had been and still were devoting so much of their valuable time, they also maintained their undoubted right and privilege of freely expressing their individual opinions on so important a matter, without the alleged imputation of opposition. When the votes were ultimately taken, it appeared that a majority of one only was recorded in favour of Mr. Saunders' proposition, and but for the forced retirement, through illness, of one of the staff during the debate, the votes would have been equal. The result of the discussion by the medical staff was, of course, reported to the managing committee, who, after due deliberation, determined in favour of the hospital being removed. When this was known the medical officers cheerfully accepted the resolution, and with a unanimous feeling resolved to work with increased energy to make the scheme a success. They all felt that, whatever their private or expressed opinions might be, the locality in which the institution was placed could not possibly affect their sincere desire for its permanent and increasing prosperity. From the report which the building committee returned to the committee of management, by whom it had been appointed, it appeared that, taking all contingencies into account, the annual rental of the new premises for the first five and a half years would be some £370.

This, however, could only occur under the most unfavourable circumstances. On the other hand, the Odontological Society undertook to become tenants of the Dental Hospital committee, and the building itself had, in the opinion of many, very distinct if not numerous advantages over the premises in Soho Square. Extensive frontage, a north light, good ventilation, and other similar benefits were enumerated. The expense attendant upon the enterprise would be considerable, but in the early part of this year, 1873, some £1600 had already been received, and a guarantee fund had been organised for the purpose of meeting any and all probable expenses in connection with the Soho Square hospital—the lease of which had not expired—the contributions to which at that time represented the sum of £200 per annum, secured for a term of five years, if required. At the annual general meeting of governors of the Dental Hospital of London, Mr. Ash proposed another plan. His idea was to build suitable premises rather than convert old ones into the nearest approach to convenience they would allow. At considerable trouble he had procured plans and drawings in connection with sites to be obtained from the Metropolitan Board of Works, on which a hospital could be erected, adapted in all points to the requirements of the managing and medical staff, the students, and also the Odontological Society. By estimates he had procured, it appeared that such a hospital could be built for the sum of £4000 inclusive, and he generously undertook to meet any extra expense which might be incurred. His proposal was discussed, but eventually the decision was given in favour of the original plan. Mr. E. Sercombe, as treasurer to the building fund, continued to receive encouraging support in subscriptions from the profession generally. In July the sum in hand was announced to be £2144, which was further increased by the following September to £2428, in October to £2529, and in December £2929 in all had been received.

The next year, 1874, was not to be allowed to grow very old before the new Dental Hospital could be said to be completed. Every effort had been made to do all that was necessary to this end, Mr. Saunders having been unremitting in his exertions and influence with the contractors from the first. The programme was that the President of the Odontological Society, Mr. E. Sercombe, should postpone his inaugural address, so as to deliver the same in the new premises. On Monday evening, March 2d, the society met as arranged to receive the remarks of the president; after which, at nine o'clock, a conversazione was held—the rooms being decorated for the purpose with many valuable paintings lent for the occasion by friends of the movement. There were the usual objects of interest which accompany such gatherings, exposed for the gratification of the visitors, who in large numbers thronged the various rooms. A general feeling of satisfaction was evident at the accommodation which the new building afforded; and the promoters of the enterprise were gladdened by the prospect of an immediate and entire renovation of the hitherto ugly and disreputable Leicester Square gardens. Altogether a very pleasant and highly-satisfactory evening was spent. On the 12th of March it had been determined that the formal possession of the new premises should be taken; and Mr. Thomas Arnold Rogers, who had consented to act as dean, invited the students to meet him at nine o'clock of that day, to inaugurate the beginning of operations there. With the house-surgeon most of the pupils responded to Mr. Rogers' invitation, and had the pleasure and profit of listening to the words of kindly welcome and instruction which that gentleman was so well able to offer. Among many excellent observations, Mr. Rogers said in conclusion: "Well, I am urging you to cultivate these habits—thoroughness, accuracy, system, and to begin to cultivate them here as an essential part of your professional training. And I may tell you without, I think, violating the secrecy of the council-chamber, that the medical committee have under their anxious consideration several matters upon which their decision will be made with the sole object of promoting your welfare. I feel sure you know the medical staff of this hospital have your interests warmly at heart, and I hope their deliberations will result in the promotion of those interests, by giving you increased opportunities of cultivating the habits I have alluded to. But you yourselves may sometimes be able to make valuable suggestions of improvements in our way of working, and I shall be very pleased indeed to receive them from you, and to give them my best thoughts; and should they appear practicable, to recommend them to the consideration of the medical committee. You know what a favourable reception your wish for clinical lectures had; and I know that both the medical and managing committees were much pleased by that instance of your earnestness; and you may rest assured that any such suggestion coming from you will be welcomed, and, whether it can be adopted or not, will, at all events, be received with interest.

"And now I think I have said all I have to say in welcoming you to your new hospital; and yet I think I should like to say one more word. Gentlemen, we have a rare opportunity before us. We begin, as it were, a new life to-day; and I am not going too far when I say that the eyes of the whole professional world are upon us, and that upon your teachers and upon you—you who are present in this room and at this moment—the future of our profession in this country depends. Gentlemen, let us rise to the level of this demand upon our energies; let us resolve here and now that we will, with God's help, do our utmost to benefit our fellow-men, to qualify ourselves to take the highest positions in our calling, and to make our school the first school in the world."

The dinner took place in the evening of the same day

at Willis's Rooms, when, under the chairmanship of that untiring friend of the profession, Mr Campbell de Morgan, a numerous company assembled, including among them many men of mark—Sir Wm. Fergusson, Bart.; T. B. Curling, F.R.S., President of the Royal College of Surgeons; and T. H. Hills, Esq., President of the Pharmaceutical Society. Among sentiments of congratulation and expressed wishes for the increasing prosperity of the hospital and all connected with it, and the society and school also, the company at length broke up, all alike feeling that the Dental Hospital of London had been thoroughly inaugurated under its new circumstances, and launched, as it were, afresh upon an ever-widening sphere of usefulness. Not satisfied with the success which had evidently attended the enterprise thus far, Mr. Saunders carried out the idea of a concert to be given in the premises, March 25th. This likewise proved a success—the proceeds being a contribution to the funds of more than £100; and Mr. Sercombe afterwards announced that the amount in his hands could be written down as £3682, 6s. 11d.

Thus, then, was the hospital, which had been since its opening in 1858 a gradually-increasing blessing as a charity, and centre of instruction to the dental students who had entered it, opened afresh for further benefit to the public and the profession alike. Among the many distinct advantages it then possessed was the undeniable one of such an officer as the new dean, Mr. T. A. Rogers. Some years before, this particular office was deemed a necessity, and was first mooted by Mr. S. Cartwright. When the decision was come to that the hospital should have such an officer, the committee of management looked almost instinctively to Mr. T. A. Rogers. Possessing all the qualifications necessary for such a post, he brought to it also extreme courtesy, large experience, and abundant goodwill, accompanied with leisure. What, therefore, could be accomplished for the benefit of the institution itself, and for the students practising there, there could be no doubt would be thoroughly done; and when that gentleman's assent was given to the proposal made to him, all interested in the success of the hospital were glad that to the list of its already zealous staff of officers could be added the well-known and universally-esteemed name of Thomas Arnold Rogers.

CHAPTER IX.

ONE of the beneficial results arising from the better organisation of the profession has been shown in the spirit which has manifested itself in other places besides London. The desire for union and progress has been very notably displayed in Edinburgh, where it has led to the formation of a society called the Odonto-Chirurgical Society. The idea of founding such a society appears to have suggested itself to Dr. J. Smith, of Edinburgh, sometime before the dental licentiateship was adopted. In the month of February 1858, Dr. Smith addressed a letter to the President of the Royal College of Surgeons, Edinburgh, "on the present position of dental surgery, and its advancement as a branch of medical education," in which the then existing condition of the dental profession was discussed. The idea for its improvement was thus epitomised, "First, that every one adopting the practice of dental surgery should be required to possess a surgical diploma or other equivalent qualification, and have any special education in dentistry superadded to this. Or, second, that at least a limited and special course of instruction, practical as well as theoretical and elementary, in dental surgery should be afforded, and considered imperative on such as might not possess, or might not feel desirous of obtaining, a regular diploma." In this printed letter Dr. Smith deprecated "partial degrees" as "in every way reprehensible," and advocated "a *bona fide* surgical diploma." Whether this address produced any result either with the college authorities or Dr Smith's *confrères*, the writer cannot say; but that gentleman has informed him that he took steps in conjunction with the late Mr. Nasmyth to establish in Edinburgh a Dental Dispensary. In this effort he was supported by Dr. Orphoot, Mr. Imlack, and others. This institution was formed and opened in January 1860, in Drummond Street. Its success and growing importance led eventually to its direction being placed under the control of a regularly-constituted committee of management, who appealed to the public for contributions for its support, instead of relying for aid, as formerly, upon the generosity of those gentlemen more or less immediately connected with it. The staff of medical officers was increased to six, and the charity had found for it a better position in Cockburn Street, where it still is. Of the beneficial results in connection with the Dispensary more will be said further on. It was at a meeting held when the institution was in Cockburn Street, January 1865, and on which occasion Mr. Nasmyth, Dr. Roberts, Dr. Orphoot, Mr. D. Hepburn, Dr. Wight, Mr. Watt, Dr. Swanson, and Dr. Smith were present, that the propriety of establishing in Scotland a Society of Dental Practitioners was mooted. A code of laws was agreed upon, by which such a society should be regulated, Dr. Smith suggesting the name, "The Odonto-Chirurgical Society." Copies of these laws were circulated among the profession for approval, with the request to those addressed that their opinion upon them should be sent in to the secretary. Difficulties immediately arose, owing their origin to the same feeling which had exhibited itself in London, on the question of qualification, and what constituted it. The result of conflicting opinions on this knotty point was not long in revealing itself. In the month of May in the same year (1865), another meeting was convened, when it was agreed that the purpose should be abandoned, the committee of organisation dissolved, and the society (?) considered as having ceased to exist. There must have been cogent reasons for this sudden collapse of such an interesting attempt to further the progress of the profession. As it was, however, Dr. Roberts felt constrained to move the abandonment of the project, which was carried all but unanimously. One gentleman, Mr. D. Hepburn, raised his voice against the conclusion, expressing his confidence in ultimate success, and belief that they could still command sufficient numbers to form a society. Of course, the majority ruled. Up to the year 1866 it had been the practice in London to celebrate the granting of the diploma in dental surgery on the day when the first examination for that degree had taken place, March 13th. On the 2d of March in that year, a circular was issued by the board of stewards for the London dinner, announcing that the result of a canvass of opinion among all the licentiates was that in future the dinner should take place in June, instead of as formerly. This being the case it occurred to Mr. Hepburn to make use of the opportunity thus created to institute a commemoration dinner in Edinburgh, to be held on the original day, hoping it would prove the means of drawing the members of the profession in the North together, and fostering a friendly spirit amongst them. To this end he consulted with Mr. Chisholm and Mr. Cunningham, who supported his views very cheerfully. The holders of the degree were written to, as well as other leading and reputed members of the profession, Dr. Roberts assisting by addressing several of them. The dinner was accordingly held, and although not numerously attended was a decided success. It was at this friendly gathering Mr. Hepburn thought he saw sufficient cordiality to warrant an attempt at the formation of the wished-for society. He stated his ideas to Mr. Chisholm and Mr. Cunningham, who agreed with him, and then, having ascertained that no effort was being made, or, indeed, seemed likely to be made by others, these three gentlemen determined to venture the attempt once more. It was furthermore agreed that with the view of securing all those gentlemen who had been engaged in the effort of 1865 to co-operate, the name and laws which had been then submitted to the profession should be substantially retained, such alterations in the rules as were thought necessary to meet the more liberal views of the many alone excepted. Acting upon these bases a circular was sent to all those members of the profession who it was considered probable would render assistance, calling a meeting for March 13, 1867, with the purpose of forming a society. This meeting was accordingly held at the house of Mr. Hepburn, and there were present on the occasion the following gentlemen, viz.:—Messrs. Hogue, Swanson, Chisholm, Wilson, Watt, A. F. Swanson, Matthews, Cormack, and Hepburn (Edinburgh), F. Thomson and Bell (Glasgow), Williamson (Aberdeen), and Campbell (Dundee).

Letters from several other gentlemen unable to attend, but concurring in the object of the meeting, were read. The circular convening this meeting had been sent to Dr. Smith, and Mr. Hepburn and Mr. Chisholm had also called upon him informing him of the purport of the gathering, and seeking his aid. On the morning of the 13th, Dr. Smith called in return on Mr. Hepburn, stating that although he could not see his way to join such a society at present, he nevertheless wished it success. Dr. Thomson of Glasgow occupied the chair. The usual business was proceeded with, resulting in the adoption of the idea that the society should be formed. The laws as agreed upon were such as to be identical with those of the Odontological Society of Great Britain, and it was decided formally to retain the name as originally proposed. The following gentlemen were then elected to serve in the respective offices:—

Honorary President—R. Nasmyth, F.R.C.S., M.O.S.

Vice-Presidents—Dr. F. Thomson, F.R.C.S., M.O.S.; Dr Roberts, L.D.S., M.O.S.

Committee—J. K. Chisholm, L.D.S., M.O.S.; Dr. J. Smith, F.R.C.S.; W. Williamson, L.D.S.; Dr. Orphoot.

Treasurer—D. Hepburn, L.D.S.

Secretary—J. G. Cunningham, L.D.S.

As in other societies it was very well, and manifested a laudable feeling, to nominate and even elect those gentlemen whom it was felt were most likely to help forward the work thus taken in hand; but it was altogether another and a different thing to secure their co-operation. The promoters of the Odonto-Chirurgical Society, like their brethren in the South, had now to pass through this mortifying and somewhat discouraging experience. Mr. Nasmyth refused to act in the office to which he had been unanimously elected, desiring his name to be removed from the records of the society; but by the strong persuasion of Mr. Hepburn, he eventually consented to allow it to remain until the end of the year. Dr. Orphoot also and Dr. Smith declined to be associated with the society. Added to these untoward circumstances, the society had to contend against difference of opinion from other members of the profession, concerning the mode of action that had been adopted, and, altogether considered, this very praiseworthy attempt to bring the scientific and social elements of our brethren in Scotland together proved no easy task. The atmosphere, however, was not entirely dark. Light streamed in from more than one point. The society was very much cheered by receiving most encouraging letters from Mr. R. Hepburn and Mr. Underwood, who were then occupying seats at the council of the Odontological Society. These came very opportunely. Then, again, the president's chair was accepted and worthily filled by the late Dr. Thomson of Glasgow. This gentleman had welcomed from the first any endeavour to strengthen the bond of union among dentists generally. His sentiments are given in the following letter:—

" 10 BRANDON PLACE, GLASGOW,
9th *March* 1867.

"MY DEAR SIR,—It will afford me much pleasure to attend on Wednesday, the 13th March, at four o'clock, as also to be present at the dinner afterwards. I quite agree in all the liberal sentiments so well expressed in your note, and have often regretted the utter want of all social intercourse between the members of our particular specialty. I sincerely hope we may be able to arrange this society, and cast aside every feeling but kindness and good fellowship.—Believe me, my dear sir, yours faithfully, FRANCIS H. THOMSON.

"David Hepburn, Esq."

Previous to the election of this excellent and warm-hearted gentleman to the president's chair, at the meeting held March 13, 1858, the vacancies occasioned by the retirement of Drs. Orphoot and Smith had been filled by the election of Dr. Macpherson and Mr. Horne.

The society thus formed and put into operation owes its name to the suggestion of Dr. Smith, who also drew up the originally-proposed laws for its regulation, and it has been felt by all the members of the society to be a matter of regret that he and others have not cooperated in this really beneficial organisation. It needs a great deal of faith and determination to proceed in any difficulty when support is steadily withheld in quarters where it might be fairly hoped for, and when success crowns such efforts the praise is doubly due to those whose perseverance has been so unremitting. Among such, Mr. David Hepburn stands worthily prominent. He has been well supported by such men as Mr. Chisholm and Mr. Cunningham, not to mention others, but the writer believes he is but stating that which many practitioners in the North would readily endorse—especially those who have been most intimately associated with him—that to his constancy and self-denial, together with his unceasing efforts, the Odonto-Chirurgical Society is largely indebted for its progress. Year by year its members have been added to, valuable papers have been produced and read at its various meetings, and published in the "Transactions" and "British Journal of Dental Science," while financially there is everything to encourage. As a rule the society's meetings were first held at Mr. David Hepburn's house, and apart from the advantage reaped in a scientific point of view, those who have thus met together have had their professional relationships much strengthened and encouraged. The profession in the North has also set their brethren in London an excellent example in the matter of celebrating the granting of the dental degree, by an annual dinner in Edinburgh. They have wisely and appropriately decided that this friendly and social gathering should be held in continuance on the 13th of March in each year. While this anniversary of the most important event in the annals of dentistry in this country has been suffered to lapse and fall into disuse by the practitioners in London —for what cause, except apathy, perhaps, it is difficult to say—the dentists of Scotland have most creditably maintained it. It would be well if their resolution could find a response in the metropolis. Allusion has been already made to the Edinburgh Dental Dispensary, but a fuller notice of that institution is necessary.

In the altered arrangements which its promoters found necessary, during the second year of its existence, the following gentlemen were appointed to its staff:— Professor Goodsir and Mr. (now Professor) Spence, of the Edinburgh University, consulting surgeons; and Mr. Nasmyth, consulting surgeon-dentist. Professor Spence still continues consulting surgeon, and Messrs. Goodsir and Nasmyth held office until their deaths. It was further resolved "to appoint a committee of medical gentlemen to aid in the formation of such a special medical institution, and for drawing up those regulations which might be necessary or expedient towards its efficient working." The gentlemen chosen were:—Dr. Craigie, P.R.C.P., Dr. Newbigging, P.R.C.S. (*ex officio*), Professor Goodsir, Professor Sir Robert

Christison, Professor Sir James Y. Simpson, Dr. Begbie, Dr. Burt, Professor Spence, Dr. James Duncan, and Dr. Omond, to whom the reorganisation might be entrusted, and the management handed over. In May of the same year considerable difficulty arose as to the eligibility of the medical officers for the daily attendance at the Dispensary, when, at a full meeting, the following resolution was framed, which afterwards formed rule 12 of the constitution and laws, viz.—" Any one engaged in the practice of dental surgery, and who possesses a medical or surgical title qualifying for registration, shall be eligible for the office of dental surgeon in the Edinburgh Dental Dispensary; and any one who, at this date, May 1862, has been in the practice of dental surgery in Edinburgh for twenty years, shall be eligible for the same office." The medical officers then on the staff were re-appointed, and Mr. Charles Hutchins, Dr. W. A. Roberts, and Dr. Hogue were elected to the office; Mr. William Kelso Thwaites, Solicitor Supreme Court of Scotland, acting as treasurer and secretary. The daily rotation of medical officers was fixed, the financial statement was examined and audited, the rules and constitution approved of and adopted, and the Dispensary fairly started under the new *régime*. Subscriptions were then solicited, and chiefly through the exertions of the office-bearers a sum of £20 was obtained, while the trustees of the late John Mackenzie, Esq., Manor Place, Edinburgh, contributed a further sum of £25. When the financial statement was submitted for approval in May 1863, the announcement was made that the Dispensary was free from debt. During the first year of its existence the number of patients seeking relief at the Dispensary amounted to 1404. At the half-yearly meeting of the institution, November 1863, the number of patients had amounted in six months to 1034, so that it was evident the benefits it afforded were well known and sought after. The boxes for donations, &c., placed on the premises yielded only the meagre sum of four shillings and eightpence; so that it was to be inferred the sufferers were either very poor, or else little disposed practically to show their appreciation of the relief they had received. The funds would not have been sufficient to meet the expenses had not the trustees of Mr. Mackenzie again come to the rescue, thus enabling the Dispensary to tide over its difficulties. The year 1864 revealed the unpleasant tidings of subscriptions coming in very slowly, when the secretary submitted to the medical committee the desirability of publishing a report of the proceedings at the public meeting, and a history of the more interesting cases, together with a list of subscribers. This suggestion was, however, postponed for further consideration, and possible adoption. The brethren in the North were adopting a similar course to that pursued by the executive of the Dental Hospital of London, viz., endeavouring to maintain their institution by the generosity of those immediately concerned. Why such a system should be followed it would be difficult to say, seeing that the public reap so distinct and direct a benefit from these charities, and, therefore, can be so legitimately and justly expected to give proportionate help. The expenses of the Edinburgh Dental Dispensary, including the purchase of instruments, furniture, &c., amounted in round numbers to £100; but by great exertions subscriptions and donations, including the house boxes—which had reached £1, 8s. 4¼d. in small sums—were found sufficient to meet this demand. About this time the subject of adding to the medical staff, or the appointment of assistant dental surgeons, was submitted to the consideration of the executive, and a committee was empowered to confer upon the matter. In May 1864 the following official statement appeared in the report, viz., that since the opening of the Dispensary the number of patients attending had steadily increased. During the first year 250 persons had received relief, while in the latter year 2028 had been entered upon the books.

At the half-yearly meeting, held in May 1865, it was stated that while the funds had fallen off by some £20, the number of patients had increased to 2750. It was in the course of that year that a correspondence was opened between the Dispensary executive and the Royal College of Surgeons of England, the object being the recognition by that body of the Edinburgh institution as a school in harmony with the imposed and regular curriculum. This resulted in the granting of the request, as the following quotation from a letter from the secretary of the Royal College of Surgeons, Mr. Trimmer, under date August 14, 1865, will show. "Resolved:—That, as recommended by the board, certificates of attendance on the practice of the Edinburgh Dental Dispensary be recognised by this college as part of the curriculum for the diploma in dental surgery, on the understanding that such certificates must only be signed by the three ordinary surgeon dentists holding one or other of the qualifications considered necessary by the council."

Further inquiries were made as to the effect of this recognition by such as might decide upon availing themselves of a connection with this institution, which resulted in Mr. Trimmer sending a reply containing the following information—" I have to acquaint you that such recognition will be applicable only to paragraph . . . of the enclosed regulations relating to such diploma. The certificates required by paragraphs 3, 4, 5, 6, and 7, can be obtained by attendance on the recognised medical schools in Edinburgh; but inasmuch as there is not yet any recognised dental school in Edinburgh, the certificates included in paragraphs . . . cannot be obtained in that city." This communication bore date 27th September 1865.

The qualifications necessary for serving on the medical staff were reconsidered, resulting in the confirmation of the terms required as agreed upon in 1862. The report for the year 1867–68 showed that between

4000 and 5000 patients had been treated, but the income of the Dispensary also showed a most disheartening decrease, the total amount raised being no more than the insignificant sum of £33. Such a state of things created a painful feeling among those who were striving to sustain a charity which it was evident was a distinct necessity, and it was resolved to publish a statement, and solicit subscriptions, especially from the employers of labour. This was accordingly done, and the result, though not what was expected as to amount, was to a certain degree encouraging, and, at any rate, enabled the financial demands of the Dispensary to be met. This was in 1870. During 1869 the appointment of assistant dental surgeons was decided upon, which arrangement still exists. Dr. Smith, who had worked strenuously in the double office of ordinary dental surgeon and honorary medical secretary, retired from these posts in 1870. Onwards to the present time, through many trials and difficulties, but invariably with a meagre exchequer, the Edinburgh Dental Dispensary has moved. The insufficient supply of funds has crippled its development, not permitting the use of nitrous oxide gas except in rare and very special cases, and precluding anything further than mere extraction of teeth. It appears to an unprejudiced mind that there is a tangible cause for the results which all connected with the institution cannot but deplore. If a public charity, which confers its benefits upon 4000 to 5000 of the suffering poor, can only obtain a bare sufficiency to meet its most modest expenditure, the question presses with great force as to the reason why. Is it from within, or from without? Can the executive improve its method? or are those who, as the general public, are, or ought to be, interested in the stability and increasing usefulness of such a benevolent enterprise, so indifferent in the matter that it is allowed thus to languish? There have been examples of well-sustained energy in connection with the Dispensary, notably in the case of Dr. John Wight, not to mention others; and it is to be hoped that some effort will be made whereby it may be relieved from the experience of past years, and placed in the happy circumstances which its importance assuredly claims. The report for the year 1875 is somewhat more encouraging, especially in the statement that the practice of filling teeth has been adopted. This, as a matter of course, is a benefit not only to the patients, but also to the students attending the institution. The following is the present constitution of the staff:—

Managers—Dr. Keiller, P.R.C.P., and Dr. Littlejohn, P.R.C.S. (*ex officio*); J. Gordon, Esq.; Dr. Omond, F.R.C.S.;* Dr. J. W. Begbie, F.R.C.P.;* Dr. John Smith, F.R.C.P.; Dr. Dunsmure, F.R.C.S.; Dr. Moir, F.R.C.P.; Dr. A. H. Douglas, F.R.C.P.; Dr. J. D. Gillespie, F.R.C.S.; Dr. Charles Dycer, F.R.C.S.; Dr. R. Paterson, F.R.C.P.; W. Walter, Esq., F.R.C.S.; Charles Hutchins, Esq.; Dr. W. A. Roberts, L.D.S.; Dr. W. H. Lowe, F.R.C.P.; Dr. James Simson, F.R.C.S.

Consulting Surgeon—Professor Spence, F.R.C.S.

Consulting Physician—Dr. Saunders, F.R.C.P.

Consulting Surgeon-Dentist—Dr. John Smith, F.R.C.S., Surgeon-Dentist to the Queen.

Ordinary Surgeon-Dentists—Dr. W. A. Roberts, L.D.S.; William Chisholm, Esq., L.R.C.P. and S. Edin. and L.D.S.; J. K. Chisholm, Esq., L.D.S.; A. Cormack, Esq., L.D.S.; Dr. John Wight.

Secretary and Treasurer—William Kelso Thwaites, S.S.C.

Liverpool has also provided a similar charity for the benefit of its poor, and a means of usefulness for the dental students there. The Liverpool Dental Hospital owes its origin to Mr. W. J. Newman, dental surgeon of that town. The first to aid him in the important work he had undertaken was the Rev. W. Banister, the late Mr. Thomas Brakell co-operating with him, and, under the influential auspices and patronage of the then mayor, T. D. Anderson, Esq., it was established in September 1860. Its first president was Laurence R. Baily, Esq., and the late Alex. Stookes, M.D., acted as vice-presi-

* Since deceased.

dent, which offices they each held until the year 1864, when John Ireland Blackburne, Esq., filled the president's chair, and Dr. Stookes became consulting physician. The institution has since been efficiently helped by the services of Lieutenant-Colonel Steble, who has acted as honorary treasurer and secretary, and since, vice-president, together with Mr. Samuel Grace, Mr. David Campbell, and others. For the first three years Mr. Newman acted as sole dental officer, and generously gave three attendances weekly, performing the necessary operations. In the year 1863 the dental staff was augmented by the valuable assistance of Messrs. R. E. Stewart and S. F. Austin, and by this step the committee of management were enabled to open the hospital daily instead of as before. Mr. Austin subsequently resigning, Mr. James B. Lloyd was elected to the dental staff in 1864, and not long afterwards Mr. W. T. Bryan, Dr. Waite, and Mr. J. Durandu were appointed honorary dental officers—so that a dental surgeon was thus secured for each morning of the week. This arrangement continued until December 1869, when Mr. Durandu resigned, and Mr. Tullius Fay succeeded him. The necessity of such an institution was demonstrated by a steady increase in the number of patients attending. The first year gave for its result 864 operations performed; while in 1869 the number registered reached 5421. Altogether, within the period of these two dates, no less than 29,650 operations had taken place. The history of this institution has been similar to that of other kindred charities, especially where they have been opened for special purposes such as dentistry. There has been struggle with difficulties, and much patient toil on the part of those more immediately concerned, which reflect credit and merit praise. The necessity of a dental hospital has, however, been thoroughly recognised by the public, and hence the practice has been considerable. Without mentioning the results given year by year in the annual reports, that of 1875 informs the friends and supporters of the hospital that the number of admissions during the twelve months amounted to 5867, being an increase of 404 over those of the year preceding. These statistics give an average of 7000 operations performed within the above time. Application has been made to the Royal College of Surgeons for the recognition of the hospital by that body, in connection with the stipulated curriculum, and this has been granted. The managing committee are enterprising enough to seek for more accommodation in better or enlarged premises. The undertaking will entail an expenditure of some £3000, but already a nucleus of that sum has been secured. That the amount of relief which this institution secures for the suffering poor of the flourishing town of Liverpool will be a strong and sufficient claim upon the pecuniary support of its many wealthy inhabitants, there can be no doubt. At the same time, the experience which such a field of practice offers to the dental student will secure for it a steady in-flow of young men seeking to become thoroughly acquainted with the details of the profession they propose to follow. Too much praise cannot well be given to Mr. Newman for having originated the Liverpool Dental Hospital. Such a charity in such a town must be an immense boon to the suffering among its many thousands of labourers, workmen, and others; and one, moreover, that the many wealthy and influential residents should very cheerfully support. As a school for the education of dental students its importance cannot be overrated, while gentlemen of professional ability give their time and attention to the conduct of its affairs. To all who have hitherto supported Mr. Newman the thanks of the true friends of the profession are due, seeing that in such methods as this the real advance in scientific and practical knowledge of dentistry unmistakably lies.

Plymouth has had its dental dispensary, that institution having been opened in July 1861. It originated through the joint efforts of gentlemen resident there, who were at the same time members of the Odontological Society of Great Britain, and practising as dental surgeons in Plymouth. These were Messrs. Coles, Spence Bate, Tubbs, and Jewers. From the first, Mr. Coles could not take the active duties connected with the enterprise, and consequently became an honorary member of the staff. After a short time Mr. Tubbs withdrew, and Mr. Balkwill, who had but recently come to live in Plymouth, took his place. Mr. Jewers was completely disabled through illness to fill the office to which he had been appointed, and under these circumstances Mr. S. Bate undertook to perform double duty as one of the medical staff. One of the first decisions arrived at was that for the future no dental officer to the infirmary could be elected who did not hold the diploma of the Royal College of Surgeons. In due time application was made to the authorities at Lincoln's Inn Fields to recognise the school which had been formed under these gentlemen's auspices. This request was at length granted, and lectures accordingly given. Owing to the necessity of two years of the students' time having to be passed in London, the lectures did not prove so useful as it was originally thought they would be. The practice at the Dispensary is very much sought after, and highly valued by those engaged in their studies there. The reason for this is obvious. There being but a limited number of students, each in his turn obtains a goodly share of work. The senior pupils attend, as a rule, when competent, and superintend the operations under the direction of the dental surgeon. There can be no doubt that the Plymouth Dental Dispensary is a boon, not only as a public charity, but also as a school of instruction to those who enter their names on its lists. The institution is conducted in a quiet and economic manner, and is another instance of what a large amount of good can be conferred at a very moderate pecuniary expenditure.

Birmingham has not only not been behindhand in the matter of establishing a Dental Dispensary, but was, indeed, the first in the field after the effects of reform in the profession were being manifested throughout the provinces. This institution, which owes its origin mainly to Mr. Samuel Adams Parker of the above town, was established in the beginning of the year 1868. The site chosen for it was in Temple Street, as being the best, because most central, part of the town. The ideas of its promoters were set forth in the statement made when the institution was founded, and were to the following effect :—" This institution is founded with the intention of affording gratuitous advice and assistance to the poor in all cases of diseases of the teeth; such advice and assistance to include the operations of extracting, stopping, and scaling, and the regulation of children's teeth. The only operation performed on the teeth at our hospitals and public dispensaries throughout the metropolis and provincial towns is extraction; and it is probable that great numbers of teeth are annually lost that might, with a little care and attention, have been rendered permanently useful. The expenses attending the working of this institution will be very small, therefore large subscriptions will not be required; sixty or seventy pounds per annum will probably cover all liabilities, including rent, instruments, stopping materials," &c.

It is but right to record the names of those gentlemen, both lay and professional, who, seeing the importance of such a dispensary, associated themselves in the effort to fairly launch the new enterprise. The following is a list of the names of the first office-bearers :—

President—John Ratcliff, Esq., Mayor.
Treasurer—Henry Marshall, Esq.
Secretary—George Warden, Esq.
Consulting Dentist—T. R. English, Esq.
Dentist—Samuel Adams Parker, Esq.
Committee—Samuel Berry, Esq.; P. H. Chavasse, Esq.; T. B. Fletcher, Esq., M.D.; J. J. Hadley, Esq.; G. H. Marshall, Esq.;

Langston Parker, Esq.; Oliver Pemberton, Esq.; Thomas Plevins, Esq.; J. N. Solomon, Esq.; W. F. Wade, Esq., M.B.; C. Warden, Esq., M.D.; T. W. Williams, Esq.

That there was a necessity for such a public charity was soon to be made evident; the first report, delivered in the month of August in that year, showing that 350 patients had taken advantage of the opportunity thus afforded them, and that the total number of distinct operations that had been performed amounted to 420. During the twelve months between January 1858 and the same month in the following year (1859), it appeared that 645 patients had attended the charity, and 755 operations had been performed. Onwards from that time the usefulness of this Dental Dispensary has been made very clear and palpable, as may be seen by consulting the pages of the "British Journal of Dental Science," where the reports have been systematically published. There have been those changes in the staff of the institution which, during the course of years, are naturally to be expected, and in other matters connected with the Dispensary; but Mr. Parker has up to a short time since unremittingly held to the offices which have been assigned him, and has done good work in the direction of promoting its stability and success. The author would have been pleased to have given a longer and fuller account of this provincial dental institution had he been able to obtain information from headquarters. From some unexplained cause, however, his two applications to that effect have not met with a response; he therefore refers the reader to the "British Journal of Dental Science," where he may find through the published reports sufficient evidence to prove its utility. There can be no doubt but that dental dispensaries or hospitals will eventually be established in all the large and important towns of the three kingdoms. When efficiently directed, and strengthened by the countenance and support of the leading local medical practitioners, they will prove in the highest sense of the word beneficial, not only as public charities, but also as schools for the proper education of the young men proposing to practise as dental surgeons. Their recognition as schools by the Royal College of Surgeons depends upon the established reputation and acknowledged position of the gentlemen on their various staffs and every true friend of the dental profession must not only hope but expect, that the demands of the authorities in Lincoln's Inn Fields in this direction will be sufficiently plain and uncompromising. Looking at what has been already effected in this department of reform, and the general desire evinced in some of the principal provincial centres to have such institutions in their midst, there can be but congratulation experienced by all who have, in years that are past, laboured so indefatigably to promote the true interests of the dental profession, and by every honourable and high-minded practitioner and student throughout its ranks.

CHAPTER X.

To record some of the names and mention the services of those gentlemen who have taken so honourable and prominent a part in the cause of dental reform in the United Kingdom, since it was commenced in earnest in the year 1856, is a very pleasant part of the author's work. It has its difficulties, however, as the least reflection on the reader's side will show. One of these arises from the fact that, happily, many of these same gentlemen are still living amongst us. So to speak as that invidious distinctions shall not occur, and the proper and honourable susceptibilities of good men may be respected, is no easy task. The object the writer has in view is to mention the names and refer to the acts of some of the true friends of reform, as from time to time they have been brought under his own personal observation. To give a biographical sketch of all who have warmly and disinterestedly wrought for the profession's advancement would far exceed the intended limits of this work. If, therefore, the curtailment of the list of benefactors should cause disappointment to some, the reason of it lies beyond the writer's control. One of the most interesting facts bound up as an integral part of the struggle for the profession's elevation is the cheerfulness with which many members of it, strenuously and to the full, aided in its accomplishment. There were those whose position and power were alike limited, but who, nevertheless, contributed their utmost, and throughout the entire campaign, too, for the welfare of their brethren and the general good. The many denials which these real friends of the profession submitted to, and the sacrifices they made to secure the desired end, can only be imperfectly known. Without them, however, that which has become the rich heritage of the rising generation of dentists in this country could never have been hoped for, much less obtained. Having been so closely associated with the entire movement, the author has seen much of that devotedness and self-denial which constitutes the chief charm and brightest grace in every benevolent enterprise, and willingly pays his tribute of praise to all who have thus characterised themselves. The major part of their good offices has, though felt, been of that nature which is not calculated to meet the open gaze of general observers, and, indeed, is of a purely private and personal character. To trench, therefore, on such a domain would be as unwise on the one part as it would be unwelcome on the other. To escape from the perplexities of the task before him, the writer takes refuge in the simple but safe resort to alphabetical order and arrangement of names. Following this method, therefore, as one which is open to the least objection, the first name to be dealt with is that of Mr. Arnott.

MR. J. M. ARNOTT.

This gentleman, as is well known, is not a member of the dental profession. Eminent as a surgeon, influential as a former president of the Royal College of Surgeons, and universally respected, Mr. Tomes had the good fortune to be on terms of close intimacy with him at the critical time when his power could be of the highest value if exercised on behalf of dentists and their interests. When the now well-understood "memorial" had not yet come into existence, the *use* of such a means for the attainment of the object which the eventual signataries of that document were formulating, was suggested to them by Mr. Arnott. He was at that time occupying a seat on the council of the Royal College of Surgeons, and was, therefore, well acquainted with the feelings of that body towards the dental profession, so far as they may have been expressed. If, therefore, Mr. Arnott advised that particular method of approach to the council, those who were anxious to gain the ear and obtain the help of that influential body had every reason to place implicit confidence in the mode itself. There can be no doubt that the strong feeling of trust in Mr. Arnott's counsel which all the memorialists had was that which accounted for their indifference to the assaults made by so many of their professional brethren—for this same memorial, and all concerned with it, received a terrible amount of buffeting as soon as it became generally known. Mr. Arnott was able to judge of the character of Mr. Tomes by his official connection with him at the Middlesex Hospital, and feeling that he was capable of only such sentiments as, if practically realised, would advance the interests alike of the public and the dental profession, he had no difficulty in giving attention to what that gentleman sought to advance. When the scheme of dental reform as it existed in Mr. Tomes' mind was submitted to Mr. Arnott's notice, it appeared to him of such importance that he demanded time to think it out for himself. This was not done, as is too often the case, to delay the matter, or even, from the prudential point of view, to test the sincerity and ardour of those more immediately concerned. At that time Mr. Arnott not only had his seat at the council of the College of Surgeons, but held several other important offices which brought him an immense amount of mental labour to perform, and fully occupied his time. When, therefore, it has to be recorded that Mr. Arnott not only considered Mr. Tomes' plan, but considered it well, turning it over and over again in his mind, and endeavouring to take such a comprehensive view of it as to be able fully to understand what it would involve, so that he might be prepared to take it up or let it drop as he concluded best, enough has been said to call forth the thankfulness of every well-wisher to the dental profession. By adding this extra duty to all the other duties pertaining to him just then, Mr. Arnott quietly fostered the infant effort which has subsequently grown to such excellent and admirable proportions. His kindness was another exemplification of that which is apparently so paradoxical in itself—namely, that those whose time is absolutely and already full are the very men who can, nevertheless, accept yet something else to do, and do it well. When once Mr. Arnott had acceded to the request thus made to him, he had abundant opportunity of knowing the pertinacity of Mr. Tomes' disposition. In a conversation which the author had with Mr. Arnott lately on this very subject, that gentleman very quietly remarked—" Tomes gave me but very little rest in the matter; he plied me incessantly with his reasons why I should adopt his idea." The motive for all this is distinct enough, especially now. Once let Mr. Arnott see his way clearly, and then his powerful influence would be used to the utmost in the desired direction. His opinion was at length made known to Mr. Tomes, to this effect, that if the project were ever realised at all, it would only be accomplished after a considerable length of time. This might have been, and probably was, discouraging; but the truth is the difficulties in the way were enormous. Rightly to understand this, it needs that the subject be viewed from the Surgeons' point of view, or, more properly speaking, from the council table, if not the president's chair at the Royal College of Surgeons. If we can occupy mentally such a position, and endeavour to feel as the surgeon of that day felt, we can somewhat enter into and understand such a conclusion by such a man as Mr. Arnott. The question may be very significantly asked, "What was dentistry?" Beyond what has been sketched in the first chapter of this book, there were deeps of ignorance and heights of brazen effrontery in connection with it, and those who pretended to practise it, which made the whole subject a most uninteresting and uninviting one for contemplation. The process of purification needed boldness to make it effectual. How many practitioners at that time were worthy either of recognition, help, or advancement? Verily, few indeed. Mr. Tomes was not at that time a member of the college, and so was not to be considered as capable of quite feeling what members of the college were supposed to feel towards dentists. But Mr. Arnott's high position brought him, or would bring him, into contact with men who, in the consideration of the subject, even if they inclined to consider it at all, might be expected to exhibit supreme indifference. There was very little, if indeed anything, that could be adduced, as from the dentists' side, which would be likely to interest surgeons of the first rank. Nor could those gentlemen be legitimately blamed for their apathy in the matter. It was evident, therefore, that Mr. Arnott had concluded rightly when he said that, "if realised at all, it would only be after a considerable time." The main point, then, to be decided was, whether, supposing the plan proposed to be the right one, on the whole it would be well to persevere? Mr. Tomes resolved to wait and watch, never relaxing a single hour when he thought effort should be made, but still guarding carefully against "hurry," lest a rash or premature step should endanger success. On Mr. Arnott's side there were all the skilful tactics which the best generalship could supply. Gradually, and at the most favourable opportunities, the opinions of his colleagues were carefully sounded. Perseveringly and with laudable prudence each step was taken; and from time to time results either probable or accomplished were talked over and further advance considered. But all this, and much more, was unknown to the profession generally. The matter was being quietly worked by two individuals, one of whom had been instigated to act in the most important direction by the other. At length the time arrived when Mr. Arnott advised the presentation of the memorial in order formally to bring the subject under the notice of the Royal College of Surgeons. This, therefore, was accordingly done. The document was placed in Mr. Arnott's hands, he having kindly consented to place it before the council. On the 13th of December 1855 the petition was presented by him, and a copy of it ordered to be entered on the minutes. It was further considered on the 10th January 1856, and mainly through the cogency of Mr. Arnott's reasoning it was referred to a committee composed of the following influential gentlemen:— Messrs. Green, C. Hawkins and Arnott—president and vice-presidents of the council—Lawrence, Travers, and Stanley. This was to be accounted good progress. The attention of Messrs. Green and Lawrence had been already directed to the subject by the repeated solicitations of Mr. Arnott in private, consequently it was to be fairly hoped that, when their notice was to be thus officially brought to it, they would give it their favour and sanction. This hope did not prove itself illusive.

Having espoused the cause, Mr. Arnott left nothing undone which he could effect to bring about the result so much desired by Mr. Tomes and the party he was working with. To this end he enlisted the sympathies of Mr. Belfour, the secretary of the college, in the cause, who, as far as his assistance could avail, rendered it very cheerfully. It may here appropriately be said that in this, as in many subsequent matters connected with the reform movement in its various stages, Mr. Belfour proved himself to be, up to the time of his lamented death, a most valuable friend to the dental profession. There were frequent occasions when the formal and strictly official duties of this gentleman, if carried out to the letter, might have become serious hindrances to advance, but he ever availed himself of the power he possessed to promote the true interests of dental practitioners. With the agency of this committee prepared to be put in operation, Mr. Arnott saw that the first step to be taken was to ascertain the legal bearings of the project as they touched the Royal College of Surgeons. On the legal adviser being consulted, he gave it as his distinct opinion that the Crown would have to be applied to for a charter, which would empower the college to institute a dental department in connection with itself, and by such a measure alone could the idea of the memorialists be carried out. The difficulties attendant upon this were many and formidable, as the statements in the body of this work have shown. Throughout them all, and with untiring effort and kindly feeling, Mr. Arnott cheerfully brought his influence to bear. Much that he has done cannot well be recorded here, but one thing is absolutely certain, that his share in the labour of bringing about the beneficial results which the profession enjoys at this moment has been very considerable. What renders these quiet but efficient efforts more valuable still is the extremely modest estimate which Mr. Arnott himself places upon them. Like a true benefactor, as indeed he has been, he prefers giving the praise in every other direction except his own. But those who know what were the obstacles encumbering the path of progress, especially in the earlier portion of the movement, will fully appreciate what Mr. Arnott did when only such an influence as he possessed could have been instrumental in removing them. The profession stands deeply indebted to Mr. James Moncrieff Arnott, and there can be no doubt that the mention or recollection of this honoured and honourable name will always be accompanied with its most just meed of thankfulness and esteem.

MR. S. CARTWRIGHT.

Inheriting a name which is more widely known, not only in England, but abroad, than, perhaps, any other connected with the dental profession in this country, Mr. Cartwright has ever held a foremost place among his professional brethren. Like others who, from the first, felt the deep and pressing necessity which existed for improvement and advance, he lent the power of his acknowledged position and the energy of his disposition for the general good. His opinion as to the method by which this could be best secured was identical with that of those who formulated the "memorial," and hence we find his name appended to that document. Mr. Cartwright was a Fellow of Trinity College, Cambridge, and has been medically educated; and, as a member of the Royal College of Surgeons, knows the importance of a thorough knowledge of the various departments of medicine and surgery to all who propose to practise dentistry in a proper and legitimate manner. He never could see the advantages which those who strove for an independent position asserted would accrue by the adoption of that method, and, therefore, from the commencement, was firmly opposed to Mr. Rymer's scheme. This was evident by his repudiation of the connection which had been ardently hoped for by the College of Dentists' party, when they ventured to put his name on the list of those who, it was felt, would be the best directors of that movement, when it was in what may be termed its incipient state. Mr. Cartwright wrote to the author at that time, and, in unmistakably plain terms, said so. Although so few members of the profession were then known to each other, there was a general admission that which ever side had on its list of supporters Mr. Cartwright's name had thereby secured that which would tell largely in its favour. This was in itself perfectly true. Several of the meetings of those gentlemen who had resolved to petition the Royal College of Surgeons were held at No. 32 Old Burlington Street—where the generous hospitality of Mr. Cartwright's father had been so often dispensed—and on those occasions Mr. Cartwright had himself taken an active part in advancing and maturing the memorialists' scheme. His voice was very distinctly heard for the union of dentistry with surgery, according to the terms of that proposal, and he was a powerful advocate and supporter of it on every occasion. Those who knew him well anticipated that he would use his best energies to carry out the idea he had espoused, nor were they disappointed. Valuable as his time was, he very cheerfully gave it whenever it was demanded, and this was by no means an unfrequent thing. Many were the questions on the all-important circumstances taking place in connection with the movement generally which he had to answer by letter, and many also were the interviews he had to grant to his anxious and inquiring brother practitioners. As one of the accepted heads of the profession, his opinion justly and necessarily carried great weight, and the counsel which, in his own quiet but forcible way, from time to time, he gave to those seeking it, added no small number of names to the gradually increasing list of his party. The author can testify from his own personal experience to this fact. When any new aspect of the subject of reform presented itself, many times over the query was put to him, "What does Mr. Cartwright think?" The very decided shrinking from anything like undue prominence—which Mr. Cartwright has ever displayed, would tend to make an impression on the mind of the casual observer that he had not contributed much to the cause of dental reform. Exactly the reverse of this, however, has been the case. He has all along been opposed to the showy display of help, and has found more satisfaction in quiet perseverance in the promotion of the good cause. Another characteristic also belongs to him, and that is his strong dislike of any effort being made with "self" as its centre. He is for doing as much good as possible with the smallest amount of notoriety and observation. This is a high quality, and is justly esteemed by men whose judgment is of any worth. While very willing to co-operate with his fellow-practitioners, Mr. Cartwright, nevertheless, invariably thinks for himself. With an astute mind, and long and varied experience on which to rely, he has always an independent opinion to offer, based on his own views of the subject in hand. It is not a matter of surprise that he has not always subscribed to the propositions of others, nor felt it his duty to act in the closest accord with them. Mr. Cartwright is not demonstrative, but is, nevertheless, exceedingly resolute. He is not to be shaken from what he conceives to be a sound position because those around him do not actually agree with him. He can well afford to be now and then in a minority upon a popular question, waiting patiently until time and circumstance concur to substantiate his views. Whatever may be the matter under consideration, Mr. Cartwright cheerfully gives it his best attention; and all concerned can rely upon his scientific and thoroughly practical knowledge being brought to bear upon it with precision and discrimination, and the question discussed with courtesy and kindly spirit.

Mr. Cartwright was one of the first honorary secretaries of the Odontological Society, acting in that capacity in conjunction with Mr. Tomes and Mr. T. A. Rogers. In the year 1863 he was called to the president's chair, and under his auspices the society passed through a most pleasant and useful session. When the Dental Hospital of London was proposed to be founded, Mr. Cartwright was one of those supporters of the scheme who willingly gave both time and money to mature and launch it. He became the first lecturer on dental surgery and pathology, and the value of his contributions to the education of the students cannot be overstated. As one of the dental surgeons to that institution, the young men intrusted to his care soon found in him a careful scientific teacher and skilful operator. In the extracting-room, the extraordinary facility with which, under proper circumstances, the "elevator" could be used was frequently demonstrated. As far as the writer has had the opportunity of seeing, this instrument has never been more adroitly employed than by Mr. Cartwright. From the first until the present time the office of treasurer to the medical staff has been filled by him, and always with business-like ability and urbanity.

When the testimonial to Mr. Tomes was decided upon, Mr. Cartwright was chairman of the committee for organising the presentation of the gift, and worked for its complete success in a most energetic and laudably unselfish spirit. It was an occasion when, with many, an entirely opposite disposition might have easily manifested itself; but Mr. Cartwright set himself entirely on one side, and with admirable disinterestedness laboured to focus all honour upon his brother practitioner. Those who were present at the public dinner which preceded the presentation, and subsequently listened to Mr. Cartwright's remarks prior to the gift being offered by him to Mr. Tomes, will not easily forget the manly sentiments and high praise which characterised his entire speech. Without the faintest tinge of flattery, he said all that could be said in testimony of the appreciation he and others felt of Mr. Tomes' efforts to benefit the profession, and said it, moreover, well.

In the same quiet, unselfish way Mr. Cartwright has worked whenever and wherever he could for the general benefit throughout the reform movement. If he could have his will, no retrograde step or compromise with those who may be content with present attainments should be made. He is a firm believer in a thorough professional education in every department. His motto may be said to be, "Onward and Upward." The high position which Mr. Cartwright deservedly occupies has been the result of steady persevering diligence. There has been no "royal road" with him, and consequently he has no faith in short cuts, or bye-paths either, in professional life.

As soon as the curriculum in connection with the licentiateship was established by the council of the College of Surgeons, the authorities at King's College Hospital took action, and determined to appoint a professor of dental surgery in their institution. Mr. Cartwright had for many years acted as dental surgeon at King's College Hospital, and the council were wise enough to appoint, and fortunate enough to secure, this gentleman to wear the professor's gown, and fill the professor's chair at their hospital. It was an honourable and exceptional post, and, it need hardly be added, was thoroughly well filled by Mr. Cartwright. King's College was to be congratulated on being the first to inaugurate such an office, and Mr. Cartwright on being so unhesitatingly chosen to it. In the year 1864 he was requested to deliver the usual introductory address on the opening of the session in October. The student of to-day would do well to take heed to the advice given then. The concluding remarks of that speech are sufficiently interesting, true, and instructive to bear quotation in this place, not only for the benefit of the young learner, but also as throwing a clear light upon Mr. Cartwright's character and sentiments. "If you," he said, "at the end of your probation have taken wise advantage of the opportunities for acquiring information, practical and otherwise, afforded you here and at the hospital, you will find that the terrors of examination will be softened, if not altogether lost upon you, and you will not be of the number of those who complain of questions put by, or the manner and address of, those who have to examine. But study terminates not with student life. As the youth at a bound changes to man, as he passes from school to college—where the sterner and real duties of life begin, of which his school days were but preparatory foreshadowings—so will you all find, when your work is ended here, the ordeal of examinations passed and diplomas and degrees obtained, that much is still to be learned; more, indeed, than could be learned in a life infinitely longer than that which is permitted us. Science never stands still, and never will be exhausted. Thousands of intellects have been at work, adding their mite to the great end of unravelling the mystery and difficulties which surround, and in making understandable the laws which rule this world of ours and all that is in it, upon it, and about it; and yet when they have succumbed to the immutable laws which in life they had been so busy endeavouring to comprehend, how much remains for those who succeed them to think upon, to discover, and to write about! Well may we exclaim, 'These are Thy glorious works, Parent of good, Almighty!' It is our mission to maintain and increase our store of knowledge, for our own good, and for the benefit of our fellow-men. In the endeavour to fathom the secret and mysterious phenomena which give life, vitality, and animation to all around us, and to arrive at a comprehension of inanimate things which are above, beneath, and about us, we are wending our way nearer to Him whose wisdom fashioned and arranged them all so perfectly as no human artificer ever fashioned anything. And when the day shall arrive when the hidden secrets shall be revealed—and it may be long ere such a revelation is permitted man—*will* the harmonious simplicity, which may probably be found to govern animate and inanimate creation, cause a doubt as to the majestic nature of the design, or on the divinity of the Designer? I cannot conceive a reason why the inquiry into natural laws and the endeavour to reconcile to our understanding things at present difficult or impossible of explanation, should tempt any one for a moment to doubt fundamental truths which have been handed down to us from age to age for ages, and which our instincts tell us must be true, and which alone can form the bulwark which ensure our happiness here, and give us hope for that which is to be hereafter. It can in no way improve or conduce to social happiness or the world's benefit to allow hasty theories or metaphysical speculations, which mark some modern investigations into the world's existence or prehistoric evidences of the origin of man and animals, to disturb our religious faith, or to bring down the majesty of the Most High to the level of the notions of earth. Doubts, indifference, or total disregard or disbelief, will not be likely to make man better, or tend to the fostering of those qualities which, from the highest sense, make us do and act well towards one another. No; let us all use the intellects God has given us to investigate to the utmost His works, for that is our province and our duty—a duty we owe Him, and in our sphere of science we owe to suffering humanity. But let me warn you never to be carried off your balance by any false notions or subtle doctrines, for they have surged to the surface periodically for centuries past, and been as often proved and condemned as worthless; or in an over-estimate of talent and eager search into material science, be tempted to lay aside belief or ignore religious responsibility; but ever remember that the one, properly estimated, will conduct nearer to the other. And let us one and all bear in our minds the significance attached to the three words which, in so small a sentence, convey so much meaning, and which constitute the college motto—*Sancte et sapienter.*"

This was, and still is, healthy food for young, and, to an extent, untainted minds. The dental profession is fortunate, and ought to consider itself happy, in having such a teacher in its midst, whose whole professional career has been an exemplification and practical illustration of the sentiments, which he thus courageously invited others to accept and apply.

Mr. Cartwright was duly appointed one of the examiners at the dental board of the Royal College of Surgeons, and, with faithfulness and kindness blended, performed his duties during the allotted term. Some time since he relinquished the lectureship at the London School of Dental Surgery, and also his post as dental surgeon at the Dental Hospital of London; but there is not another member of the profession more deeply interested in the daily progress achieved by the body at large, or more willing to give valuable assistance in promoting its true interests than he. Mr. Cartwright has done much, in his own unostentatious way, from the commencement of the movement which has resulted in the present recognised status and corresponding privilege as its sequence, and there can be no doubt whatever that he will continue to be its true and sincere friend as long as power and opportunity may last.

MR. DE MORGAN.

If patient continuance in well-doing be recognised in professional as in social life as an evidence of worth in the individual so acting, then no one who is or has been connected with the progress of dental reform, at least since the Dental Hospital of London was established, can hope to have a larger meed of grateful recognition clustering round his name than can Mr. Campbell De Morgan, unhappily for the medical and dental profession alike, now removed by death. This indefatigable and untiring friend to the latter body was first identified with it through his joint scientific examination on the structure of bone with Mr. Tomes. For many years past eminent as a surgeon, Mr. De Morgan came to be well known to the dentists of this country on account of his connection with the above-named hospital. He was the first appointed chairman of its managing committee in 1858, and with but a slight exception retained that post up to the time of his lamented decease. The amount of benefit that has thus been conferred upon the charity is not easy to calculate. The value of clear and comprehensive judgment in the direction of the affairs of a public hospital needs no enforcement. Safely to guide it through any and all crises it may be compelled to undergo is a by no means easy task. Conditions of this sort, the Dental Hospital, in common with all others, has had to sustain, and those who have held official positions in connection with it are fully aware of the permanent good which has accrued from the fact of Mr. De Morgan having been at the helm of affairs. His foresight and exemplary prudence were alone equalled by his assiduity and excellent qualification for direction. Men of high position in all the departments of science and art have ever and anon shown breadth of sympathy with the collateral branches of the profession with which they have been engaged, and, therefore, the fact that Mr. De Morgan gave so much time and attention to the Dental Hospital of London is not here mentioned on account of its singularity. The statement that he was so persistently helpful to this branch of surgery is made in order that his kindness thus manifested may be duly recorded, and that the dental profession may know that he was one of its substantial benefactors.

Mr. De Morgan was one of those quiet, unobtrusive workers in a good cause whose valuable assistance was of all the deeper worth from the method he employed in rendering it. The very opposite of so many who propose to confer benefit, but claim the sound of trumpet or some general recognition as they take each step, this worthy and generous-spirited friend gave time and influence, through a succession of years to an effort which could neither expect nor claim either the one or the other from him, contented with the conviction that he had been enabled to contribute to the success of an enterprise which he felt merited it. When the names of showy benefactors have faded from the memory, or perished altogether, that of Mr. De Morgan will be held in fresh and fragrant remembrance by all whose judgment is of any worth. His appearance at the committee of management of the Dental Hospital of London was always an occasion of warm and respectful greeting. His genial disposition invariably shed brightness all around him, while his quiet wit was always sure to tell. With marked urbanity, but with equal firmness, he directed the propositions and discussions coming before him in his official connection with that institution. His views on difficult questions were remarkable for their soundness, and under his presidency there was an admirably skilful pilotage of the hospital affairs.

In the conviction that he was enabled to contribute something to the success of this institution, he found both the stimulus to work and the satisfaction of labour. He was distinguished throughout his entire career by a peculiar reticence concerning himself; what might, indeed, be fairly called an unwillingness to do or say anything which might in an overt way contribute to his own advance—a sort of lethargy in regard to his personal interests. But what his friends could not succeed in inducing him to do in this direction, they had no trouble in effecting when the benefits accruing from his efforts would fall to the lot of others. Hence his unwearied exertions in connection with the dental profession. With such a leader as his close and familiar friend Mr. Tomes, he seemed to derive a constant pleasure in the work in which that gentleman was so ardently engaged.

The profession is indebted to Mr. Tomes for the influence he exercised upon Mr. De Morgan, and through which his co-operation was secured. That which still further enhanced the value of the aid he gave so cheerfully, and for so long a time, was the fact that his health was by no means strong. His conduct throughout was an instance and exemplification of a circumstance often seen, that where the vigorous and robust fail to confer any palpable and permanent benefit upon their generation, the feeble and weak frequently succeed simply by their self-denial and devotion. Every office and act which Mr. De Morgan undertook and performed was marked by the unaffected courtesy which distinguishes the true gentleman. However any sitting at the same council-table might feel constrained to differ from his views, no one could for a moment suspect or fear anything to offend the most sensitive spirit. It indeed was pleasant to watch his presidency in this direction, so different from many who, when " in the chair," make the authority of their position felt.

He was a warm supporter of Mr. Saunders in the matter of the transfer of the hospital, and in every other circumstance which seemed likely to promote its permanent efficiency. When Mr. De Morgan passed away for ever there was a feeling of deep sorrow in the hearts of all who had been privileged to know him.

MR. C. J. FOX.

Although Mr. Fox has taken an active part in dental affairs from the year 1856 up to the present time, his name is better known, perhaps, as that of the editor of "The British Journal of Dental Science" than in any other way. Mr. Fox lays claim to an hereditary connection with the medical profession, and, with a by no means unjustifiable pride, points to the fact that he is the eldest son of Charles James Fox, M.D., whose father and grandfather were also medical practitioners. When Mr. Rymer summoned the first meeting of the dental profession at the London Tavern, in September 1856, Mr. Fox was one of the members then present. He subsequently was elected to, and held the offices of curator and librarian to the College of Dentists of England, and was also chosen one of the honorary secretaries of that institution, in conjunction with Mr. Rymer and the author. When the Odontological Society of London was in process of formation, he was of the number of the first fifty gentlemen invited by the executive to associate themselves with it, and was duly elected a member. It is due to him to state, that as this invitation came to him at a time when he had already identified himself with the rival institute or college, he wrote a frank and explanatory letter to the council of the Odontological Society, setting forth his views concerning the objects and aims of the promoters of the Dental College, affirming his concurrence therewith, and expressing his wish to be connected with it as a thoroughly educational institution. His statements on this subject were considered by the Odontologists not to necessarily invalidate the proposed membership, and the result was his election by that society. Since that time Mr. Fox has served in the society as a member of the council, as honorary secretary during three years, and as honorary foreign secretary for the same term. Up to the time when the celebrated amalgamation question was brought forward, he fulfilled the offices allotted to him at the College of Dentists, and threw a considerable amount of energy into the departments he was called to superintend. When, however, the important attempt at union with the Odontological Society failed, and some sixty members of the Dental College resigned their connection with it, Mr. Fox identified himself with the seceders. From that moment he felt that the original intentions of the founders of the College of Dentists were being set aside by the council and the members together, and very zealously protested, on several occasions, against many of the acts of the college party, endeavouring by these means to test the legality of the various proceedings in Cavendish Square, and this to the utmost of his power. It is needless to say that, with this particular section of the profession, under such circumstances, Mr. Fox was in bad odour. He was very resolute, however, in the steps he then took. Not only by his personal public remonstrance in the midst of the college meetings, but also by protests printed in the "British Journal of Dental Science," and by pamphlets as well, he endeavoured continuously to neutralise the various acts of which he so loudly complained. It would be difficult to say how much or how little these efforts amounted to when considered as the instrumentalities of an individual member against the College of Dentists at that time. They served to make both the council and the members of the college think with more caution upon what was then being proceeded with, while the opposite party felt that internal dissension boded no good for the independent institution. One thing was very evident, namely, that Mr. Fox had decided views upon the matter then in hand, and, moreover, possessed sufficient determination to make them known. Eventually these attacks ceased, and when in due time the Dental Hospital of London was about to be founded, Mr. Fox became interested in it as a public charity and school of instruction to dental students, and when the managing committee of the hospital resolved upon appointing assistant dental surgeons to a place on its staff, Mr. Fox applied for that office, and was one of the first six gentlemen appointed. After some years of service in this subordinate capacity, he became one of the senior medical officers, which position he still retains. Not very long since Mr. Fox, believing that the full membership of the Royal College of Surgeons gave an improved social status to its possessor, submitted to the necessary examination, and obtained that degree. Although holding this distinction, he is, nevertheless, one of the most strenuous advocates of the licentiateship, which he maintains should be the first qualification sought for by the dental surgeon, as the truest evidence of the holder's fitness to practise as a dentist. Mr. Fox is a licentiate himself, having passed his examination at the Royal College of Surgeons to that end in the year of the inauguration of the degree (1860). He holds several public appointments, esteeming that of dental surgeon to the Great Northern Hospital—which he received on that charity coming into existence in 1856—and his present position as honorary secretary to the medical committee of that hospital very highly. The circumstance of a dentist acting in the latter capacity is certainly rare, if not absolutely unique, among the hospital arrangements of the metropolis.

Throughout the many phases which the reform movement has taken, Mr. Fox has invariably had his place and position, which, if not so prominent as some, have been nevertheless very useful. He has willingly given both time and energy to promote the cause in hand and the prospective and permanent benefit of his professional brethren, and considering that he labours, unfortunately, under more than one physical difficulty, the activity he has displayed, and the amount of work he has been able to accomplish, must be accounted all the more creditable to him. His pen has not been suffered to be idle, for he has used it on several occasions, publishing his views upon passing subjects in pamphlets issued from time to time, as he considered necessary and useful to others around him.

Mr. Fox has also edited the "Transactions of the Odonto-Chirurgical Society of Edinburgh" since the establishment of that society. It is now several years ago that he succeeded to the management, and eventually to the proprietorship, of the " British Journal of Dental Science." With the columns of this periodical at his disposal and under his control, he has availed himself of them as channels or avenues by which he could state his views to his readers at least. He has been ever ready to champion the cause of charity where there has been a necessity for its practical exemplification — and instances in this direction have not been absent — or when suggestions and counsels in its administration have been wanting. As has been stated elsewhere, the purpose of the author has been not to include any mention of the "Manchester Movement," as it is familiarly called, and, therefore, Mr. Fox's part in that movement is not alluded to here. Journalism, with which Mr. Fox is so closely identified, will be found under review in the closing chapter of this work, and, therefore, that subject is not further noticed in this short sketch. It will be sufficient, perhaps, to say here, that in Mr. Fox the dental profession in this country has a warm and earnest friend, and to the extent of his power he has proved his willingness to serve, through a succession of years, in the endeavour to promote the best interests of his brother practitioners. While all may not approve or endorse his several views and acts, none can deny him the tribute of a strong desire to help forward the beneficial cause of substantial and real reform in the dental profession.

MR. W. A. HARRISON.

It was on the occasion of the meeting of the founders of the Dental Hospital of London at the Medical Society's rooms that the author first met Mr. Harrison. His tall, spare figure and extremely courteous demeanour were very impressive. Even his dress was noticeable—adopting, as he did, the straight-cut coat with its broad roll collar of the time of George IV. When he addressed his brethren in the profession, his language was well chosen, strictly correct in general and scientific phraseology, sometimes didactic, and always precise. Although full as to his matter, he avoided verbosity, habitually spoke to the point, and scrupulously avoided pedantry and display. Whenever he rose he always commanded the immediate attention of his audience, and was invariably listened to with the patience and respect he so fully deserved. Peculiarly thoughtful, his forecast and prudence displayed themselves on every occasion. No one could convict him of loose or speculative ideas. What he advanced was invariably the result of close study or well-attested experience, and his counsel could always be relied upon for soundness. One who knew him gave the writer the idea that he would find him in official matters tedious to deal with. This, however, so far as his experience went—and it was very considerable—never once proved true. When seated at the council or committee table, he ever proved a kind and courteous adviser; and no one could be brought into contact with Mr. Harrison without feeling that he was in the presence of a highly-educated gentleman. He had much to do with the drafting or otherwise preparing the various documents which came under the notice of the profession in connection with the Odontological Society and the Dental Hospital of

London, and in all of these might be clearly traced the impress of his careful and thoughtful mind. His notions of order and correctness amounted, perhaps, at times, to punctiliousness. If that can be considered a fault, assuredly it was a good one, especially under such circumstances as starting new and altogether untried institutions. His opinion and advice upon many matters were frequently sought, and a large amount of correspondence consequently came before him. Woe to the writer of any manuscript intended to meet the public eye who used a comma instead of a semicolon, or flourished his flowers of rhetoric before his eyes. One dash of his pen disposed, in a moment, of all redundancy and rhodomontade. A ruthless cutting down of all superfluity was the invariable result in any faulty sheet submitted to his critical consideration. He was patient to listen to any and all reasons why this or that sentence should stand as written, but if he thought such reasons unsound, never hesitated, kindly but faithfully, to adduce his own for its abandonment. Whatever he suggested or proposed was always introduced with true and becoming modesty, and the result generally was a willing deference to his judgment.

As an instance of his frankness the following circumstance may be mentioned. It had fallen to the writer, as honorary secretary to the Dental Hospital managing committee, to correct an erroneous statement which appeared in the public press concerning that institution. The letter sent had been despatched between the sittings of the committee, and, therefore, on the occasion of its next meeting it had to be read for the approval, or otherwise, of those present. Being very fatigued at the time, the writer imagines the reading may have been somewhat slovenly. Mr. Harrison, in his turn, spoke concerning its purport ; and his opening remarks were to the effect that he congratulated the committee on the letter sent to the journal in question—" a letter," he added, " infinitely better written than *read*." A quiet look towards the individual alluded to, and a good-natured smile, effectually disarmed one of any irritation likely to be produced. The kindly criticism was doubtless both true and just. Not only was Mr. Harrison's judgment valuable, but his unsparing trouble and willing sacrifice of time also were of great worth.

For some years he was part proprietor of the "British Journal of Dental Science," and he cheerfully devoted both time and labour towards making that publication a success. One day out of the seven in each week was invariably set apart for the purpose of carefully going over the various papers and contributions to its pages, correcting errors, and making the "copy" ready for the printer's hand. Those who, like the writer, had to meet him for the purpose of projecting any new arrangement, or modifying or carrying out the plans already in existence, could not but notice his sagacity and excellent common sense.

In his turn Mr. Harrison occupied the honourable post of president of the Odontological Society; and his year of office was characterised by the stately and dignified conduct necessary to the fulfilment of the proper duties of the chair. Every one felt that his ardent love for order would secure a series of sittings wherein each member would have ample opportunity given him for the due expression of his opinions upon any subject before the meeting, while his scientific and thoroughly practical knowledge would effectually prevent discussion from drifting into the region of the frivolous, or desultory chit-chat. To say that he was not only earnest but ardent in the promulgation of every measure having for its object the advancement and elevation of the profession is to assert the merest truth. His unremitting attention, for years, was cheerfully given to every subject which was connected with the society and the hospital alike, and to the last he was of the number of those who laboured energetically for success in both these directions. The true charm in all real labour was distinctly manifested in his entire career, namely, unostentatiousness. Mr. Harrison never once evinced a desire to thrust himself in front, but when called to that rank and place, he occupied it willingly and with modesty.

For some time after the lamented decease of his friend and colleague, Mr. Arnold Rogers, Mr. Harrison held the office of treasurer to the Odontological Society. He was one of the first elected dental surgeons to the Dental Hospital, and the students there at that time had every reason to be grateful for the instruction he was so ready and pleased to impart. His pride and ambition were to lay the foundation of things both deep and strong. Although he was aware that much of such effort, both on his own part and that of other real friends to the movement, would be doomed to remain unseen hereafter, he nevertheless freely worked in this all-important direction with admirable zeal. The younger members of our profession, who are now in the enjoyment of the privileges which the improved condition of things has brought to them, must be told, and invited ever to remember, that to Mr. Harrison and his unflagging assiduity they are deeply indebted.

In whatever position Mr. Harrison was placed, whether as examiner at the dental board of the Royal College of Surgeons, president of the Odontological Society, treasurer of the same, trustee and dental surgeon to the Dental Hospital of London, or connected, as he was, with the management and proprietary of the "British Journal of Dental Science," his energy and disinterested devotion to the cause of professional progress were remarkable. His decease, therefore, can only be accounted as a very severe loss. The writer most willingly testifies to the worth of the late Mr. Harrison as a coadjutor and friend, knowing as he does, from his intimate association with him in so many departments of varied labours for the durable benefit of the profession, that his valuable assistance was of the highest order. Over and again, when in private and friendly intercourse with him, he had the fullest opportunity of realising the deep interest which Mr. Harrison felt in the progress of dental reform, and with what anxiety he watched the different indications of success or failure in the steps which were being taken towards securing for his brother practitioners, and especially the younger members, a substantial and elevated status. There was no occasion, when his counsel or co-operation were required, that he refused to yield them; and with the greatest cheerfulness he would work out dry, and, to many, distasteful details of the plans then in hand. His place at the committee of management at the Dental Hospital of London was never vacant, except, indeed, when illness precluded him from taking it; and those who had occasion to meet him there felt that his presence and support were a distinct gain, especially when difficult measures were before them.

He was peculiarly apt at logical sequences, and that which in any proposition did not bear the trace of a due effect being likely to follow upon a given cause he made short work with, dismissing it from the region of argument as a waste of valuable time. On the other hand, no one could be more patient in investigation, or more moderate in discussing any subject under consideration. If he erred, it was in the direction of a too close and critical sifting of all that constituted the case in hand. This caution told against him with the more impulsive around the table; but one of the results of Mr. Harrison's many decisions was, that what he had advised or effected required little or no alteration, and never needed to be done over again. Mr. Tomes, in alluding to him in his second inaugural address, has remarked that he "was born for public work," and this is a concise but correct description of him. Certain it is that, throughout the earlier stages of the reform movement, when every step needed to be taken with the utmost caution, few men could have been found to do either the kind of work, or the amount of it, which Mr. Harrison did so willingly, and, withal, so well.

MR. R. HEPBURN.

Throughout the entire effort to raise the status of the dental profession, and among its truest workers and supporters, there has been no more candid worker, and no more sincere and disinterested coadjutor, than Mr. Robert Hepburn. This warm-hearted friend to the dental body was among the number of those who attended the public meeting called by Mr. Rymer in September 1856. He was deeply interested in the steps then proposed to be taken, and cordially identified himself with the college movement. A seat at the council was accorded to him, and the wisdom of this course was soon manifested by the excellent advice and moderate but sound counsels he was at all times so ready to offer. During the many discussions on the multiplied and various subjects which were brought before the council, Mr. Hepburn was always to be relied upon in advocating such a course as would ensure the advance of the profession without endangering its dignity either socially or otherwise. That which savoured of rashness, or had a tendency to set aside the just claims of the less-favoured members of the body, Mr. Hepburn steadily and calmly opposed. While that which was illiberal met with a distinct protest from him, there was never the least occasion to fear that he would support any measure which, either in its letter or spirit, would lead to the acknowledgment of the unprofessional. He ever desired to make the very best of such opportunities as were then occurring to secure for the profession which he had so long and honourably practised all the benefits which, through patient and properly sustained effort and enterprise, could be obtained. His appearance, therefore, in his proper place was always welcomed; and those who laboured with him in those early days of hard work and self-denial felt their hands strengthened by his presence and kindly spirit. His influence was cheerfully lent to every just and honourable course, and no one who was associated with him could avoid feeling that his permanent and persistent desire was so to act that, in after years, each step then taken could be recalled to memory and reflected upon without self-censure or chagrin.

The aspect of dentistry prior to the plan proposed by Mr. Rymer was a great discomfort to him, and he therefore very willingly lent his aid to what he conceived was a very laudable attempt to place it on a proper footing. He was one of those who considered an independent institution was not only possible, but highly beneficial. As the scheme in its earlier career developed, Mr. Hepburn felt sure that by its ultimate completion an opportunity would be given to the future dentist of qualifying himself properly to practise in this useful and honourable department of surgery. No one more than he realised the degradation which dentistry was suffering from by the want of accurate knowledge by those who had so largely entered its ranks, and none more than he felt the reflection upon all true practitioners which comes from the impudent assumption of the charlatan. His advocacy, therefore, was always strongly for education. That which seemed to him the true remedy for the many evils apparent to all, was a full acquaintance on the part of every dentist with the principles on which dental practice, in its highest and truest sense, should be conducted.

With these views he energetically associated himself with those who felt with him in the joint effort to establish the College of Dentists of England, that being in his opinion the best method of the hour for their practical realisation.

In due time, when the amalgamation of the two societies was under consideration, Mr. Hepburn was unanimously chosen as one of the college delegates to negotiate that important measure. The council of the college and the members generally were confident that in his hands their honour and their interests would be inviolably secure. Whatever course events might take, there was no reason to doubt that that which was beneficial, just, and to the point, would have in him a most strenuous advocate. Mr. Hepburn was not a member of the Royal College of Surgeons, but as a practical and successful member of the profession he was fully qualified to speak on all vital questions, and fitly represent the large number of dentists who practised without the diploma of that body. The rejection of the terms which had been arrived at, and duly submitted to the College of Dentists, left him and his colleagues no other choice than to resign, with them, his official position. The failure in the attempt which he and they had made was a great disappointment to him; he justly considering that it was the only opportunity likely ever to occur for the mutual blending of the divided interests of the profession. His services, however, were fortunately not to be lost. By a very natural process Mr. Hepburn became associated with the Odontological Society, which, under the circumstances, he believed would eventually bring about that order of things for which from the first he had been contending. He foresaw that the Dental College, deprived as it soon was of a large number of influential supporters by the adverse vote on the amalgamation question, would ultimately fail to command the support of the profession. It was evident to him that the success of the Odontological Society's scheme, as set forth in the celebrated memorial, was simply a matter of time.

Although not agreeing with the memorialists in the manner in which they had endeavoured to obtain the ear of the council of the College of Surgeons, he yet preferred using such means as were likely to secure the important educational advantages their plan proposed. If those advantages could not be obtained by an independent institution, rather than sacrifice them he would identify himself with another method. This he accordingly did when the proper opportunity offered itself. Through all the various stages which, since the year 1856, the dental profession has been called to pass, he has taken an active and influential part. No time or energy which he has had to bestow have been withheld by him. Hardly one occasion when the dental body has been called together has he been absent, and the opinions he has had to offer have ever been such as every gentleman wishing well to the practitioner of dentistry has been glad to hear and accept. He was one of the founders of the Dental Hospital of London, has sat frequently on the committee of management, and was elected to the office of Dental Surgeon and Lecturer on Mechanical Dentistry from the first. In both these departments Mr. Hepburn admirably filled his post. As lecturer on the above-mentioned subject no one could have been better selected than he. With an immense experience in this department, and with a most pleasant method of imparting instruction, the students, during his term of office, had abundant cause for thankfulness as from themselves, and of congratulation by others. His comprehensive lectures were followed up regularly by practical demonstrations in mechanical dentistry. At his suggestion the upper rooms of the hospital were fitted up as a laboratory, and there, with his own private assistant to aid him, he called the young men together around him, and personally instructed them in all the departments of the dental workroom. He ever held that the student should pass a definite term at the bench. A most skilful workman himself, he knew the great value of an adroit use of the tools and instruments of the laboratory. He aimed at perfecting his pupils in the correct manipulation of the materials before them, and if they did not succeed in producing artificial dentures of the best construction, and wrought upon the truest principles of mechanism, it could not be said that they lacked the necessary opportunity and teaching. At considerable personal and pecuniary expense he placed within the students' reach every article with which they had to become familiar, and led them forward in all the details of true mechanical dentistry.

It was a pleasant sight for any friend to the profession to go and see these gatherings at Soho Square. The young men, attired in true workman fashion, were actively engaged in every conceivable part of dental work. Metal, bone, vulcanite, each and all in turn were placed before them, and some very admirable results were from time to time presented as the effect of their skill and his supervision and direction. To Mr. Hepburn all this was a labour of love. Nothing seemed to give him more pleasure or real gratification than witnessing these embryo dentists endeavouring to perfect themselves in their art. His sentiment appeared to be "Knowledge is not how much is known, but how much is thoroughly understood." He strove with a ready cheerfulness to impart instruction in such a way that the learner might be able, not only to work well, but also intelligently. The result of his connection with the students at the hospital was a feeling on their part of more than respect for such a teacher. On his part there was a constant and unvarying demonstration of the deepest interest in their progress. The warm shake of the hand with each and all whenever they met, and the readiness which was so constantly evinced to answer any question on the subject before them in the most practical way as those inquiries were put to him, served to knit together both teacher and taught in the pleasantest of bonds.

A prominent characteristic in Mr. Hepburn is his belief in the power for good which lies in the direction of social intercourse. Singularly free from all ostentatiousness, he is always ready to mingle with those who have not yet trodden the path of experience, and cheerfully to impart to them out of his knowledge acquired by many years of practice. It may be safely said that no young man has ever applied to him for guidance in professional matters without receiving, both promptly and fully, that which he sought. The united testimony of all who have had to meet Mr. Hepburn in these relationships is to prove that he is not only a thoroughly capable instructor, but a friend to every honest and honourable practitioner. As soon as the charter of the Royal College of Surgeons had been altered so as to admit dentists to examination, he submitted himself to the new ordeal, and received his degree. This same proof of efficiency he, with many others, has firmly held to be the distinguishing mark of capability for every dentist. Whilst not ignoring any other distinction, he affirms, and rightly, that the licentiateship in dental surgery should be first possessed, whatever else may follow.

For many years Mr. Hepburn was chairman of the medical staff at the Dental Hospital of London, and under his genial and prudent guidance the affairs of that department have been conducted in the most pleasant and profitable manner. From the time that several gentlemen, who had formerly been on the executive of the College of Dentists, thought it best to secede from that institution and join the Odontological Society, his connection with the latter has been unbroken. Mr. Hepburn has sat at its council, been on the list of vice-presidents, and in the year 1870 was called to the honourable position of president.

Throughout the entire movement in the direction of professional reform, he has steadily laboured for union and advance. Division and strife have been to him a source of unfeigned regret; and whosoever seeks to loosen the ties already effected, or by whatever means the bonds of union are sought to be shaken, neither the individual nor the purpose can ever hope to receive sympathy from him. The abandonment of the Licentiates' annual dinner was a matter of regret to Mr. Hepburn, for he ever felt it to be an opportunity for the renewal of old friendships, and the pleasant formation of new ones, among a profession which, by its constitution, does not possess a redundancy of means whereby practitioners can personally become known to one other.

His kindly disposition has more than once shown itself towards the students at the hospital by his generously entertaining them at his own house. He availed himself of these opportunities to speak to the young men on the duties of professional life, giving them much excellent counsel as to what should characterise honourable practice, and encouraging them to persevere diligently in their studies, that they might be thoroughly qualified to fill the various positions to which they might eventually be called. Having had to contend with the disagreeableness which beset the profession when it was in its isolated and subsequently divided state, Mr. Hepburn is one of those who heartily rejoice in its altered and amended condition. He has made sacrifices to enable him to take his part—which has been no mean one—in the general advance; and no one can outvie him in the desire to see dentistry in this country thoroughly consolidated in the elevated position to which it is fairly entitled. The writer can say that with Mr. Hepburn he has passed some of the happiest hours, both in private and official life, and that in a very large circle of professional friends he is highly and deservedly respected.

MR. J. H. PARKINSON.

The name of Parkinson, as it stands connected with the practice of dentistry, is one of the oldest, if not actually the oldest, in the profession. This worthy member of a thoroughly worthy and highly-respected family of dentists had long been in practice when his name began to stand forth more prominently on account of his public association with the reform movement. Although representing the "old school," he had sagacity enough to perceive the indications of progress, and energy sufficient unhesitatingly to identify himself with it. He set an example in this direction which it would have been well for some others at that time to have followed. Mr. Parkinson was not a member of the Royal College of Surgeons, doubtless from reasons cogent enough to himself, but he was one of the signataries of the celebrated memorial, his name standing at the foot of that document next to that of the late Mr. Cartwright. His deep interest in the result of that petition was evinced on all occasions when the meetings connected with it were held; and no sooner did the College of Surgeons grant the request therein contained, and open its doors to dental practitioners, than he came forward, on the first day when examination was to be held, and submitted to the ordeal. At that time the addition of such a name was of great value, showing as it did his hearty concurrence in the new *régime*, and exemplifying his faith in the beneficial results so likely to accrue from it. The writer remembers the fact of this step on Mr. Parkinson's part being pointed to and quoted as a stimulus to the hesitating and faint-hearted. When, in due course, the Dental Hospital of London was established, Mr. Parkinson became, by unanimous request, the treasurer of that institution, which office he filled to the time of his much-regretted decease, with all the courtesy coupled with business ability which was to be expected from him. Of a singularly modest spirit, and quiet, kindly heart, those who had the pleasure and privilege of association with him felt constrained to show him the greatest respect. He was verily worthy of it. His long standing in the profession, together with the position accorded to him there, secured for him a deferential hearing whenever he had a communication to make to his brethren, and all alike felt that the true interests of the profession were safe in his hands. The author had many opportunities of knowing Mr. Parkinson's views on the subject of the profession's prospects of advance, about which he entertained no doubt. Whenever it was possible for him to take part in any of the meetings held for this purpose, he did not fail to unite with his brethren; and although fully sharing the views of the party with which he had identified himself, he still spoke kindly of the other side, and had firm faith that sooner or later the general confusion and conflict of opinion which for so long prevailed would eventuate in a clearer atmosphere, and a distinct benefit to every honourable practitioner. In the year 1858 Mr. Parkinson was called to the president's chair of the Odontological Society, and his term of office was marked with both urbanity and efficiency in the post thus filled by him. Up to the time of his decease, which took place in 1865, he fully associated himself with the strenuous efforts to improve the status of the profession he had so long and successfully practised, and to the end of his career was acknowledged and felt to be a true, disinterested, and warm-hearted friend to all around him. He lived to see the pacification of the opposing parties in the amalgamation of the College of Dentists with the Odontological Society, and fully shared in the general feeling of contentment which that event produced.

MR. JAMES ROBINSON.

More than once this gentleman's name has been mentioned in connection with the dental reform movement, and in referring to it again specifically there is a difficulty in selecting a characteristic to begin with. Mr. Robinson was one of those men who have much of the paradoxical about them. Hence he puzzled many who were not actually in the closest association with him. He possessed a fiery temper, yet he could stop in the streets and stoop to relieve a little child crying in its poverty and distress. He had the most resolute of wills, yet he was open to conviction, and could be guided by those who knew how to exercise prudence with their counsel. The practice of his profession was pursued by him with all the energy and ardour of one who made gold the great idol of his heart, nevertheless, possessing ample means, as the result of his indefatigable industry, few could vie with him in liberality, and none could surpass him in the joy springing from hospitality or any act of benevolence. There are those still living who can testify to the cordial welcome he frequently extended to them as brother practitioners when sitting at his well-spread table. To see him hurrying into town from his charming home at Kenton, near Harrow, during the season, he might have been fairly classed as the keenest of business men, one to whom occupation afforded the only congenial method of spending the whole of his time; but throughout the entire profession it may be doubted whether one could be found who put off the harness at the close of the day more eagerly, or enjoyed the freedom from the demands of practice with more boyish hilarity than he. His position had been for a long time an acknowledged one, but he did not—as some have done—repudiate the means by which he had attained it. He frankly spoke to his immediate friends upon the way which he had taken, and how he had been able to succeed in elevating himself to what he then was. To the writer, at least, he often opened his heart, and, if it were necessary, much of the struggle of his early days could be given here in minute detail. Certainly his path had not been strewn with flowers.

Mr. Robinson had succeeded in obtaining a *clientelle* which included persons of the highest rank, but he nevertheless thought of, and acted kindly to, the humbler classes, whether in his profession or out of it. It could not be said that it was the abundance or the brilliancy of his talents which secured him so much success. He had neither the one nor the other of these. It was rather the diligent use of the moderate qualities which he possessed that brought his name so prominently to the front. In this respect he was an example which the young aspirant to a recognised professional position may hopefully imitate. As a rule, he was quick to perceive what he considered his opportunity, and equally prompt to take advantage of, and act upon it, with all the force he had at his command. Mr. Robinson was a good dentist, and knew it, but was not reticent on the subject of how he had been helped in his career. Conversing on this on one occasion at the writer's house, he took the opportunity of describing a difficult case for gold filling, and then said, "Now, Hill, if you cannot make such a plug as that, I am not the least surprised: there was a time when I could not have done it to save my life; but I can do it now, and if you choose to learn, I will show you how to do it too. The truth is, an American dentist taught me to put in gold plugs; ever since I have been very thankful to him for his instruction, and I do not hesitate to tell you where I got it." This was a candid and manly admission.

Mr. Robinson was an eager searcher after information, and was glad to obtain it, from whatever quarter it came.

His frankness in investigating, and then giving his opinion on any case before him, were noticeable features in his character. If some considered it correct to throw a veil of mystery over their proceedings in practice—press their fingers on their lips, knit their brows, fix their gaze on nothing, and appear profoundly thoughtful—to give a fictitious importance to the case in hand, not so with him. He was free to explain all that needed explanation,—tell how, why, and where, and make himself the personal friend of the patient seeking his assistance. Nor was he lacking in judgment or practical skill in conducting difficult cases to a successful result.

As has been already mentioned, Mr. Robinson made an effort in the year 1842 to introduce a new order of things in the profession, but failed. He inaugurated a journal called the "Forceps," the first number of which appeared in January 1844. This was a mistake. The spirit manifested in its pages was satirical, and in many instances offensively personal. There appeared from time to time short biographical sketches of some of the then leading dentists, which were more caricatures than delineations of character, and were altogether to be condemned. The "Forceps" could never have achieved any good, and was calculated to irritate many, and produce much hostile feeling against the writer. Happily, the journal had but a short existence; yet it lived long enough to bring about a spirit of antagonism to Mr. Robinson from many quarters, from which he suffered for years afterwards. To this cause, perhaps, and this all but alone, was to be attributed the isolated position Mr. Robinson held among his brother practitioners. It is pleasant to learn that, though tardy in its appearance, yet at last regret on his part concerning this journal came not only certainly, but with force to Mr Robinson's mind.

On one occasion, when the writer was spending an evening in his company at his house at Kenton, the subject was alluded to.

"I have written," said Mr. Robinson, "many silly things in my time, and I am afraid many unjust things too. As to the 'Forceps,' I heartily wish I had never had anything to do with it; and I should like to know that not a single copy of it was now in existence."

It was very evident that he felt the utter inutility of the method he had employed to compass the result intended; and, furthermore, that he realised, by a disagreeable experience, that the pen which is dipped in gall sooner or later becomes an instrument to wound the conscience of him who uses it.

This subject is reluctantly introduced, but it permits the revelation of the truth that Mr. Robinson was sorry for his sin. This fact may have been communicated to others, but the author has never heard that it was.

Allusion has been made to the commencement of Mr. Robinson's efforts in direct connection with the reform movement. Whether as first president of the College of Dentists, or in any other capacity, he displayed a remarkable amount of energy. His inaugural address was undoubtedly clever, and showed considerable acquaintance with the history of dentistry in the long past. The delegates chosen by the Odontological Society to represent that side of the profession had no fault to find with him as a representative of the opposite party. He was thoroughly in earnest when he fought for the College name, but contact with his brethren had the usual influence upon him as upon others, and led him courteously to listen to the expressed sentiments of those who differed from him. He believed that the conclusions arrived at by the chosen delegates of the two contending bodies were the best that could be then obtained, and hence his resignation from the official position he had been holding with the College party when those conclusions were nullified by the adverse vote in Cavendish Square.

His subsequent conduct in not only returning to the College of Dentists, but in accepting office there, created some surprise; but only those who knew his disposition were capable of divining his reasons for so acting. There can be no question that, whatever other motive was then operating, his ardent love for prominence and influence was not extinguished, or indeed extinguishable. When the step had once been taken, he seemed animated with fresh devotion to his former College acquaintances, and resolved to show that he would do his best to promote their interests. Certainly the students there should not lack incentive to work heartily, if, by offering prizes to the most meritorious of them, he could stimulate them to close application in their studies. Hence his generosity in this direction.

His desire to carry out his own views led him to inaugurate the National Dental Hospital; but the method he employed in getting quit of his position in and connection with the Dental Hospital of London, to say the least, was not to be admired, and many considered it altogether inexcusable. When, however, he had formed the resolution to take action in that direction, his force of character, as usual, displayed itself. With unremitting ardour he set about the new enterprise, and left nothing undone that could be accomplished to compass his ends. The institution in Great Portland Street was very largely indebted to Mr. Robinson, not only for its establishment, but also for its support. He gained for it many adherents and subscribers, and took the liveliest interest in its success. The Metropolitan School of Dental Science was also taken up by him, and assisted to the extent of his power.

To a large number of his brother practitioners the energy he displayed, especially in these latter directions, appeared to be dictated by a spirit of opposition. His capriciousness deprived him of the countenance of many who could not but admit the great zeal and love of work which he so constantly displayed. No enterprise with which he was connected could ever flag in his presence; but there can be no doubt that his lack of judgment on many occasions outbalanced his activity, and liberality as well.

What result a longer association with those who were working for the general advance of the profession might have produced upon his habit of thought and mode of action it is difficult to predict; but up to the time of his lamented death Mr. Robinson had not succeeded in winning the esteem and securing the co-operation of many of the leading dentists of his day. To some he appeared an enigma, to others his impulsive nature presented a formidable obstacle to concerted action, and thus, while drawing to him those of a kindred spirit, he nevertheless repelled all those whose temperament was opposed to vehement, resolute action, and there were many at that time—perhaps too many—who could be brought under this particular classification. His death, which was purely accidental, and took place at his country house at Kenton, cut short a career which no doubt would have been useful, and robbed the profession of one whose mind would, doubtless, have felt sooner or later the change which prolonged contact with other minds is so sure to produce. His principal influence for the general good was exerted at the commencement of the reform movement, when, as has been already mentioned, he courageously stood where others either declined or feared to stand. It is, indeed, very questionable, whether the College of Dentists of England would have been able to take the firm position it did in its earlier days but for him. As a private and personal friend, James Robinson exceeded in kindness, of which the writer had many undeniable proofs; and his death, so sudden and lamentable, was very keenly felt both by him and many of his professional brethren besides.

MR. ARNOLD ROGERS.

The subject of this notice, like many others, was not originally educated for the dental profession. Endowed with many excellent qualities, and gifted with a clear and intelligent mind, when he at length turned his attention to the profession he subsequently and for so many years practised, he soon acquired an acknowledged position, and won for himself universal esteem. His frank and genial disposition, together with his courteous and dignified bearing, attracted many to him, and his circle of friends and admirers was, consequently, a very large one. When he had once espoused dentistry his entire energy was given to practise it upon the highest principles. In the second chapter of this work his name is found in connection with the attempted reformation of the year 1843. The evidence is there given of his strong desire to do all that lay in his power in that direction; could he but have carried out that enterprise, even alone, his will was to achieve it, and none more than he felt grieved at its ultimate collapse. During the agitation dating from 1856, Mr. Rogers worked heartily and continuously with the party whose views he considered most likely to obtain the best interests, and secure the best and most permanent results for the dental profession. There was no lukewarmness in his service. What he did was done heartily and with excellent judgment, while his kindly spirit was distinguishable from first to last. He regretted that there were those around him who felt tamely in the matter, and condemned those who could, but would not, work in the good cause.

As an evidence of Mr. Rogers' deep interest in the

affairs of the profession, and as a specimen of his earnest spirit the following letter is introduced:—

"16 HANOVER SQUARE, *December* 3rd, 1861.

"DEAR MR. HEPBURN,—First, as Mr. Twyning's old traveller used to say, 'to business.' Thank you for your cheque for you and your friends' subscription. I send you an acknowledgment for each; you may wish to enclose a scrap; but I am sorry that we have lost Mr. W——— and Mr. O———. I cannot afford to lose members, or my balance-sheet will tell badly against me. However, I have £500 in hand, and as the publishing committee have had near £200 this year, we have no reason to complain. Hereafter the library committee will pull upon me I suppose. Never mind that; we shall have something to show for it, and also something worth seeking by the members. Now, having disposed of that part of my business, let me assure you how comforting a thing it is to me that my brethren are all so kind and well disposed to me as an individual member of the profession. It reconciles me very much to the long five months' solitude of my winter ailing-months: but I long to be amongst you, and am as anxious to hear how every meeting and everything goes off as if my bread depended upon it: it is, in fact, a necessary part of my existence. I could have wished, and did wish, to partake of your hospitality—it went off gloriously I hear. It is the commencement of a new era in our science. The great responsibility of the teachers and officers towards the pupils and patients is, I have no doubt, a source of contemplation for your daily thoughts. The benefit to patients, the advantages, so bountiful, to the pupils, but, above all, what are you not doing for the future public? Why the public, aye, the rich public, will, in after times, be most profited by the movement. They will have young men well qualified to practise, instead of as formerly. Then a man began to know a little just as he was leaving the world. I hear that you have a goodly number of pupils entered. Good speed to you! And, forsooth, we have another Dental Hospital! If it be as well conducted as yours, then I say it will be a boon also; for if ours were to go on at the rate of the last three years, it would be impossible to do with your present staff—if even with your present accommodation. The more I reflect upon Mr. Robinson's measures, the more I am bothered to know what more *he* would desire to be done than we have accomplished; and, also, why he could not have taken his proper position with us as others have done, and so formed one substantial and united body. I cannot understand him, but I pity him. Now, farewell! Thank you for much kindness, and believe me, my dear Mr. Hepburn, yours very sincerely,

ARNOLD ROGERS."

Such a letter not only reflects credit upon Mr. Rogers' straightforward views of the business demands of the society of which he was the treasurer, but also proves his deep anxiety concerning its progress, and the means by which that could be secured. As to the warmth of his generous disposition, too much could not be easily said. To those who had the privilege and the pleasure of his acquaintance this characteristic was positively paramount. Whoever might elect to be cool or indifferent to the forward movement of the profession, this genial-spirited friend could not do so. His heart was palpably thrown into the efforts being made for the general good, and his interest therein was simply unceasing. Quiet, but very telling instances of his generosity have come to the author's knowledge, which, if related, would further prove that something more than mere sentiment actuated him throughout.

Whenever his state of health permitted, Mr. Rogers was present at the council of the Odontological Society and the Dental Hospital committee meetings, where his good sense was invariably shown, while the urbanity and courteousness of his manners greatly endeared him to all with whom he acted. When the attempt to improve the status of the profession was being made in the year 1843, Mr. Rogers not only manifested a noticeable anxiety for its success, but took, with Mr. Tomes, the most active part in endeavouring to bring to a practical issue the scheme which lay before him. It is almost needless to say that its failure was to him a great disappointment, if not a positive grief. His hope, however, did not once fail him; and when the subject was subsequently revived, we find him appearing on the scene, with renewed ardour and enlarged experience, ready to take that part in affairs which his brethren considered most advisable. His time, influence, and purse, were all pressed into service, and placed so as to be available when and where they might be required. His sympathy with the less fortunate members of the profession was very strong.

The author, at Mr. Rogers' invitation, spent many evenings in the winter time with him at his house in Hanover Square, and had full opportunities of knowing his thoughts upon such subjects. Although never reticent, yet on these occasions he spoke with great freedom, and related, with evident feeling, his own early career, and touched upon many things which could not be mentioned under the more formal circumstances of official interviews. It was on one of these occasions the author took the opportunity of submitting to him a scheme which he had been projecting for the formation of a "Benevolent Institution," for the purpose of providing means of support for aged or infirm members of the profession, or those who by sudden affliction could not continue in practice. Mr. Rogers not only listened to the proposal, but warmly entered into the project, but considered the idea at that moment a little inopportune. "My dear Hill," he said, "you must put your plans into your pocket for the present; not but that the thing is right enough, but the profession is not ripe for it just yet. We may fairly hope to see it carried out by and bye; now, however, it would be expecting too much." * His intense interest was concentrated on what had then been originated, and although evidently prepared to second and support such a scheme, he was fearful lest in attempting too much we should fail in other things.

It was after a meeting at the Medical Society's rooms in George Street, Hanover Square, in the year 1858, that he threw open his house for the meetings of the provisional committee of the newly-determined-upon Dental Hospital of London. The founders of that charity gathered together there, Mr. Rogers generally presiding, and under his hospitable roof the fundamental laws were carefully considered, and eventually framed for working purposes. It was on one of these occasions that, in discussing what were the necessary views to be held by gentlemen qualified to hold office in the charity, that a good friend to the profession and an excellent representative man, Mr. A. J. Woodhouse, was lost to the institution. By a rigid insisting upon absolute allopathic views by Mr. W. A. N. Cattlin, as the *sine qua non* with all concerned in the management of the Dental Hospital, Mr. Woodhouse felt that he was ineligible, and retired from the meeting. Mr. Rogers was one of the first to regret the issue thus arrived at, and all who know Mr. Woodhouse share that regret to the present time, for although the latter gentleman was elected to the committee of management at the first, the institution has not since reaped the benefit of his presence and counsel at its meetings.

In the year 1859 Mr. Arnold Rogers was duly chosen to act as president of the Odontological Society. It need hardly be stated that he filled the chair admirably,

---

* Could not the idea of a Dental Benevolent Institution be now considered, with the idea of its speedy formation? Such a charity would be worthy of every effort which might be given to make it a success.   A. H.

and throughout the period of his office conducted the affairs of the society with excellent tact. His position in the profession ensured him the respect of all the members; while his urbanity and courteous manner won for him universal esteem. As treasurer to the society, he had displayed from the first thorough business qualities, and the various duties of that office could never have been placed in abler hands. And when the highest post in the society was intrusted to him, his long and extensive experience gave him the necessary power to fulfil its functions to the satisfaction and delight of both the council and members alike. Mr. Rogers was singularly devoid of all acerbity, ever anxious that the discussions that might come before the society, should be conducted with moderation and due attention to the laws which operate amongst gentlemen.

It can easily be understood that, with such a president, a year of pleasant and profitable meetings would be secured to the society. Mr. Rogers' professional career had been such that, at this period, he could claim to be possessed of a very large amount of knowledge. While the scientific side of the papers submitted to the society received from him the attention they necessarily demanded, the real and practical aspect of things was much encouraged during his administration. The president was, in fact, a thoroughly practical dentist. The author remembers the interest with which Mr. Rogers showed him, when on friendly visits to him at his house in Hanover Square, his method of making for himself some of the finer and more delicate instruments in daily use, explaining the method he adopted in fashioning them to his purpose. He insisted that there was a necessity for every dentist being instructed in the art of working the metals employed in his practice, maintaining that there were occasions when special instruments became necessary, and also that few, if any, regular manufacturers could be got to produce them with the required exactness. Certainly, those which were made by him evidenced his accurate discernment of the quality of the material demanded, the form it was to take as applied to the case in hand, and also his manipulative skill in the finish of the instrument. Some of these having been kindly given to the writer, he can testify experimentally concerning them.

The office of treasurer to the Odontological Society had been held by Mr. Rogers for a period of seven years, but his failing health during 1856–57 had prevented his attendance at the council meetings during the winter months almost entirely. This was to him a source of deep regret, involving as it did the extra duty to the secretaries of keeping him informed of those matters which concerned him as treasurer. Considering this, coupled with the medical advice he had been compelled to seek, Mr. Rogers decided upon the, to him, regretful step of resignation. His letter was, with equal regret, reluctantly accepted by the council, who accompanied their letter of acquiescence in his wish with an expression of their high sense of the efficient manner in which he had conducted the financial department of the society, together with its relative duties, and also their affectionate desire for his speedy restoration to health. To one so warm-hearted as Mr. Rogers, this letter was very acceptable, and by him highly prized. But a still more gratifying announcement was in reserve. Such was the general feeling of the members of the society towards Mr. Rogers, that it was felt some appropriate manifestation of it should be made. Accordingly a committee was formed to consider what form the expression should take. A testimonial on vellum, with illuminated heading, and bearing the autograph of every member of the society, was decided upon. This, it was arranged, should be enclosed in a chased cylinder of massive silver, on which an inscription was to be engraved.

The necessary sum for carrying out the project was immediately subscribed, and when completed, a deputation, with Mr. Ibbetson at its head as president of the society, was appointed to present the testimonial. The day selected was Friday, August 23rd, 1867. In a very feeling and appropriate address, Mr. Ibbetson expressed the sentiments of every member of the society towards Mr. Rogers, their gratitude for the great assistance he had rendered it, and their deep regret that the state of his health deprived them of his future services. The testimonial was then gracefully presented, and with much emotion accepted by him. The following is the text:—

"*Odontological Society of Great Britain to Arnold Rogers, Esq., F.R.C.S., L.D.S. Eng., &c. &c.*

"DEAR SIR,—We, the undersigned members of the Odontological Society of Great Britain, desire to express to you, on your retirement from the office of treasurer to that society, our high appreciation of the zealous, careful, and able manner in which you have discharged the duties of that office during the period you have held it, and of the kindly manner in which you have at all times exercised the various contingent duties which have devolved upon you in connection with it. We, therefore, beg you to accept our cordial thanks for the services which we consider you to have rendered to the society in these as also in many other ways, accompanied by our sincere wishes that the quiet which we understand you are about to seek may speedily restore you to your usual state of health."

Two hundred and sixteen signatures were appended, arranged in chronological and alphabetical order, in harmony with the organisation of the society. The design and execution were alike creditable to all concerned.

On one of so warm and susceptible a disposition such an expression, and thus made, could not fail to produce a very deep effect. It was with great difficulty that Mr. Rogers replied, and in fact more than once he was completely overcome. It was very evident that this altogether unexpected demonstration of respect and esteem by his brother practitioners was highly prized by him. His own words fully demonstrated this, as his closing remarks amply testify:—

"I have not language, sir," he said, "to convey adequately the high estimation in which I look upon this diadem, this heirloom, presented to me in this respectful way, as it will often recall to mind, with all its endearments, this most gratifying epoch of my life; but be pleased to accept, in the depth of sincerity, my most grateful thanks."

A sumptuous entertainment at the conclusion of the ceremony was given to the deputation, when reiterated sentiments of esteem for Mr. Rogers, and hope for the future of the profession of which he was such a distinguished member, were again and again expressed.

There were others who had laboured arduously in the good cause of dental reform, and to whom the lasting thanks of every practitioner are due; but no one better deserved such a tribute of admiration and good-will than Arnold Rogers. For many years he had been looked up to by the younger men, amongst whom his name was a household word. His position had been attained by indomitable perseverance, and all around him appeared to concede, and that willingly, the honour to him of being a highly-respected and thoroughly-representative man. Conducting, as he had done for a long period, a large practice, and with his time, therefore, fully occupied, there was nothing which could be fairly considered as tending to the elevation of the profession which he was unwilling to give both time and attention to secure for it. He was noticeably free from the angularity and eccentricity which are sometimes so painfully perceptible among leading men. Ever courteous and kind, he had the happy method of drawing to, instead of driving from him. The writer yields his most willing testimony to the urbanity of Mr. Rogers throughout the many occasions he had to consult and converse with him, and he feels sure that, to all who really knew him, Mr. Rogers stood as the Nestor of the profession.

His retirement from office, in connection with the Odontological Society, produced no abatement of his intense interest in all professional matters. Whenever his health permitted, his well-known face was to be seen at its sittings, as also at the committee meetings of the Dental Hospital of London. He was one of the trustees of that charity, and from the first had given unceasing effort to secure its permanent success. His carefulness and forethought were prominent characteristics, and constantly displayed themselves, but never more prominently than in the formation of the laws, &c., by which that institution was to be governed.

On the occasion of these rules being drafted, the writer remembers that attention was drawn by him to certain clauses which appeared very stringent. Mr. Rogers' reply was illustrative and worth recording: "We must make our laws," he said, "as though we had to deal with dishonest men; good men and true will not object to their severity; *they* do not feel their application, and therefore do not fear them."

He was very active in obtaining supporters to the hospital, and the funds of the charity were in no small degree augmented through his instrumentality. In accordance with a suggestion made by Mr. T. G. Palmer of Cheltenham—another excellent and untiring friend to the hospital—Mr. Rogers had a subscription-box at his house, which periodically yielded its contents to the treasurer for the time being.

In speaking of this worthy member of the profession, it is most difficult to say where his energy was not directed, or its beneficial influence was not felt. His advice was constantly sought by many, especially by the younger members of the profession, and often, too, by those who were in practice at a distance from the metropolis. It need hardly be added that, to the utmost of his power, this was ever most cheerfully given, and, doubtless, with the most salutary and excellent results.

Amongst other important positions Mr. Rogers was called to fill was that of Examiner at the Dental Board of the Royal College of Surgeons. He was one of the first three gentlemen elected to that office, and performed the duties assigned him there with all the courtesy and candour for which he was so well known.

A very noticeable feature in his character was the persistent hopefulness concerning the future of dentistry in this country. Even when the conflict of opinions was at its highest, and appeared so likely to result in utter confusion, he never gave way to despondency. Out of the gloomiest and most mortifying circumstances he had the happy art of extracting comfort. Whatever he could do to help to a better understanding all round was most cheerfully done, and words of encouragement were ever on his lips. Every one having the privilege of his acquaintance was constrained to feel that entire dependence could be placed upon him in the direction of personal effort for the general welfare, and substantial help whenever that was needed.

MR. RYMER.

This gentleman's name has been so frequently mentioned, and his acts and intentions recorded in the body of this work, that there remains but little more to be added to give the reader a just view of what the dental profession owes to him. His courage in publishing his own ideas concerning the condition and necessities of the profession, so far back as 1855, merits praise, for at that particular time, as is now well known, such a step as even that was more than liable to misinterpretation. Such, however, was his deep conviction of the importance of a substantial effort being made with the object of general advance and improvement, that he hesitated not in stating them where they would most likely be read, namely, in the pages of the most influential medical journal, the "Lancet." But a still more courageous act was his summoning a public meeting of his professional brethren in London as the readiest and most efficient method at his command of testing the soundness and practicability of his own personal views in the matter of dental reform. That Mr. Rymer felt this to be so is very certain, for he admits it in the preface to a pamphlet he published in the year 1857, entitled, "The Dental Profession: its Present Position and Future Prospects, considered in Relation to the Recent Reformatory Movement." His own words were to the following effect:—"My own share was, after all, not a great one, although its results have been important. The step of calling the public meeting at the London Tavern was a bold one, and would have laid me open to undying ridicule had it failed; and it was in braving this possibility—which might have been done by any one else—that all my credit lay." This was Mr. Rymer's own estimate of the matter: but it is needless to say that, with regard to the last part of the statement, many took a very different view. Credit was most certainly due to him for *much more* than calling his brother practitioners together, and those who were most intimately acquainted with him, and were best able to watch his actions, found ample opportunity for giving him their unqualified commendation. To him most certainly belongs the credit of first, and both practically and publicly, arousing the dentists of this country from the wretched apathy into which, as a body, they had sunk. It is highly probable that there were many gentlemen practising the dental profession who deplored, as Mr. Rymer deplored, the condition of things around them. But while others thought, he resolved to act; and this resolution of his, carried out in the way it was, was certainly beneficial in the highest degree. But for him the quietude of those days might have continued to an indefinite period. There was much discussion, as soon as the intentions of Mr. Rymer were made known, as to who was first in the field as champion of reform—he or the memorialists of that day. The general feeling, however, was that Mr. Rymer had the priority of claim in the matter. But whether he or the memorialists made the first advance, no one can dispute the fact that to him, and to him alone, belongs the praise of publicly endeavouring to ameliorate the many evils by which the profession was hampered and disgraced, by the proposal of inagurating an educational institute for dentists in this country.

When he came before his brethren, it was very evident that he had something more than a crude, unmatured notion of what was required. His own views were very clearly and succinctly given to the five or six gentlemen who met him in response to his public invitation, just prior to the general meeting of the profession about to be held. These views were still more fully stated when he met the first publicly-convened assembly of dental practitioners on the evening of September 22, 1856. If reference be made to Mr. Rymer's letter to the "Lancet," published a year before this meeting took place (August 1855), the original conception in his mind will be seen to partake largely of the prophetical character. "If," said Mr. Rymer, "the College of Surgeons were to appoint a properly-constituted board of examiners, whose duty should be to hold periodical examinations of such candidates as were desirous of obtaining such a distinction, for instance, as might well be termed 'Licentiates in Dentistry,' I believe that, on the one hand, the public would be spared a vast amount of injury, and that, on the other, dental surgery would take its just position by the side of other liberal professions." It cannot be actually avowed that the memorialists, and subsequently the Odontological Society, borrowed this idea when they pressed for recognition by the Royal College of Surgeons, or that the latter body made use of it as a suggestion ready to hand, when about to accede to the petitioners' request, or formulate the consequent and necessary curriculum; but seeing how events have thus far developed, Mr. Rymer can be well excused if he congratulates himself now the past and present can be looked at together. It is one thing to be the means of inaugurating a new movement, but it is altogether another and a different thing to manifest such qualities as will carry the scheme to a practical and acknowledged result. As the first idea of the profession, or rather that part of it which agreed with Mr. Rymer, began to take form, the test was applied to him as the recognised leader of the "independent" party. Had he been simply a self-opinionated and consequently an obstinate man, his troubles would very soon have proved overwhelming.

It only needed that he should come face to face with others, and he would discover the truth of the old saying, "Many men, many minds." The "independents" were first to have an "association" or "society," then an "institute," at length a "college." It was while the professional mind, identified with himself, was thus in transition that Mr. Rymer gave ample evidence that he did not desire to force his personal opinions upon his brethren. He was perfectly willing to be ruled by the sense of the majority of those who were discussing the scheme, and, although having a voice of his own on the subject, he very cheerfully conceded his views so long as those which were intended to supersede them did not militate against the object immediately before them, namely, improvement and advance. This same excellent spirit of conciliation and concession in things non-essential characterised him all through. The author can speak from close and personal experience of Mr. Rymer's conduct in this direction. At the many council meetings, which were the order of the day in the early history of the College of Dentists, all who sat around the table of the inner chamber at Cavendish Square had ample opportunity of judging, not only of Mr. Rymer's disposition, but of his ability to direct and sustain the movement he had inaugurated.

One of the most prominent features of his character was his earnestness. He was intensely earnest in his desire for professional improvement; in seeking for the best means for the accomplishment of this object; in promulgating his own ideas concerning it; in utilising such material as he could command; and in resisting any and all attempts to frustrate him in his avowed intentions to endeavour to bring about a better state of things. This same spirit of earnestness displayed itself very unmistakably when he came to hear of the secret action of the "memorialists." He did not hesitate then to become aggressive. When he was assured that these gentlemen were moving in that direction, and in a secret manner, and that the great body of practitioners generally were not permitted to know what was being done—although that which was sought thus to be accomplished would so distinctly affect them—he was thoroughly aroused, and made no disguise of his indignation. Whoever chose to submit to such proceedings, he at least would not do so in silence. In fact, the method chosen by the memorialists seemed to act as an extra, and very powerful, incentive to him to persevere in the opposite direction in all his doings and dealings with the profession. There can be no doubt that the contrasting of the two modes of procedure—the secret and the open—one with the other, made political capital accumulate rapidly for Mr. Rymer's use as he proceeded. That which he had from time to time to propose, he strongly insisted ought to be submitted in what he termed a public and constitutional manner. He thoroughly believed in the accepted English feeling in such matters, and resolved always to appeal to his brethren on that particular ground and foundation. His tenacity of opinion that the College of Dentists of England was the best and surest method that could be adopted for the upraising of the profession as a body, was strenthened through the fact that the dentists of this country, to say nothing of many of the medical profession here, and the dental profession generally in America, agreed with him in the end proposed, and the means whereby he sought to accomplish it.

Having obtained the concurrence of so many around him, he devoted himself with the most commendable promptitude and unflagging exertion to the carrying out of his own and his friends' desires. It must be remembered that Mr. Rymer did not live in London; and that, for the seven years through which the College of Dentists was sustained, he had to travel from Croydon to London on every occasion of the college meeting either in general assembly, or in council, or in committee. As the chosen honorary secretary to the council of the college, every paper and document of importance had to come before him; while, in numerous instances, he had to prepare for sudden and imperative action to be taken in order to counteract the tactics of the college's opponents. His duties were not light or nominal, as the author can personally testify.

To this also must be added the statement that Mr. Rymer was not generally in robust, vigorous health. So thoroughly imbued was he, however, with the importance of the enterprise then in hand, that he very cheerfully laid aside all personal considerations, and laboured to the full extent of his power in the cause of professional redemption and progress. He stood in strong and remarkable contrast to some who had both health and wealth at their command, but whose voices were either not heard at all, or heard only very cautiously, to commend, or else to condemn outright, the effort he was determinedly making. It is an instructive, and sometimes a very amusing and suggestive study to notice the extreme sensitiveness with which some people are pervaded under similar circumstances to those in the midst of which Mr. Rymer found himself. How quiet and self-possessed such individuals are at the critical moment, when the delivery of an opinion is asked for from them. With what commendable prudence do they patiently wait until the course the stream is likely to take becomes clear to all around them; and when the toil is about to be consummated in triumph, with what painstaking ingenuity do they become identified with the earnest workers of the past, and seek to share with them the honours and reward that have been so fairly earned by others.

Certainly the dental reform movement did not prove an exception to such a rule as this. However, despite the wavering, the faint-hearted, and the reticent alike, Mr. Rymer determined to persevere until it was undeniably demonstrated that his proposals were not capable of being practically and permanently utilised. Not only from without, but also from within, was Mr.

Rymer tested and tried. By the unavoidably different views of his colleagues at the council table, or among the members of the college generally; by secession; by protests almost *ad infinitum*; and many other matters and things inseparable from such an undertaking, not only was the ingenuity and determination of Mr. Rymer put to the proof, but his courtesy and good temper also. These latter qualities he fully possessed, and on no single occasion could even his opponents convict him of any breach of etiquette.

Not only with the college, but with the Metropolitan School of Dental Science and the National Dental Hospital was Mr. Rymer intimately associated, and all three institutions were indebted to him for a most liberal support. Whatever lay within the compass of his ability in the direction of assistance and counsel he very generously did for their general good.

Although the acknowledged leader of the party endeavouring to set up independence in the dental profession, he was singularly devoid of ostentatiousness. A great lover of truth and justice, he strove hard to make these the basis of action with himself and those working with him. Convenience, or mere policy, had no attractions for him; he sought to do rightly for right's sake. As a result, he often found himself face to face with many stern difficulties, on account of so much demoralisation as then so largely obtained throughout the profession. When the subject of advertising was under consideration, with a view to its suppression, no one showed more anxiety to prevent it in the future, and none felt more chagrin and vexation than he, as the thousand and one forms of subtlety and deception came before the "scrutiny committee." In the weary conflict of opinion between the Collegians and the Odontologists, Mr. Rymer steadily adhered to his original views, and defended the position he had assumed when the necessity arose, either with his voice or his pen.

X

The eventual eclipse of the college scheme has been already recorded, and, therefore, no further allusion need be made to it here. When the inevitable arrived, Mr. Rymer accepted it, and strove to make the best possible terms for those who had so long and strenuously supported him. He subsequently showed his good sense in submitting to examination at the Royal College of Surgeons, and obtained the licentiate's degree. His example was speedily followed by several gentlemen who had been formerly associated with him. His term of office in connection with the council of the Odontological Society was faithfully served, and since then Mr. Rymer has been resting upon the good opinion formed of him by all with whom he had been so conspicuously allied. His American brethren, having watched his career, and the many unselfish attempts he made to institute a similar order of things in England as obtained on the other side of the Atlantic, conferred upon him the honorary membership of one of their dental colleges.

Apart from this, and the recognition of his services by his own colleagues and countrymen, as has been recorded in a former chapter of this work, Mr. Rymer has certainly won for himself the good opinion not only of his friends, but of those also who for a time were ranged against him. His name is indissolubly connected with dental reform in Great Britain, and to him unquestionably belongs the credit, not simply of long and disinterested labour in a most honourable cause, but also of having first instigated a thorough and complete movement in the dental profession, the ultimate beneficial results of which cannot easily be predicted even now. Those who are now either in the actual enjoyment of the very distinctly marked improvement, both legally and socially, which the dentists of this country possess, or are on the high road to that enjoyment, must look back to twenty years since, and see to whom in a very large measure, indeed, they are indebted for that impetus which, so efficiently and perseveringly employed, has been mainly instrumental in securing to them the privileges they hold or may hold to-day. If they read past events impartially, there can be but little doubt that they will instinctively and most justly conclude themselves deeply indebted to Mr. Samuel Lee Rymer.

MR. E. SAUNDERS.

When the idea of memorialising the College of Surgeons was first mooted, Mr. Saunders was one of the eighteen practitioners who appended their names to the document eventually drawn up. As, however, that since celebrated paper was not known at that time to have been in existence except by those who formulated it, the gentlemen who, in September 1856, met to originate the Dental Society, College, or Institute, looked very naturally to Mr. Saunders for his support to their scheme.

When the election of a working committee took place, the voice of the meeting was given for his name to be inserted on the list, and it was accordingly placed there. A correspondence which ensued immediately afterwards between Mr. Rymer and Mr. Saunders on the subject of the memorial gave evidence that the latter gentleman had little faith in the ultimate issue of the proposed movement. Mr. Saunders wrote: "It is quite true that a movement was made to obtain a separate examination and diploma for dental surgery from the College of Surgeons, and a memorial was hastily prepared and signed and presented to the council. . . . . I agree with you that it is to be regretted that the profession was not more extensively made acquainted with it; there was, however, no intentional exclusiveness, nor was the scope of the measure other than most catholic. My share in the business amounted simply to affixing my signature, being of opinion that if the college were disposed to receive us in this way, it would be better than to attempt to erect an independent institution. I am sorry to miss many names of note and influence in your working corps." In another letter to Mr. Rymer, written on 15th October, four days after the preceding one, Mr. Saunders, after stating his regret that Mr. Rymer's project did "not appear to have enlisted the support of those members of the profession who by their position and acquirements have a large and legitimate influence," counselled Mr. Rymer "to wait for the reply of the council of the College of Surgeons to the memorial;" and then enumerating several names of well-known practitioners, added, "Your committee are doubtless men of talent and respectability; but are they the recognised and legitimate representatives of the dental body?"

From such expressions of sentiment it was inferred that although Mr. Saunders would not disavow his interest in the attempt Mr. Rymer and his party were making, he nevertheless leaned towards the memorial scheme, not perhaps simply on the score of its inherent merits only, but because it was connected with names of gentlemen with whom he could better afford to be associated. This was, after all, but to be expected from Mr. Saunders' official position. The result, however, was, so far as the promoters of the independent institution were concerned, a feeling towards him of coolness, and a disposition of quiet unconcern. Although the friends of Mr. Rymer were, so far, disappointed in Mr. Saunders not co-operating with them, it would be very unjust to conclude that he was not friendly to the profession's elevation and advance. He was thoroughly entitled to his own opinions on the subject, and as much entitled as others to select for himself the time and method of dental reform, and also to choose the particular gentlemen with whom he would work. The result was the selection of the influential and accepted heads of the profession as his party. Whatever influence Mr. Saunders had was exerted, if at all, in a quiet manner during several years from the commencement of the new era in 1856. He was, of course, one of the members of the Odontological Society from the first, and in the eighth year of its existence (1864) occupied the presidential chair. When the Dental Hospital of London was founded, Mr. Saunders became one of the trustees of that charity. It was expected by some that the students would have received the benefit of his instructions either as one of the dental surgeons, or as lecturer on some of the subjects forming a part of their scientific education, but these positions Mr. Saunders has not occupied. He has, nevertheless, taken a warm interest in the hospital and school, and has frequently attended the meetings of the hospital managing committee. What has been considered by a large number of his brother practitioners to be a mistake was his not taking the licentiateship degree, he having petitioned, with others, the College of Surgeons for the granting of the examination which led up to that degree. Reasons sufficiently strong, doubtless, Mr. Saunders had for abstaining from this step, but it is to be regretted, nevertheless, that his name is not enrolled on that particular list, which includes so many members of the dental body, and among them the leading practitioners both of that day and this also. It must be remembered that when that degree was first granted it met with a great deal of disrespect from some and disdain from others, but this did not prevent many of the best men from offering themselves as candidates for examination, and now that it is the *sine qua non* for every aspiring and honourable practitioner, those whose courage displayed itself thus are all the more to be commended. Some time before the lease of the premises occupied by the Dental Hospital of London expired, Mr. Saunders expressed himself anxious to secure for the staff and the students there increased accommodation. He considered the site not sufficiently prominent or public. When the subject of a further lease and alterations in the building was under consideration his feeling was distinctly against the project. He was ready with his purse to aid in obtaining a larger building and one better placed, and it was felt that Mr. Saunders' influence among the wealthy would materially help towards the necessary funds being contributed. As the time of occupancy in Soho Square drew near to its close, Mr. Saunders occupied himself assiduously in searching for another site. In such a metropolis as London the task was a difficult one; but perseverance conquered the obstacles, and in due time he was prepared to submit an outline of his ideas in connection with premises in Leicester Square. Mr. Saunders found coadjutors in the work, but the main stress certainly lay with him, and through his instrumentality the preliminaries necessary in all such undertakings were made, and he was in a position to lay them before the managing committee of the charity. The opinion of the medical officers was deemed absolutely necessary, they being so closely concerned in the adaptability of the suggested building to the purposes for which it would be required.

The proposed removal of the hospital was an event not only of interest, but of importance to all. It was much to be regretted, therefore, that a division of opinion should arise, especially among the medical officers. That there was a divided opinion in the staff, however, is true, and it arose principally from the way in which the whole subject had been submitted to them. The proposition came hampered with what was felt to be restrictive and quietly coercive ideas. Mr. Saunders, it appeared, had most generously offered to give the sum of £500, under certain conditions; and the medical officers were informed that if, through their refusal to accept these terms, the project should fail, the whole *onus* of a lost opportunity would rest upon them. From the constitution of the two committees (the managing and the medical) the latter body could not well be acquainted with what took place in the councils of the former. To some members of the medical staff the subject was comparatively if not altogether new. Its crude mode of presentation did not at all help its acceptance by them. Whatever their individual opinions were, not one of the dental surgeons or their assistants had any other than the most earnest desire for the permanent and increasing success of the institution to which they were devoting so much of their time and energy. All admired Mr. Saunders' liberality, and were ready to applaud it, but they claimed the right to differ from him and his proposition; and when the subject was discussed in their committee that right was used.

Although subsequently altered and vastly improved, Leicester Square was at that time a byword and reproach to London. Its disreputable condition was the subject of constant comment and jest in the columns of the daily press. The premises which Mr. Saunders with so much difficulty had selected were in a condition to necessitate their having a very considerable sum of money expended upon them, apart from what would be necessary to adapt them to the requirements of a dental hospital. All this, however, had been thoroughly considered by him, and with praiseworthy determination he still pressed his scheme.

Nevertheless many of the medical staff could not see things in the same light as he did, and the result was that when the question was before that committee for their decision, those of their number who supported the removal obtained a majority of only one vote; and even this would not have been secured but for the sudden indisposition of one of the opposite side, who was compelled to leave the meeting. The expression of opinion thus given was construed into opposition to Mr. Saunders, but it is difficult to discover in the thoroughly English and free statement of sentiment among gentlemen of equal position one with another the suitableness of the particular term.

It need not be added, that when it was finally decided by the managing committee that the removal to Leicester Square should take place, "contents" and "not contents" accepted the verdict, and entered heartily into the work of making Mr. Saunders' enterprise a thorough success. All felt that, whatever their private or expressed opinions might be, the locality of the institution could not possibly affect their sincere desire for the true utility and development of the Dental Hospital of London. Not only was Mr. Saunders' contribution large, but his influence was freely given to secure the necessary funds—his efforts in this direction proving very successful. No one could have shown more devotion to a cause he had espoused than did Mr. Saunders; and to one whose time is necessarily valuable, the demands in this direction must have been heavy. This matter of the Dental Hospital was the means of bringing the name of Edwin Saunders into prominence. He had from the commencement of the movement been little heard of—in fact, his position was felt by many to be one of more or less isolation from his brother practitioners. Beyond his official connection with the Odontological Society, and his trusteeship of the hospital, Mr. Saunders has not been conspicuously placed in the profession. From want of time, perhaps, he has not added to the literature of dentistry except by a little treatise published several years ago, entitled, " The Teeth a Test of Age." But that which has fallen within his province, namely, the bestowment of money for a truly professional purpose, and that with no sparing hand, Mr. Saunders has done. The profession has been laid under obligation to Mr. Saunders for this his commendable act, and in return it has subscribed to a fund which, when completed, took the form of a testimonial, which was subsequently presented to him. The original idea in connection with this testimonial was that it should be a marble bust to be placed in the hospital, but on the advice of his friends Mr. Saunders determined that he would devote the sum subscribed to founding a scholarship in conjunction with the hospital. This was a generous and wise resolve, and has commended itself to all really thoughtful persons. Latterly this proposal has taken practical shape, and thus a fresh stimulus is offered to the young men pursuing their studies there.

There may have been insuperable difficulties in the way of Mr. Saunders obtaining a numerous following in the dental profession, and he may, in fact, have never desired to occupy the position of a leader; but with the opportunities which, apparently, at least, encircled one who is appointed to wait on royalty, it was felt, especially twenty years since, that he might have taken the initiative with his brethren, and have been powerfully instrumental in guiding the destinies of the profession. This, however, has not been the case; and the leadership consequently fell into other hands. Fortunately for all concerned, those who did lead proved fully equal to the important and onerous task, and it may be safely said that, concerning the happy result of what they have been able to accomplish for the general good, no one rejoices more heartily than Mr. Saunders himself.

MR. J. TOMES.

Throughout the entire movement towards reform the name above written has been one of power. It is associated in the minds of those who have been intimately acquainted with its possessor with the ideas of science, professional success, integrity, and hard work. As far back as 1849 the writer remembers the influence it exerted among such as himself, who were then young and inquiring men just beginning their professional career. Mr. Tomes work on dental physiology and surgery had not been long published, and was making its own mark on the minds of the embryo dentists of that day. After studying Hunter, Blake, Fox, Bell, and others, it was felt that the scientific facts given by those writers were not all that might be known on the subjects treated by them. The valuable truths which Mr. Tomes by his patient research had elucidated were hailed as a great advance in scientific dental knowledge, and, therefore, his name became not only familiar, but full of force. It was in the above year that the author became acquainted with Mr. Tomes in the relationship of pupil to instructor in the operative department of dentistry at the Middlesex Hospital. Mr. Tomes was then acting as dental surgeon to that institution. The first impression of the writer was, that he was eccentric and capricious, with a decided leaning towards the severe. Very few words passed between Mr. Tomes and his pupils at that time, and in fact no one can accuse him of ever being guilty of verbosity. What was said had its import and necessity, and all that the hearer had to do was to listen respectfully, and endeavour to retain in his memory the facts that had been mentioned. Whatever others might have felt, this the writer can testify concerning himself—that he could not escape from the feeling that he was listening to the words of one who *knew* what he was speaking of, and was aiming directly so that the exact truth, neither more nor less, should be presented to the listener's mind. A great reverence for such a teacher was the result, and considerable happiness was experienced in knowing that there was a rich mine of information thus opened up and offered to him, or any other pupil at the hospital, if the desire to take advantage of it were manifested.

Mr. Tomes was ever ready to impart knowledge when he perceived that the questioner or student was, like himself, thoroughly in earnest. The author's earliest acquaintance, therefore, with Mr. Tomes was grounded deeply and firmly in respect and admiration. It was some years after this, however, that he had occasion to meet Mr. Tomes, and then under somewhat unpleasant circumstances.

The meeting in public assembly of the profession, under the auspices of Mr. Rymer, in the autumn of 1856, had, in the flush of its first success, nominated several gentlemen to a seat on the council of the institution then being formed. They were well known names, and such as the friends who were then gathered together felt inevitably necessary to anything like permanent success in the direction of professional progress. In the public record of that event, which was published immediately afterwards, these names appeared on the list without an asterisk or other mark opposite to such as were not personally present, or had otherwise signified their intention not to act, if thus proposed by their brethren in the profession. Mr. Tomes saw the announcement, and wrote a very sharp note repudiating his connection with the movement altogether. The author having, through his official connection with the movement under Mr. Rymer, been the unwitting cause of the offence to Mr. Tomes, thought that, as he personally knew him, it was due to that gentleman that a personal explanation should be offered him. Accordingly Mr. Tomes was waited upon, and received the writer with his usual quiet demeanour. The explanation was given, by which it was shown that the error was an omission, and not intentionally made; whereupon the subject of the reform, and the method of bringing it about, came to be somewhat freely discussed, Mr. Tomes prophesying then that the movement could not possibly succeed. The writer thought differently, and said so, with all the respect due to Mr. Tomes' better knowledge. The interview ended with a suggestion that before venturing to make any gentleman's name public for the future, it would be well to obtain his unqualified sanction of the same. The young official had, evidently, his ear pinched by fingers which could have pinched it much harder had they been disposed, and he has ever felt that his former acquaintance with Mr. Tomes saved him from that very unpleasant procedure. The firm conviction held by that gentleman concerning the non-success of Mr. Rymer's project may have been produced by many different circumstances, yet there is little doubt that the unbounded faith which he had in the scheme which had been advanced by him and the eighteen memorialists, but which was at that time unknown to any save themselves, made him stronger in the belief of the truthfulness of his utterances.

As events proceeded, the author had very many opportunities of consulting with Mr. Tomes on matters connected with the agitation which existed throughout the profession. Few, indeed, are aware of the terrible demands which were, from one cause or other, constantly being made upon Mr. Tomes' time and attention. In his inaugural address, delivered on the occasion of his being called for the second time to the president's chair of the Odontological Society (1875), the fact is modestly alluded to, but in such a way as—if the author may be allowed to say so—to produce the inference that these interruptions had to be borne principally by others.

Although many gentlemen, especially Mr. S. Cartwright and Mr. A. Rogers, were subjected to these ordeals, it is but just to say that Mr. Tomes was more open to them than any besides. The writer can testify, from personal as well as other experience, to the absolute willingness of Mr. Tomes to receive visits from all parties at all times, when the object in view was to push forward the work of reform. To those for whom especially this work is written, the bare mention of such a fact is quite enough to elicit a feeling of thankfulness for this exhibition, at a most critical period in the history of the profession, of such unsparing devotion. If Mr. Tomes had never contributed pecuniarily towards the sustentation of the labour of reform, the constant demands thus made upon his time, when he was conducting an excellent practice which called for all his energy and attention, must be put down as representing a very large sum of money. He never failed to set aside his own interests in this direction; and in looking back upon the past from the present happy position of the dental profession, this fact must not only not be forgotten, but be held in very grateful remembrance, as infinitely to his credit and praise. Many were the occasions when minutes became of the utmost importance; and had Mr. Tomes, when his advice or co-operation were sought under these circumstances, pleaded his many engagements as an excuse for his inability to give them, it is a question whether what has been effected would ever have been accomplished at all.

The inner workings of the reform movement have only been made known to a very few amongst us, but from the author's official position on both sides, and from the first, he is, perhaps, as competent to speak concerning them, at least, as many. From the commencement to the present time the profession has had no one member of it more willing to help, or more able to do so, than Mr. Tomes. Full of quiet determination, and peculiarly gifted with both foresight and the faculty of administration, he has never once failed to use these qualities for the interests of the profession at large. Many circumstances have occurred by which he has been able to bring very valuable influence from without to bear upon the object he had in view. He was incessantly placing his hands upon what may be termed secret springs, by which very many important results were obtained, and without which the progress of events would have been either materially slackened, or in some cases, to the writer's knowledge, brought to a standstill.

The opinions which Mr. Tomes held concerning the necessities of the profession, especially during the period of its most violent agitation and excitement, had been arrived at after long and careful thought. He therefore held to them tenaciously. It is but just also to record that what has been achieved is in exact accordance with the views he expressed to the author at the outset. He never could be brought to believe that an independent institution, as proposed by Mr. Rymer and his party, would, even if consummated, be beneficial, or in any way advance the status of the dental profession.

A proper connection with the Royal College of Surgeons Mr. Tomes considered the best guarantee for the public and the profession alike, although he himself was not, until the year 1859, a member of the college. This fact, among others, although appearing to be somewhat incongruous with the views he advanced, was utilised by him for the general benefit. It enabled him to speak as from the ranks of the unqualified practitioners, and this power he largely availed himself of in his many communications to the Royal College of Surgeons authorities. So much so, indeed, was this the case, that the then secretary—the late Mr. Belfour—plainly told Mr. Tomes that he was the source of considerable embarrassment—to use no stronger term—to the executive in Lincoln's Inn Fields. When Mr Tomes asked how this could be, Mr. Belfour replied: "You write upon physiology and surgery, and are quoted as an authority on these subjects, and yet you are not a member of the college. If," continued Mr. Belfour, "the council will grant your request in forming a dental department, as you desire, will you promise to become a member yourself?" Mr. Tomes agreed to this proposal, and accordingly, when the licentiateship was about to become a fact, he redeemed his promise and took the degree at once.

While the great body of dentists was separated—at least representatively—into two hostile camps, Mr. Tomes came in for a large share of blame from the college party for what was then considered quiet and gratuitous action against their project. A great many facts oozed out concerning him and his untiring exertions in maturing the Odontological Society's plan, but only those who were most intimately acquainted with him could hope to become cognisant with all that he was so constantly doing. There was not a single circumstance or individual whose influence could be made available for furthering his views but was pressed into the service. Not only with Mr. Green, Mr. Lawrence, and Mr. Arnott, as gentlemen of influence and authority on the council of the college, but with Mr. Belfour as the secretary also, he used his constant exertions in endeavouring to make plain to them the manifold benefits which he believed would accrue from the reception and adoption of his plan. It was the same with Mr. A. Beresford Hope, Lord Robert Cecil, and others, whose word and counsel in the House of Commons could further assist him.

There was not a meeting convened upon the important subject which was then engrossing the earnest attention of the profession at large but Mr. Tomes was one of the principal, if not the principal speaker.

There were gentlemen of determination and spirit among the executive of the College of Dentists of England, as even their opponents freely acknowledged, but certainly not more largely endowed with these faculties than Mr. Tomes. His energy and determination were immense, although they were never displayed ostentatiously. Apart from his admittedly-deserved high position in the dental profession, these qualities told marvellously upon the progress and ultimate result of the movement. There never seemed to be a time when he was inclined to relax the smallest effort. Thoroughly impressed with the importance of the subject, and believing that the time had arrived when, if ever, the object could be achieved, he simply resolved not to put down his pen or be silent and at ease until it was accomplished. The cost of this resolution was, in more than a pecuniary sense, dear. He, nevertheless, cheerfully paid that cost, although health itself had to be included in the account. Although money has not been withheld, and in some instances freely given, yet useful and necessary as that is, it can never be considered as approaching the value of such contributions as Mr. Tomes and others beside him have so liberally bestowed to bring the profession where it is to-day.

The difficulty with the writer, in attempting to record the eminent and unflagging services which this true friend to education and advance has rendered, is to find out where his name and influence cannot be seen. The Odontological Society has been deeply indebted to him, not only in its origin but throughout its entire career; and this has been most appropriately acknowledged by his being called twice to the president's chair. When the Dental Hospital of London was founded, he was one of its most energetic helpers. As a matter of course he became one of the dental surgeons on its staff, and when the London School of Dental Surgery had been formed, he was appointed lecturer on dental physiology and surgery, fulfilling the duties of that most important post with acknowledged ability.

As was to be expected, Mr. Tomes was appointed to

the office of examiner at the board instituted by the Royal College of Surgeons in connection with the dental department of the college. He, with Mr. T. Bell and Mr. A. Rogers, formed the dental portion of the first examining board. In that office he acted with the most honourable impartiality. It was the opinion of many, especially among the opponents of the licentiateship degree, that the examination to which candidates were required to submit would be of the most nominal kind. Whatever the outside opinion at that time was, Mr. Tomes had his own views and his own resolutions in the matter. The author had occasion to call upon him shortly after he himself had passed the ordeal at Lincoln's Inn Fields, and the opportunity was taken advantage of to state these resolutions.

"You," said Mr. Tomes, "see a large number of men in the profession, and I wish you to tell them that I am determined not to write my name upon their diploma unless they show a thoroughly fair acquaintance with the several principles of their profession. They must give me good proof of their ability to practise, or I, for one, will not endorse their degree."

The request thus made the writer accordingly fulfilled. If, therefore, any presented themselves under the idea that the examination was contemptible, they soon had their notions refuted. The whole bent and bias of Mr. Tomes' mind has been opposed to shallow and superficial knowledge. The effort which had thus culminated in the establishment of an examining body, had been engaged in by him with the express object of securing a class of dental surgeons who possessed real knowledge, and were, therefore, worthy to represent the profession in the immediate future. Like many others, he deplored the ignorance which abounded. He stood out resolutely against *shams*, whether they were manifested in "high places," or among the lowly and the low. To see good work in any of the departments of practice appeared to give him great delight.

His contributions to the surgery of the dentist all exemplify his intimate acquaintance with the necessities of the practitioner, not only in ordinary everyday cases, but in exceptional ones also. Many years ago he employed the well-known instrument maker, Evrard, to carry out his designs, and, if report speaks truly, has more than once tested not only the quality of that individual's material, but his mind also and patience too. Mr. Tomes, as a rule, gets a very clear and definite idea of the object or subject occupying his attention, and will not be content with any agency or instrument unless he feel morally certain of its adequacy to the occasion. It was this proclivity, or rather habit of mind, which was in constant operation with him when he, with others, projected the idea of affiliation with the Royal College of Surgeons. When connected with the College of Dentists the author had frequently to come into contact with Mr. Tomes, and in discussing the relative merits of the two plans which were in such fierce opposition to each other, had not the above characteristic been very plain, he might easily have concluded that Mr. Tomes' resolute antagonism to Mr. Rymer's scheme was based upon nothing more than dogged partisanship. The truth is, however, that he had been thoroughly investigating the tactics and the aim of the other side, and failed to see either in the means or the end that which he felt would be a permanent benefit to the profession.

Looking at the reverse of the medal, there was in it that which commended itself to him, and hence the pertinacity and perseverance exemplified by him all through. Since the cessation of hostilities Mr. Tomes has employed all the means at his command to sustain in vigorous operation that which has been already effected. He has displayed an unflagging interest in the present and future well-being of the dental profession, and is never weary of urging forward thorough reform, through education and self-culture, on all who propose to practise as dental surgeons. His pen has not been suffered to rest, as the work which he first published in his own name, and also the enlarged edition of it, with which was associated the name of his son—Mr. C. Tomes—will testify.

Not only in the matter of the removal of the Dental Hospital of London to its present position, but in other matters subsequent to that event—which it is not within the province of this work to deal with—Mr. Tomes has given many and vigorous proofs of his unabated desire to benefit the dental profession, as such, and help forward every member of it honourably conducting his practice. He still adheres to the opinion of so many around him, that the licentiate's degree, which he was so mainly instrumental in obtaining, is that which denotes the holder's fitness to practise as a dental surgeon. Even the loss of private friendship cannot alter his settled conviction upon this important point. Whatever new aspect the revolutions of time may produce in the dental profession, there can be no shadow of a doubt but that Mr. Tomes' views will be eagerly sought for, and as highly valued when obtained, as they certainly deserve to be. All that has transpired in the past clearly confirms the idea in the minds of the really impartial that the present acknowledged position which Mr. Tomes holds among his co-practitioners has been most fairly earned by years of devotion to the general good, and by a series of services the cost of which no one would for a moment either question or deny.

MR. J. UNDERWOOD.

From the time of Mr. Robinson's associating himself with the movement originated by Mr. Rymer, Mr. Underwood, who was then in professional partnership with Mr. Robinson, has been identified with the progress of reform in all its principal aspects. He has been one, among many others, who has both hoped and striven earnestly for true advance, and whenever and wherever he has found, or even hoped to find, by resolution and perseverance, an occasion or opportunity for raising the professional status, he has very willingly identified himself with those he believed were labouring for that desirable object, and supported such measures as he considered most likely to lead up to it. Mr. Underwood throughout the many phases and ramifications which has, the agitation of the last twenty years has developed, always shown himself both thoughtful and prudent in the various steps he has been led to take, and his judgment has been singularly clear and sound. He was amongst those who were first elected to a seat at the council table of the College of Dentists of England, and his value as a member of that body soon made itself evident. Of an independent spirit, he generally spoke distinctly from his own point of view, and being one of those, whose number is by no means large, who can express themselves publicly with good effect, his utterances always commanded attention.

In the earlier days of reform, when meeting followed meeting in such quick and constant succession, and in the midst of which there was so much of conflicting opinion, the advantage of this particular gift was considerable. Those who have had occasion to meet him under such circumstances have been constrained to feel that what Mr. Underwood had to say and submit to their consideration was said without prolixity or redundancy of words, and withal in thoroughly intelligible language. He from the first felt keenly the degradation which so widely overspread the profession he was practising, and was most anxious that some efficient measures should be taken to bring about the amelioration which others also with him regarded as so essentially necessary. He believed firmly that a sound, thorough, and comprehensive education was the best means for accomplishing this. It was because he conceived that Mr. Rymer's scheme was highly conducive to that particular end that he, when solicited, gave it his sanction and, presently, his assistance.

Once elected to the council of the Dental College, he threw all his energy into the undertaking, was constant in his attendance at the many meetings which took place, and was counted upon as one of its firmest and most influential supporters. When the action of the memorialists in petitioning secretly the Royal College of Surgeons became a certified fact, it aroused his opposition, and he did not hesitate to express his disapproval of the step on all occasions when the subject was under consideration. He felt that, in order to neutralise such action, the complete organisation of the College of Dentists, and its speedy and effective operation as a centre of instruction, was the best method to be adopted. To effect this he unhesitatingly lent himself to everything likely to promote such a course and consummation. In due time, however, as has been recorded, the idea of amalgamation became prominent, and when this idea could only be carried out by the leading men of the two opposing factions being brought into personal contact for the purpose of discussing the project, it was very natural, and, withal, appropriate, that Mr. Underwood should be chosen as the representative of the Dental College to meet Mr. Tomes.

Although Mr. Underwood was the personal friend of Mr. Reid, who had first thought of this particular method of calming the angry strife which then existed, it was not solely on that account that he was selected. There was at that time an opinion, as if by common consent, that he would be the best expositor of the views and feelings of those with whom he was so earnestly working, and that they could very safely rely upon the quality of his mind and the clearness of his expressions for a fair, faithful, and firm exposition of their principles and the objects they sought to obtain.

It is but right to say that Mr. Underwood had honestly earned this confidence of his brethren. The hope they entertained was certainly not disappointed. By the constitution of his mind, and his method altogether, he decidedly was the best representative the college could have selected. There can be no question or doubt of Mr. Underwood having argued the matter in such a way with Mr. Tomes as most thoroughly to commend himself, if not his colleagues or their scheme, to that gentleman. At any rate, from the interview which thus took place, a warm, lasting, and hitherto unbroken friendship may be said to have sprung up between these two practitioners, who before had been thorough strangers to each other. The same qualities which had led to this official duty eventually dictated the subsequent appointment of Mr. Underwood to the more delicate and difficult position of delegate upon the subject of amalgamation. In that ordeal he acquitted himself thoroughly well; and from his own keen sense of honour, and feeling that at the termination of that conference all had been yielded and done which honour and justice required from the delegates of the Odontological Society, he felt he could no longer hold office in the College of Dentists if an adverse vote were given upon the result of their joint deliberations.

The rejection of the terms of amalgamation which had been arrived at consequently necessitated Mr. Underwood's retirement from the college council, and accordingly he was one of the sixty gentlemen who seceded at that juncture of affairs. His next step was, when all hope of amalgamation with the Odontological Society by the College of Dentists had faded away, to join the former association; and he was accordingly admitted a member. That membership has continued to the present time; and during the period that has elapsed he has served in the most important offices in connection with it, and has occupied the presidential chair. As soon as the object of the society's petition to the Royal College of Surgeons had been attained by the establishment of the licentiate's degree, Mr. Underwood sent in his name to the authorities in Lincoln's Inn Fields as a candidate for examination, and on March 14, 1860, obtained his diploma.

When the idea of instituting the Dental Hospital of London was mooted, Mr. Underwood was among the number of those first connected with the enterprise, and was one of the six gentlemen elected to the office of dental surgeon to the charity. As one of the medical staff he has continued connected with the hospital, with great benefit to the institution itself, and to the students as well, ever since. His present tenure of that office is by special request of the managing committee. Since the retirement of Mr. R. Hepburn from the chairmanship of the medical committee, that post has been occupied by him, and, it is needless to say, with excellent results. As an operator Mr. Underwood is bold and successful, and the students coming under his instruction may never hope to have meanly executed work slurred over, or passed without reproving notice. Mr. Underwood does not hold the full membership of the Royal College of Surgeons, but he is an instance among many others of what education, perseverance, and real practical knowledge can effect. No one would deny the position he occupies as a thoroughly efficient practitioner. In this sense he is a representative dentist. Although he by no means disparages the membership of the College of Surgeons, yet he cannot but notice the pretentiousness of some who assume a superior position in virtue of being able to place the initial letters of membership after their names, but who cannot demonstrate that superiority in any practical way, and he makes no disguise of his opinions on such conduct. Whatever the membership of the College of Surgeons may do towards improving, or being thought to improve, a dentist's social status, he for one—and there are many besides—is firmly impressed with the conviction that, alone, it cannot endow its possessor with the power properly to practise as a dental surgeon. He holds that all who take this latter position are qualified to fill it only by a special education, such, indeed, as the licentiate's degree includes and demands.

With the several matters which have occupied the attention of the profession since the year 1856, Mr. Underwood has been invariably more or less officially connected; and his appearance at the various committees seems to be expected almost as a matter of course. Certainly in him the profession has a zealous worker, an intelligent and prudent supporter, and an ever firm and sincere friend.

It would not be just to omit the mention of other names, besides those already dealt with at greater length, as those of real workers in the cause of professional advance, although a full record concerning them is not practicable. Some did not become officially or otherwise prominently connected with the reform movement until it had taken definite form, and had become largely developed. Among these may be mentioned the late Mr. E. SERCOMBE, whose early death formed a subject of deep regret to all who knew him. He attended one or two of the public meetings called together by Mr. Rymer, but did not associate himself with the party that gentleman represented. For several years he contented himself with being a member of the Odontological Society, and continued as such up to the time of his deccase. Just prior to that sad event he was called to the presidential chair of that society, and throughout his term of office carried its affairs forward with the vigour which was so prominent a feature in his character. He was identified with the movement for re-opening the College of Surgeons to those who had not availed themselves of the privilege of seeking the licentiate's degree as it originally offered itself. He was also very active in the design of Mr. Saunders for removing the Dental Hospital of London to its present site, and also in the measure which was taken for obtaining for that gentleman the testimonial which was eventually presented to him. There can be no doubt of his strong desire to see a better condition of things in the dental profession firmly established, notwithstanding his abstinence generally from the earlier attempts made to secure this.

Mr. ALFRED COLEMAN also has devoted much time to the important movements as they have arisen, and has brought to every question under discussion, with which he has been concerned, the powers of an educated and well-ordered mind. When, through severe illness, the author had to resign his position as honorary secretary to the managing committee of the Dental Hospital of London, Mr. Coleman succeeded him in that office for some years, and, it need not be said, to the promotion of the best interests of that important institution. He has been officially connected with it as a member of the medical staff, to the great benefit both of the charity itself and the young men pursuing their studies there. He has also held important offices in the Odontological Society, of which he is still a member, and although his ideas concerning the licentiate's degree as contrasted with the full membership of the College of Surgeons, as shown in the steps which he and a few other gentlemen have recently taken, may not be endorsed by the bulk of his brother practitioners, yet there can be no doubt as to his sincere and ardent desire that the dental profession should rank higher than it already does. It is, in fact, to such members of the dental profession as Mr. Coleman fitly represents that others may fairly look, in the well-grounded hope that no retrogression shall by any means take place.

Mr. KEMPTON also deserves honourable mention for what he has done in connection with the Metropolitan School of Dental Science, his official position with which he has so disinterestedly and for so long a time filled to the satisfaction of all concerned. When that enterprise was first launched, it was surrounded by many difficulties—among others, that which arose from the idea which then obtained, that it was to be a rival to the London School of Dental Surgery. He persevered, however, in the post and department to which he was elected by his brethren who had established the College of Dentists and then the school, and has had resolution and energy enough to surmount the various obstacles which lay across his path.

Mr. HOCKLEY, as a colleague of Mr. Kempton, did good work in connection with the College of Dentists, having, from the time when the author resigned his position as honorary corresponding secretary to that institution, succeeded to that office, which was indeed no sinecure, and maintained the post to the period when the college itself was dissolved. He also undertook to deliver a course of lectures on mechanical dentistry at Cavendish Square, for which he was well qualified; and in more directions than one, and on all occasions, gave ample evidence of his readiness and ability to serve the cause of the profession's improvement.

Mr. THOMAS ARNOLD ROGERS has been one of those quiet but substantial coadjutors in the work of reform of whom it would be difficult to speak in too high terms of praise. Inheriting all his lamented father's excellent qualities, he has ever shown the deepest interest in all that concerns the welfare and real progress of the dental profession, and has displayed a most cheerful alacrity to help whenever and wherever he has perceived the slightest opportunity of doing so. Not only with the truest courtesy, but also with keen perception and discrimination, has he held himself in readiness to take his part in the general effort which has been going on throughout the last twenty years. He has been identified with the Odontological Society from the first, and has held important official connections with it, not omitting the honourable position of president.

In every department of his varied usefulness Mr. Rogers has brought to bear both scientific and practical knowledge, and, moreover, has readily and liberally contributed pecuniarily to the many objects which dental reform has comprehended and included in its progress.

The qualities of his mind were quickly demonstrated when he kindly consented to become the dean of the Dental Hospital of London. Under his careful supervision, the house was soon set in order, and new and wide-reaching regulations introduced and established, which all but revolutionised the former state of things, but always for the palpable benefit of all concerned. He undertook and rapidly completed a dental calendar for the special use of the students—in itself a laborious task, and one which involved a close and clear conception of the students' needs, and the best method of meeting them. His interest in their progress was practically demonstrated by his donation of "The Dean's Prize," and in all his efforts, which have been so unremitting, there has been an unmistakable desire to secure to the future dental practitioner every benefit that the present improved condition of the profession can offer him.

It cannot be a matter of surprise to any one knowing Mr. Rogers that the young men by whom he is surrounded entertain for him high esteem and a feeling of warm regard, and have endeavoured to show this in a very pleasant, and, moreover, practical form.

To find a gentleman of Mr. Rogers' experience as a dental practitioner occupying a seat at the board of examiners at the Royal College of Surgeons is so natural, and by all means such an expected thing, that his appointment to that important office caused no surprise. To him the credit must be given of first suggesting the desirability of every candidate for the dental diploma passing the preliminary examination. Such a step was certainly one in the right direction, narrowing as it does, by a most proper and comprehensive measure, the gateway which leads to the possession of the licentiate's degree. Unobtrusive and deferential to the opinions of his colleagues as Mr. Rogers is, and always has been, there is not, and, indeed, cannot be, a truer or more sincere friend to the dental profession than he, or one more instinctively ready to offer all the help which it is in his power to give.

Looking away from the metropolis, and turning the thoughts due north, energy and unflagging effort are perceptible there as well. In Edinburgh these qualities have been evinced in the cases of several gentlemen there, notably so in that of Mr. DAVID HEPBURN. With the tendency to question and protest which seems to be indigenous to some of the best of men, the establishment of the Odonto-Chirurgical Society, together with the institution of the annual dinner of the licentiates in dental surgery, and the maintainence of both alike, is not a matter which could be made succeed by a simple wish in that direction. It has needed a great deal of self-denial and perseverance to effect what has been thus accomplished, and Mr. David Hepburn has had both these qualities somewhat severely tested. Believing, however, as he has done from the first, that there was a necessity and an opportunity for a scientific society, and an annual commemoration of the most important event in the annals of the dental profession within the last twenty years, he has cheerfully given time and attention to the securing of both these matters. Misconceptions and misinterpretations are the almost certain concomitants of all such undertakings, and he has not been without his experience of these things. Those, however, who know him best esteem him most, and are certain that he acts in a really disinterested and thoroughly unselfish spirit whenever he puts his hand to a work such as that which he has been so largely instrumental in accomplishing.

When the hopes of unity and progress seemed to all but die out with others, Mr. Hepburn still held tenaciously to the belief that such things were possible, and in this belief he had found a pleasure in working on. Possessed of a kindly nature, he is not very easily ruffled by unkind words from others, and certainly does not pale before obstacles which to some would be formidable, nor shrink at the prospect of plenty of hard, unthankful work. He has been many times cordially supported by the countenance of his brethren both around him and at a distance, and is one of the last to appropriate any share of praise which may result from the success of enterprises with which he, in association with others, has been engaged. His desire has been, and still is, to contribute what he can to the profession's real benefit, and is never better satisfied than when that object—either by his colleagues or others—is likely to be accomplished.

In the establishment of the Dental Hospital at Liverpool there is another instance of real devotedness to professional advance, with which Mr. NEWMAN's name is so distinctly associated. That charity is an evidence of what may be accomplished by determination and perseverance. If all were known which concerned the enterprise, and tended to check or divert the intentions of those who with Mr. Newman laboured to have such a charity established, there can be but little doubt that many disheartening circumstances would have to be recorded. When, however, the result proves such a successful accomplishment of good desires and sustained effort, there is but one thing left for all true friends of the profession to do, namely, to accord to those who have laboured so long and so well, the just meed of praise which so evidently belongs to them; and here Mr. Newman stands foremost.

The same remarks apply to Mr. PARKER in connection with the Dental Dispensary of Birmingham; for long services rendered and unselfishly discharged surely command commendation.

Mr. SPENCE BATE, F.R.S., of Plymouth, by his efforts, now long sustained, in regard to the inauguration and maintenance of the Dental Dispensary in that town, must be justly considered as one of the many who have contributed to the consolidation and true progress of the dental profession. He, too, has had his difficulties, but the increasing usefulness of the charity which has been set up in the town where he practises, and the certainty that it works well in the direction of benefiting the students who enter it, are doubtless sufficient atonement for any disappointment he and others working with him may have been called upon to undergo.

The author feels that the distinct mention of the kindness and interest shown by the late Mr. BELFOUR formerly secretary to the Royal College of Surgeons, to those who had to associate with him officially in regard to the dental reform movement in its earlier and more important stages, is but an act of the simplest justice, and but a feeble tribute to his memory.

It would be difficult to say how much and how far his co-operation contributed to the ultimate success of the undertaking which the memorialists first of all, and then the Odontological Society, had taken in hand. Certainly with some persons in such an office as that of Mr. Belfour the result, if not actually marred, would have been materially delayed. As it was, however, he proved a true friend to the dental profession, and by many acts outside the category of officialism contributed in no unimportant measure to the end desired so ardently by those more immediately concerned in the effort to obtain recognition by, and affiliation with, the Royal College of Surgeons.

In his successor, Mr. TRIMMER, the profession will find one of a similar disposition; and it is a great pleasure to the author to state, that from the kindness and courtesy he has himself personally received, he can certainly assure those of his readers who will have to know more of Mr. Trimmer than at present they perhaps do, that in him they will find a gentleman ready and pleased to assist them in those directions in which they will be only too glad to find kindness and help.

CHAPTER XI.

THE dental profession in this country now stands on broader bases and a more solid foundation than have ever before belonged to it. The realisation of this is, of course, vastly more palpable and vivid to some connected with it than to others. It needs, in fact, to have been of the number of those whose lot was cast some twenty or thirty years ago, and whose training, surroundings, and expectations were tinged by the murky professional atmosphere which then prevailed, to thoroughly feel and duly appreciate the many advantages which now exist for the profession at large. No doubt to the younger men it seems all but incredible that dentists, who, as a class, have common interests—and always did have them, whether the fact were recognised or not—should have been so short a time since absolutely estranged from each other, and all working, not only in the dark, but working thus pre-eminently for themselves, and themselves only. To them it must appear passing strange that practitioners in London were, to all intents and purposes, as far from each other as any widely-separated city or county is from the metropolis itself. That such an isolation did exist it has been part of the object of this work to prove; and in this, the concluding chapter, it is a pleasant and grateful thing to write it down as a condition which has passed away, and, as the author believes, for ever. Estrangement may, like a spectre, appear again; its unwelcome visit is not among the impossible things which beset a body of men like the dental practitioners of this country; but such a reappearance is highly improbable, and certainly may be prevented, or at least held in check, should it come, by those who really represent the profession seeking to fulfil the position thus assigned to them.

Compared with its former state, the dental profession is now certainly, to a large extent, organised. The opportunity has been given many times over for the varied and conflicting opinions of those who desired to make them known to be laid open to the general gaze and submitted to the general scrutiny. In this sense the long-sustained hostility of the once rival parties was an admirable medium or vehicle. It was only as the many and multiplied phases of professional requirements became known, through the agitation which once prevailed, that what was necessary, and even imperative, came at last to be distinctly seen. Upon that protracted and somewhat painful experience the representative dentist of this epoch takes his stand.

If there is not a College of Dentists of England for the present generation of young men to flock to and call their *Alma Mater*, it is because such a method, with its principle of independence, has been found, by trial and proof, not to be the method best calculated to meet the wants or accord with the proclivities of British dentists. If, on the other hand, a close and distinct affiliation with the Royal College of Surgeons for every respectable and honourably-practising dentist is the recognised law, which all such are encouraged and expected to acknowledge and accept, it is because, after years of trial, this method commends itself most clearly to those who have the formation and direction of the professional mind generally.

To annihilate estrangement, disorder, and selfishness, a standard around which men may rally is a necessity of the first importance. Those who laboured so strenuously in the past for the amelioration of the many evils which then obtained saw this plainly, and hence the unremitting efforts which this work has chronicled, and hence, after the two methods have been so vigorously sifted, the choice of that which every true friend to the profession does not hesitate to acknowledge as the best. To have expected an improvement throughout the ranks of the dental body without having earnestly searched for, and, when found, tried, to the fullest extent possible, the standard to be upraised, would have been sheer infatuation and egregious folly. But the workers of the past have an acquittal from all such charges, and a proof of their correct judgment, in the results which have followed their earnest thought, and their then decided action. Not impetuously, but, on the contrary, slowly—even, as some think and assert, too slowly—have men gathered around the standard erected for the general benefit. Those who, among the older members of the profession, were inclined to disregard and do without "the degree," have gradually felt their way towards obtaining it. The selfishness which led some at the first to be content with the diploma they possessed—in the confidence of their patients and the public generally—eventually gave way before the just perception that there was something they owed to the generation which would succeed them. And consequently, as that and similar sentiments asserted themselves, they came forward, and lent the influence of their name to the promotion of a general advance, and thus, not only performed an act of justice to themselves and the younger men about to practise, but added their contribution of testimony to the wisdom and prudence of those who had wrought on so energetically to secure the degree for future aspirants to dental name and fame. As the result of this course of procedure by gentlemen for long established as dentists, the students themselves were led to see that such a step was, of all others, not only the most necessary, but the best for them to take. Gradually, therefore, the list of names of those who coveted, and at length obtained, the licentiate's degree increased, and the profession now stands with this particular diploma regarded as the *sine qua non* of the qualified dental practitioner. Thus, then, has organisation not only become a reality, but a reality in a sense which, twenty years ago, seemed so impracticable as to fill the minds of some of the most enthusiastic well-wishers of the profession, and not a few of the most ardent and indefatigable workers in dental reform, with dismay, if not with despair.

Health, time, money, exertion, and much more besides, have been laid heroically on the altar of the profession's welfare, and such sacrifices render that which has resulted from them, in a certain sense, sacred. Such a statement may appear, perhaps, to some mere sentimentalism; but there can be no doubt that those who would lightly esteem the labour of others, or seek to overturn or neutralise the result of their self-denying efforts, are they who have not contributed much out of their own mental, moral, or material wealth; and, perhaps, have not thought it worth their while to study the motives and actions of those who have.

Not only has organisation been, happily, to so large a degree accomplished, but that which all true friends throughout the dental ranks must certainly desire as its sequence, namely, consolidation. With the isolation of former days was weakness, instability, uncertainty. When men stood apart from each other, how was it possible for them to know what was passing in each other's minds, and how nearly their common needs and common desires approached to a common level? The inevitable result of such separation was discoverable in the general tendency to concentrate all thought and effort upon the individual's own interest, and make every act to rotate on "self" as on a pivot. Organisation, which has come at last, has brought with it in its train friendliness, mutual interest, the recognition of right, submission to higher principles, desire for progress, and many other things which may be classified under the one suggestive term—consolidation.

The dental body in this country is more worthy of itself now than ever it was before. No individual member need now complain of a forced isolation and estrangement if he only practise as an honourable member of an honourable profession. This is not only true as a statement coming from within the profession, but it is true also as an acknowledgment already distinct, and gradually growing more so, from those who are outside, and have the best opportunity of observation, and who are, moreover, more or less interested in the stability and progress of the profession—the medical practitioners in particular.

The establishment of the Odontological Society was an excellent and appropriate step in this direction. It afforded an ample opportunity and provided a large arena for the discussion of the many subjects and scientific theories which dentistry, as such, embraces. To it might be brought any and all new discoveries which required discussion and analysis, with the undoubted prospect of a free and full investigation of their respective merits. Encouragement was offered to every one having new views to promulgate or exceptional experience to submit, with the certainty that what was necessary to, or promotive of, the general welfare would receive a fair and impartial hearing, and an authoritative endorsement. An admirable stimulus to contributions of scientific and practical interest has been given by that society, and so long as it rigidly adheres to its first principles, and maintains firmly a high standard, it will continue to be an incalculable benefit to the whole profession.

Should it become lax in the administration of its laws, no effort should be spared to cause its executive to respect both the letter and the spirit of its constitution; and if the rules which govern it prove inadequate to the progressive action of the profession and its increasing enlightenment, new regulations should be made more in accordance with the spirit of the present time, so that it may ever be looked up to by the profession generally, and the younger members in particular, and all occasion and ground of reproach by its adversaries, if there are such, completely removed. As a corrective to what in this country are considered unprofessional practices it has been, and still is, of great worth. To name only one will show how this purifying influence may be exerted by it. From the first it has discouraged and discountenanced the secret acquisitions of knowledge. No member of the Odontological Society is permitted to hold a patent.

In this respect the present position of the profession stands out favourably, and in strong contrast as well, to the accepted order of things not many years ago. A reference to the "British Journal of Dental Science," under the heading of "Patents," will enable the reader to see with what eagerness many men in the past availed themselves of the protection which the Patent Office supplies to inventors. The series of papers furnished for the above journal by Mrs. G. Owen tell their own tale. The Odontological Society has insisted all along, and still insists, that in a liberal profession, such as dentistry, the hoarding up for the inventor's own pecuniary benefit of any discovery he may make is altogether an unworthy and undignified proceeding. Whatever, therefore, is ascertained and proved as a step in advance must be cast into the general fund of knowledge for the general good, or membership with the society is forfeited. In like manner it has dealt with the difficult subject of advertising and advertisements. By its laws it would infuse into the mind of the profession the necessity of standing aloof from everything which savours of the mercantile and tradesmanlike.

There can be no possible doubt that the light and flippant ideas which formerly obtained concerning public announcements have, through this society, received a wholesome check. It has corrected much of the erroneous notions which once existed as to what constituted canonical conduct; and no individual who, either openly or surreptitiously, attempts to win the attention of the public by parading his name, may hope to have that name enrolled upon its list of members. Whatever may be done in the direction of educating the public on this head by gentlemen who properly practise their profession, the Odontological Society has been, since its formation, an admirable instructor of the profession itself. It is of high importance to the younger men in particular to know that what, through the disintegrated condition of the profession, was tolerated twenty years since, cannot be permitted now.

The temptations which an uninquiring and unreflecting public offer to the would-be advertiser must be sternly and steadily resisted by all who claim to be considered dental surgeons, and desire to be in reality worthy of the name. It is of the last importance that the Odontological Society should be so constituted and so directed as that a high and healthy tone should be its prominent and prevailing characteristic. In the selection of its presidents hitherto this feature has been very distinct. There has not yet been a single instance of any gentleman who has been called to this important position the mention of whose name has not commanded immediate respect. The many papers read at its meetings have, as a rule, been of great utility, and some of the highest interest, conferring the greatest benefit upon the profession generally. To have a society the immediate tendency of which is to impart scientific and practical knowledge to all concerned, is surely an advantage which cannot easily be overrated. Its power for good in the direction of further organisation is, or ought to be, considerable. That such has been its influence is certain. Gentlemen from all parts of the three kingdoms, the Continent, and distant countries and the colonies as well, have flocked to its standard, and felt themselves to be honoured by being in association with it. It will be an evil day when this state of things pales down from any cause; and every member of the society should so conduct himself as to make any diminution of its high and proper influence impossible. Hitherto, the dental profession proper of the United Kingdom has been focused in the Odontological Society of Great Britain. Its earliest aim and original effort and object was to offer a recognised centre of science and practical knowledge to the general body of practitioners through its own elected members. This it may be justly said to have accomplished. With the accession of so many gentlemen of influence as its earlier list of names in particular displayed, political power was accorded to it, or, more properly speaking, was found in it. This, as has been related in the body of this work, it freely used. Hence the obtaining of the licentiate's degree. Hence, also, the Dental Hospital of London, with its natural and most appropriate sequence, the London School of Dental Surgery. To say that these two most important institutions are a complete success is to utter the merest truth. They have been from the first, and still are, an ever-increasing success. To think of the state of the profession a couple of decades back from this point of view, and then to compare that condition with the many and multiplied advantages which now exist, must be a great reward to those who have endeavoured, through so many vicissitudes, and with such manifest disinterestedness and self-denial, to confer palpable and lasting benefit upon the present and future generation of dental practitioners. Instead of having to gather up meagre crumbs of information under many difficulties, and endeavour to profit by them with little or no assistance from others, as was formerly the case, the student of to-day has innumerable opportunities of becoming familiar with and well practised in all the departments of his profession. The field of observation opened up and made accessible to him at the various centres of instruction, both in London and elsewhere, is an immense one, the value of which cannot well be exaggerated. It is a time of reaping for him, following upon, and the natural result of, the patient sowing of others.

To speak only of one institution—the Dental Hospital of London—the general good done may be understood all the more plainly from the statement of the fact, that since its opening in the year 1868, no less a number than *two hundred and fifty thousand cases* of treatment have been entered upon its books. To have an opportunity of inspecting and studying from fifteen to twenty thousand cases each year of his pupilage is a gain which, although the student himself may not accurately estimate or appreciate its value, those who know, from a long experience, what dental practice demands will unhesitatingly admit. Not only at the above institution, but at the National Dental Hospital as a special centre, and also at the many general hospitals where dental practice is far more closely pursued than was formerly the rule, the student of to-day may find occasions for increasing his practical knowledge which were altogether unknown a generation ago. The carefully-prepared lectures delivered to the young men at their studies at the different schools now in operation, both in the metropolis and the provinces, are channels through which they may receive instruction that will be the means of furnishing their minds with the most valuable knowledge, the results of which will be clearly visible to them and others in their future life and practice. The benefits now so freely offered to a student do not terminate with the mere observation of a very large number of patients at the hospital or hospitals which he attends. Confining the attention of the reader mainly to the institution in Leicester Square, the advantages which it offers may be briefly thus alluded to. For a long time it has been the place where every novelty sought to be introduced to the profession is, almost as a matter of course, sent, in order to its being submitted to a full and impartial test of its merits. Inventors of dental appliances and materials for daily use in the operating room unhesitatingly forward samples to the committee of management, or to the medical officers, requesting their opinion of them. Whenever it is deemed expedient to subject these things to trial, it is always done in the presence of the students, and results recorded, or otherwise taken notice of. The exhibition of the various anæsthetics, either alone or in combination, has been, and still is, a noticeable feature in the practice at the Dental Hospital of London. By the three able administrators of anæsthetics, specially appointed by the committee for that purpose, or by others under their immediate superintendence, as well as by some of the medical officers, the important adjunct, anæsthesia, is fully introduced to the student, its value enforced, its danger explained, and its importance illustrated. Many cases of great and special interest continue to be sent to the Dental Hospital by the authorities at the general hospitals, while in the range of its own practice instances of difficulty and complication in the diseases and affections of the mouth and teeth frequently occur, thereby offering opportunities for observation which could not fairly be expected in the course of private practice by any means so often. Another means of advancing the education of the young learner at this particular institution is open to him in his being able to witness for himself the particular methods of twelve different operators through the week. Under the personal direction of the dental surgeon, or the assistant dental surgeon of the day, the pupil is instructed how to commence, carry on, and complete, the treatment of the case before him; and the general efficiency of the pupils on terminating the period of their studies is the evidence and proof of the sort of training they receive. The clinical lectures and demonstrations, as first suggested by Mr. Thomas A. Rogers, prove most beneficial to the students; and the eagerness with which, as a rule, the remarks of the medical officers are listened to, and the various operations which at times they consider necessary to perform are watched, furnish proofs of the estimation in which this system is held by those for whose benefit it is intended. The managing committee has strenuously endeavoured to make the hospital a blessing to the suffering poor, and at the same time an efficient means of education in every department of dental practice to those who enter there for that purpose. In this effort the members of the medical staff have cheerfully and constantly concurred. The beneficial result of this is seen in the fact that a class of men is now found among the junior members of the profession, of which, as a body, their former teachers are justly proud. It may be most truly said that all who have had the important office of instructor to fulfil have been actuated by the desire to impart all the knowledge they possessed to those intrusted to their care, that, when their own career shall close, they who are destined to succeed them shall be men of stamp and quality in their profession. That these just and laudable intentions are bearing excellent fruit already has been attested over and over again. One evidence in proof of this is to be seen in the fact that such practitioners as require the services of efficient assistants turn instinctively to the hospital as their surest and safest resource. Certain it is that not a few young men occupying positions of importance and trust at the present time have been called to their various posts mainly from the fact that they had received their training at, and had been connected with, the Dental Hospital of London. Such varied opportunities as are there given to the diligent and intelligent pupil must necessarily eventuate in practical skill.

In order, however, that the treatment of the patients attending this institution should not be the result of manipulative skill alone, the London School of Dental Surgery claims the time and earnest attention of the student. To enable the young practitioner to bring to a successful issue the various cases which are brought under his observation and intrusted to his care, he is instructed in the theory of his profession, and taught upon what recognised scientific principles he should base his method of action. Carefully-prepared lectures have, from the first, been systematically delivered upon all the subjects with which the student must needs be familiar, and every effort is made by the lecturers to impart a full knowledge of all such matters as are of the highest importance. Apart from these lectures, which embrace dental anatomy and physiology—human and comparative—dental surgery and pathology, mechanical dentistry, and metallurgy in its application to dental purposes, the hospital pupils are frequently called aside from the patient's chair, or during the time of their attendance, to receive instruction on some subject of interest, the lesson being often illustrated by the use of the black-board. Any case which offers an opportunity for demonstrating in a precise and particular manner some given scientific theory or principle is never neglected, but taken advantage of for the practical benefit of the learners.

No one could become acquainted with the working of this important hospital and school through all its various departments, superintended as they are by the medical staff, the lecturers, the dean, the house-surgeon or assistant house-surgeon, without becoming thoroughly convinced of two things at least. The first is, that everything lying within the range of human capability is being done to fully instruct the rising generation of dentists in this country in the principles and practice of their profession ; and the second is, that, compared with the condition of things surrounding dentistry, as such, twenty years ago, its position to-day is as clear light to darkness. It may safely be said that the student of the present time may learn more in one month, under the present *régime*, than he could with an immense expenditure of time and trouble have hoped to learn formerly in an entire year. This has been so palpable to many gentlemen and dental practitioners visiting the hospital whilst the practice has been at its full, that the observation has been made to the author over and over again, "Is not all this instruction *too* freely distributed?" and, "Are you sure these young men appreciate what is being done for them?" Those who are engaged in the work of tuition there seem not to be too anxious to answer these questions, either one way or the other: their principal desire appears to be rather to do their duty to the full extent of their power, and leave results to speak for themselves. Certain it is that if the future dentist be not better furnished than the present, the responsibility will not lie at the door of those who have the important office of instructor to fulfil. These remarks, although made with direct reference to the Dental Hospital of London, may certainly be applied to the National Dental Hospital, and to the provincial hospitals and dispensaries as well.

One of the encouraging features of the present as compared with the past is the evident tendency which exists in the direction of these special institutions springing up throughout the length and breadth of the land. If this country is to have a larger supply of dentists than heretofore, it becomes a paramount duty with those who have any influence in the profession that they should be a superior order of men. In this lies the most certain cure for the plague of quackery. Ignorance and impudence—which inevitably go together—are best overcome by real knowledge, with its inevitable accompaniment of modesty. Not only will the public be guaranteed, to a large extent at least, against the piracy of the unprincipled pretender, but it will gradually learn to look towards the qualified practitioner, and the qualified practitioner alone, as its real and true helper in this department of surgery.

By more highly educating the upcoming race of dentists the medical profession also will perceive that dentistry, or rather the practice of dentistry, is no longer what it has been in the past to so great a degree, a sham, "a delusion and a snare." The present position of the profession is now no longer undefined. The important result which has been attained in the affiliation of it to the Royal College of Surgeons has given it a distinct position and a clearly-marked place among kindred professions. It is for every real friend to use his exertions to prevent the standard which has been set up from being lowered. The curriculum imposed by the executive in Lincoln's Inn Fields is of such an order that it is now impossible for any young man to take his degree without his being fairly, if not fully, acquainted with the principles and practice of the profession he intends to follow.

Not only, therefore, has the student of the present day various and multiplied opportunities of becoming proficient in his studies, opportunities which were altogether unknown to many of his seniors, but he has facilities in the acquisition of knowledge which should transform duty into delight. Whatever an intending dentist of the last generation might propose to himself as the object of his ambition and desire, one thing is clear—that, outside of his own determination, he had no encouragement to persevere. Even in the event of his surmounting the huge obstacles which encumbered his path, he had no position—recognised as such—offered or made possible. All that he could do was to endeavour to prosecute his work in an honourable manner, and be content with the acknowledgment which a good conscience and a slowly increasing practice perhaps might yield him.

Fortunately for the student now, there is also to be

added to the opportunities and facilities which lie thickly around him the mark of distinction and recognition as a professional man which the licentiate's degree confers. Much has been said concerning this degree, and not a little by way of detraction and disparagement; but the most absolute answer which can be made to all who would take away from its real value, and the most encouraging to such as have advocated it and continue to advocate it, lies in the undeniable fact that it is more earnestly sought after than ever, and is justly regarded by the impartial as the proper and distinguishing mark of the duly qualified dental practitioner.

Whatever deficiency may have been discoverable by the hypercritical concerning the admission of partially educated men to participation in the benefits which the possession of this degree confers, there can be no just cause of complaint in this direction now. The edict which has gone forth, which will speedily enforce the passing of the preliminary examination by all intending candidates, sets this *questio vexata* at rest. No individual ignorant of what are known as the essentials of general knowledge is eligible for examination under the new order. The wide range which the curriculum takes gives every assurance that those who seek to obtain the coveted degree have been well instructed in the details of their profession, while the high and universally acknowleged position and recognised attainments of the gentlemen forming the board of examiners at the Royal College of Surgeons alike forbid any idea of undue clemency being shown to those who appear at Lincoln's Inn Fields for examination.

Whatever has been advanced concerning the necessity of all dentists being full members of the College of Surgeons may, or rather must, be considered by the side of the results of the practice of such as are full members. There has been, up to the present, no overpowering proof that surgeons produce better examples of manipulative skill or remedial treatment than licentiates, and in many instances the very reverse has often been demonstrated. The question of the sufficiency or insufficiency of the licentiate degree is one which may be argued at any time by any one.

If it can be fairly shown that its possessors are not equal to the demands which high-class and thoroughly legitimate practice always makes, there can be no doubt that the council of the Royal College of Surgeons would be ready and willing to remedy any defect in the present order of things, but it would be difficult for those who think the present curriculum defective to show palpable reasons for their opinion. Less than twenty years may appear, in the minds of some, to be a period long enough for any code of regulations to be in operation, but unless something more than the mere lapse of time can be advanced for alteration, the advocates of change have but a feeble cause in their hands.

The legislation which has brought the dental profession into its present acknowledged position, the steady working of the accepted order of things, and the consequent advance made in the capabilities and practical knowledge of the young practitioner, are benefits so palpable, that to disturb them, without a strong and legitimate reason, may well be accounted a grave and serious mistake. There can be no doubt that improvements from time to time will be necessary, and is plain enough to even the casual observer.

Life—it matters not in what aspect it is considered—is progress. The dental profession, if it is to be worthy of the name, must not hope to escape from this inevitable law, but rather gladly accept it as that by which it seeks to be governed and directed. Yet, while all this is true, change, whenever and however it may come, must not be capricious or whimsical. Neither must it be for the gratification of the ideas of the few, but must bear upon its surface, and display all through its entirety, the manifest desire and object of its introducers, and that must be the distinct and permanent benefit of the majority. The error of the reformers of the profession—that is, so far as one side of the question is concerned—in the past, was exclusive action. Now, that the dental body is organised, consolidated, instructed, recognised, and a distinct position accorded to it, that mistake must not be repeated.

Another feature of the present position of the profession is that of enlarged experience. In the course of years it cannot but be expected that new theories, new discoveries will be made known, and, in fact, those whose life is engaged with the intimate association that it holds with both science and art are constantly on the alert, and eager to welcome the announcement that something fresh has been brought to light. The dental profession has not been exempt from these sentiments and experiences. It takes its present stand all the more firmly because of what it has been compelled to know of several matters, which have been the result of painstaking investigation in the domains of science and art alike. One of the subjects it has considered, tried, and laid aside is "Congelation" on Blundell's system. The eager desire to obtain some distinct method of obtunding sensibility made the announcement of this method a piece of welcome news to all concerned twenty odd years since. The matter was taken up, considered earnestly, tried, and by some commended, but gradually, and after a while, was laid aside. The local application of cold for the purpose of extracting teeth on Blundell's plan has no place with the dentists of the present day. Experience has taught the profession the lesson of its inadequacy to the demand made. Electricity also has had its trial, and is now relegated to the limbo of the past. In its day it pretended to be a panacea for the evils which it was considered able to remove ; but, like congelation, having been weighed in the balance, it was found wanting, and to-day no one thinks of electricity as an agent, the use of which would enable a patient to

2 A

be indifferent to the painful process of extraction of teeth. Eventually the ether spray was introduced by Dr. Richardson, and for a time, and in certain cases, greatly approved.* It had its difficulties and its drawbacks, however, and the profession, as a rule, does not depend much upon it, if, indeed, at all, now. Chloroform, as the king of anæsthetics, has been largely used in the dental profession, and the experience of some of the senior practitioners has been obtained by trying ordeals, and in some cases with terrible results. When the dental surgeon has to lay his account with chloroform, he knows that he is dealing with a giant who sometimes kills in the dark, and, therefore, this agent is not so unhesitatingly used as when it was first introduced by the late Dr. Simpson, and so largely administered by the late Dr. Snow. From ether—first applied to dental purposes in this country by the late Mr. James Robinson—all through the catalogue of anæsthetics the experience of the dental profession has gone, and the large and all but general adoption of the nitrous oxide gas, as the most appropriate agent for anæsthetic purposes in dental practice, is the result of painstaking trial and innumerable experiments and observation.

All these things make the ground firmer beneath the feet of the younger men in particular, and put into their hands much information, which only a series of years of study and growing experience could produce. However the profession may have been agitated, it has not permitted itself to be blinded to its own real interests; and what it has gathered together it now places at the disposal of all. With the impetus that has been given to education has come the natural demand for improvement in the various appliances which the dentist, both in the operating room and laboratory, daily requires. A glance at the depôt list of instruments and the articles there supplied, reveals a wonderful fulness in

* The author has found it very useful in cases of torsion of the superior central incisor teeth.

the *repertoire* of the dentist compared with the number and fitness of instruments formerly in use. Mechanism of the highest order and best kind is at the disposal of all, and admirably adapted to every sort of requirement. The manufacturers of dental instruments have kept pace in their supply with the demands laid upon them, and it cannot be said that inferior work, whether in the operating room or laboratory, is due to a lack of good implements to perform it with.

Although this country has been thoroughly alive to these particular needs, and active and successful, too, in meeting them, yet it cannot be denied that English dentists are largely indebted to their American brethren for many of the advantages they now possess. In the department of chemistry a noticeable progress has been made. It were needless to mention the many invaluable drugs which are in constant use now, seeing they are so well-known, but a large number of them were a short time since either undiscovered or not utilised by the dentist. In whatever direction the mind may turn, there is abundant evidence to prove that the dental profession is now so completely launched on the stream of improvement and unquestionable usefulness, that no fear may be entertained of its sure and steady development. The desire for knowledge is fully met in the society and schools, while the practical application of acquired skill has its opportunities before it in the various departments of the hospitals in the metropolis and the provinces. The incessant labours of the many friends of the profession since 1856 are proving their value in all directions.

Professional literature must ever be regarded as one of the most powerful helps to progress that can be brought to bear upon the minds of all directly concerned. As a specialty dentistry cannot hope to have a profuse library of works of reference; yet, as a department of surgery, and one, moreover, where art goes hand in hand with science, it has ample scope for authorship;

but it is of the last importance that when the pen is used it should be wielded by those who really have some practical knowledge to impart to others, and not employed in the production of works which contain merely, in the writer's own language, the utterances of men whose sentiments and statements they have themselves already made public. The profession requires *text* books, works to which all may refer, and that safely, for distinct guidance on given subjects. When writings such as have appeared as the joint production of Mr. Tomes and Mr. Charles Tomes are given to the practitioner and student, they are accepted as valuable contributions to dental literature. Such a work as that by Mr. Salter is of the order about which the profession can afford to be pleased, and proud as well as pleased. The promised work of Mr. Charles Tomes on Anatomy* will doubtless be a welcome addition to the store of knowledge already possessed, proving—as it is certain it will—that the subject has been efficiently elucidated by a thoughtful and well-cultivated mind. If others, besides, thoroughly capable of addressing their brethren, would undertake to do so upon these plans and principles, the benefits would be immense.

Journalism, or periodical dental literature, is another excellent channel of good. There can be no doubt of the benefits arising from journalism properly directed and thoroughly devoted to the interests of the dental profession. Such an adjunct would be of immense value, especially to the students and younger practitioners generally. At present, as is well known, the profession is said to be represented by two publications, each appearing monthly, though at different dates of issue. "The British Journal of Dental Science," now twenty years old, still maintains its position as *the* journal; but its editor would be the last person to admit that it fully meets the requirements of its readers, or answers altogether his own

* Since published.

purposes or desires. "The Quarterly Journal" has long since died out, having been followed by, or rather transformed into, "The Dental Review," which also in its turn succumbed to inexorable fate. "The Monthly Review," edited by Mr. Oakley Coles, was started in 1872, to fill what was considered by its projector to be a vacancy in dental journalism. But the same remark may be applied to it that has been made concerning its elder brother. Political articles are, happily, not a necessity, as they were in the earlier days of reform, and an occasional but well-written statement in the place devoted to "leaders" is all that is really requisite under the present circumstances of the profession. It is not simply the writer's, but many others' idea besides, that'a Quarterly Review containing, as its main feature, highly scientific and soundly practical papers on the many subjects which the profession includes in its various departments would far better meet the demands not only of the young and inquiring minds, but of the older and far-advanced practitioners as well. Some years ago an attempt was made to supply such reading for the dental profession in a publication entitled "The Archives of Dentistry," under the auspices of Mr. T. E. Truman; but that effort failed, only some few numbers appearing. The dentists of this country were not, even a short time back, in such a position as they now occupy to appreciate really scientific literature. The impetus to do so is only now becoming really felt, and, therefore, any contribution in the above direction would certainly have a far higher probability of acceptance by the profession generally than hitherto. Those who would be real friends to the younger practitioners in particular, could not do better than occupy their leisure in furnishing, through some channel or other, communications of a thoroughly superior order. Such reading would harmonise with, and add strengthening to, the teaching which the student receives in the lectures delivered in the various general and dental schools. There are many subjects touched on by the lecturer, when instructing his class, that would amply repay both him and his hearers too, if further elucidated and put before them in print. To give Mr. Fox his due, it must be acknowledged that he has many times asked for such papers for his journal, and appealed to those who are well able to write them to assist in the cause of true professional education. It cannot be said, however, that the publication he conducts has been remarkable for contributions of this kind. To be compelled to fill up a journal, which is bound to appear once every month, with clippings and cuttings from other periodicals is unsatisfactory in the extreme. Notices of subjects altogether irrelevant not only disappoint, but are apt to disgust the reader, eagerly searching for information in connection with his own immediate studies. It might be that those gentlemen who are so thoroughly qualified to give the results of their mature experience or advanced thought would respond to such a request if a longer time between the issues of the journal were allotted to them.

There is, of course, the commercial aspect of such suggestions as these, but that is a matter which the proprietor of any journal must consider for himself. What voluntaryism cannot be coaxed into conceding, a liberal pecuniary payment will seldom fail to obtain. One thing, however, is very clear—if the dental profession is to be thoroughly well represented by its journal or journals, those publications must, of necessity, be fully equal to the demands which a more enlightened and more advanced condition of things around will, legitimately and assuredly, claim. On this point there need be no reason to fear the directors of dental journalism will be either obtuse or blind. This department of literature may be made to exercise a very healthy or a very retarding influence on the dental profession, according as it is worthily or unworthily exercised. It would be well, also, if every contributor would condescend to lay aside all really unnecessary technicalities in the papers they may from time to time offer. In such matters the advice of one who was no mean authority—the late Dean Alford—might surely be accepted and followed with advantage. He said, "Be simple, be honest in your speaking and writing. Never use a long word where a short one will do. Call a spade a spade, and not a well-known oblong instrument of husbandry; let home be *home*, not a residence, a place a *place*, and not a locality; and so of the rest. Where a short word will do, you always lose by using a long one. You lose in clearness; you lose in honest expression of your meaning; and in the honest opinion of all men who are qualified to judge you lose in reputation for ability." That there should be good, clearly-expressed, practical, and scientific reading provided, especially for the student and younger practitioners, is a self-evident fact. While in former years a mere smattering of knowledge was deemed sufficient for the dentist, the happily-changed circumstances and condition of the profession, which make the object and aim of the present practitioner to be to obtain the largest amount of information, necessitate the supply of such mental food, not only in ample quantity, but in quality as well. It is not an exaggeration to say, as a sign of the distinct advance made by the profession generally, that those who have obtained the licentiate's degree are giving welcome evidence of their desire and resolve to practise in a high and honourable manner. While such a statement as this may still bear modification in some instances and some directions, nevertheless, to a great extent, it is strictly true.

The great desire of those gentlemen who have for so long a time made such strenuous efforts, and submitted to so much self-denial for the common good, has been to see their future successors fully alive to the demands of true professional conduct. By this means they believed that they would surely and firmly elevate the profession which they themselves had adorned. Their object was to raise up a generation of men, able and disposed to practise as educated gentlemen. This only could redeem dental surgery from the mire in which it had so long grovelled, and assuredly in the future wrest it from the grip of the ignorant and unprincipled. They believed that the remedy for charlatanism did not lie in the direction of any amount of pamphleteering—however that might lay bare the misdeeds of the unprincipled and impudent pretender—nor depend upon rigid, restrictive legislative enactments. Quackery had been, as it still is, their horror and constant annoyance. They have been all along humiliated by the hateful practices of men assuming to be called "professional," but who by their actions declared themselves to be ignorant of the meaning of the word, and were consequently not amenable to its recognised laws. The success of their praiseworthy efforts to erect a new and elevated status for dental practitioners, worthy of the name, has led them to hope that gradually the standard which has been set up will be thoroughly and gladly respected.

The full recognition of dental surgery by the Legislature and the Royal College of Surgeons, as a branch of surgical practice, is such an alteration for the better, so decided an improvement over that condition which existed prior to the year 1860, that those who were engaged in obtaining it may now well believe in future advance. Their arduous and self-denying labour has resulted in lifting the profession out of the low estate into which it had sunk, and placing it on a fair and level road for the time to come.

Like many other things, the future of dentistry in this country is in the hands of the young men of to-day. It will become just what they resolve to make it. A trust has been placed in their hands which it is quite competent to them to honour or dishonour. At present there is no reason whatever to doubt the proper use of the many and multiplied advantages which the junior members possess, or fear that any retrogression will ever take place. There are, of course, still, many difficulties to encounter and overcome. From the fact of their acknowledged superiority to many others, the educated race of young dentists will keenly feel the rampant empiricism which still taints and tarnishes the profession they are following. They will have to bear with this as their predecessors have done; but, being where they are, and what they are, they will be better able to exercise an influence for its suppression than was accorded to their seniors in days gone by. The power lies within their reach, and is ready to their use, to prove their superiority to, and their distinct separation from, those individuals who so unblushingly endeavour to win over, or rather entrap, the unwary public day by day. They must not expect that charlatanism will die an easy and speedy death. They may certainly look for assistance in their attempts to suppress it from the journals which so ably represent the medical profession, to which they are now completely affiliated. If these periodicals would steadily abstain from favourably reviewing the many and constantly issued pamphlets and *brochures* which are forwarded to them for that purpose, one important channel, at least, of their obtaining publicity would be broken up. It has been a matter of surprise and annoyance often experienced by the legitimate dental practitioner to see how blind some reviewers of these pretentious sheets have been to the commonest and, ordinarily, best known truths concerning dental practice.

It may be, perhaps, too much as yet to hope that the secular press will act in this direction, or that advertisements in the acknowledged place for such things, either in the medical or daily ordinary newspapers, will disappear. Money-gain still wields its powerful sway in so many directions, and in the above directions included, that the advertiser who holds a golden key will not yet despair of its successful use. However, time and perseverance may be relied on, if properly utilised, to bring about a difference at last, even there. It will be the constant duty of all who seek still further and further to elevate the dental profession, to prove that it is a real profession, and a most honourable calling, by their proficiency in practising it, and their correct conduct towards those who seek their advice and skill.

On the other hand, there may be a difficulty, or rather a danger, with some, in the endeavour to make dentistry more than it really is. While they seek to uphold it, and be proud of it, it will be well if they are upon their guard against the subtlety of this latter temptation. The part is not, and cannot be greater than the whole —the less must ever be included in and by the greater. The branch should never be mistaken for the trunk; and, after all, this is the true relation of dental surgery to the medical profession. For the dental practitioner to assume the airs of the medical practitioner would be certainly most unwise. He has a department of surgery to practise, and, if properly considered, it will soon be seen to contain in it a fulness sufficient to absorb and engross all his time and all his powers.

Whether he hold the full membership of the Royal College of Surgeons or not, if his vocation be that of the dental practitioner, let him be content with practising, and, moreover, being considered by others, as such. It may be in the future that further changes will take place in the profession which will render it advisable that every dentist should hold the full degree of member, as well as that of licentiate. Even now there can be no possible objection to such a step being taken by all who are at present prosecuting their studies. But with such a curriculum as that already imposed in connection with the licentiateship, and with such an examination as that to which all candidates for that diploma are subjected, it would be a warped and notably partial mind, indeed, that would conceive that the knowledge thus demonstrated to have been obtained by the successful candidate was a knowledge inadequate to all his future requirements as a dental surgeon.

But should this be even so, there is nothing to interfere with or prevent the test to be applied being increasingly stringent and severe. Up to the present the author, in his many conversations with those who are members of the Royal College of Surgeons as well as licentiates, has not heard one assert that when he takes up his position in his operating-room he feels himself to be a better and more practical dentist than when he was only able to add the letters L.D.S to his name. Social status may be secured or improved by full membership with the college, and for this purpose simply it has been sought for, and obtained by several practitioners of dentistry; but its practical benefit to the dental surgeon is, at least in the minds of many, a shadowy conjecture. Either the licentiate's degree is a sufficient proof of its possessor's fitness to practise the art and science of dental surgery, or it is not. If the latter be true, then those who are in the position to bring about the desired alteration must put their hands to the good and imperatively necessary work of making it so. In such an effort they might count upon the support and influence of every dental practitioner in the kingdom worthy of the name, without the remotest fear of their being denied to them. With the increasing acquaintance by all interested persons with the real and practical value of the dental diploma, facilities will also increase in the direction of gentlemen holding it being elected to positions of honour and trust in the various hospitals of the metropolis and the provinces. The insisting upon the candidates for the post of dental surgeons to these institutions being members of the College of Surgeons will not, it is to be hoped, be so dogmatically enforced as it has been hitherto. Gentlemen who hold, by the means of a special education and subsequent special examination, the degree which the College of

Surgeons itself has proclaimed *the* proof of real qualification to practise their special department of surgery, ought assuredly to be entitled to the hope that, when that particular post requires some one to fill it, they might be considered eligible. It can be but a matter of time, and this will come about. Patience must be exercised in this as in other directions, and eventually the legitimate dental practitioner will be better understood than at present, and, consequently, better appreciated.

One of the eventualities which lie away in the mist of the future—the appointment of dental surgeons, as such, in the army and navy—it may be hoped will gradually take form and reality. This idea is by no means new. It has been discussed again and again; but only as the proper treatment of the affections and diseases of the teeth and oral cavity becomes clearly apparent to those in authority will the probability here referred to assume definite form and proportions. There can be no doubt that more importance than ever before is now attached by the general public to teeth, and their proper treatment in health and disease. This feeling, it is but reasonable to conclude, will gradually ramify and extend itself until it shall reach the men in our armies and fleets.

In the meantime those who hope legitimately to represent the profession they have espoused must look well to their individual conduct and character, the eyes of so many being now directed to, and resting upon, them. Those who have lately commenced practice will not surely forget the sacrifices they have themselves made in order to obtain the knowledge they possess, nor will they, in justice to their instructors, lightly esteem the sacrifices made on their part, in order to put the results of long experience fully, and withal so pleasantly, within their reach. The future of the dental profession will be coloured, if not actually shaped, very much by their method of treating facts in their daily practice. It would be wise upon their part if they would take the trouble to register both the facts and the treatment pursued, for reference, as they might be subsequently required. Data, carefully kept and catalogued, may involve some time and trouble, but as the practitioner commencing his professional life has, as a rule, a little of this to spare, it could not be much better employed than in the above direction. From such a book of records he might speak with certainty at the Odontological Society, or write with precision when inclined to make a contribution of his experience to the journals devoted to such subjects as those he would comment upon.

There is a tendency, especially with some, in all departments of scientific and practical life, to elaborate in everything written, said, or done. The various operations on the teeth certainly present temptations in this direction. While, on the one hand, it is of the last importance that what is commenced should be properly and absolutely completed, and in order to effect this many instruments and innumerable applications of them may have to be used, yet, the multiplication of these, beyond that which is absolutely necessary, is to be condemned, and ought to be avoided. The author is led to make this remark from what, in his official position at the Dental Hospital of London, he has often been compelled to witness among the students there. A simple operation ought to be performed in a simple way, and not hampered about with complex and diversified methods. There are those, however, who fancy that the latter plan is not only necessary, but positively correct, and, moreover, "scientific." It should ever be remembered that the charm and value of every ingenuity is simplicity. To this end every artificer, constructor, inventor, properly so called, labours to attain. Nature teaches the same lesson, and art is most truly art when it is simple and plain. To enshroud a thing about to be done with mysteriousness, to employ ten times as many instruments as are necessary to its accomplishment, and then to consider or call the process scientific, is distinctly a mistake. Those who are well grounded in the principles and the practice of their profession will find it most to their credit, and certainly to their advantage, to seek to arrive at the desired end in all they attempt by means which are as little encumbered by the complex as it is possible for them to be. One of the distinct benefits accruing to the students at the above institution has been the dissemination of instruction, to a large extent, on this principle. The young men have had the reasons given for different methods being applied under the various aspects of the cases placed before them for treatment, but that which was plain, simple, and direct, encouraged as the plan most to be recommended. The showy, as a rule, always savours of the charlatan, and has, therefore, been steadily discountenanced. It is to be hoped that in their private practice this will not be laid aside or practically forgotten.

The lever now in the hands of the profession is EDUCATION. This must be sedulously employed, until the dental body in this country—and it is to be hoped in the sister island, and in Wales also—can be fairly regarded and known as men fully equipped for their professional pursuits. Self-culture will bring self-respect; and this, in turn, when properly manifested, will secure the co-operation of the medical profession, and that part of the outside public which is given to discernment, in establishing the reputation of the dental surgeon, and according to him his rightful position among the scientific gentlemen of his time.

The hope of "registration" for licentiates in dental surgery is, at present, and possibly for some time yet may continue to be, a faint one. The enthusiasm of the more ardent on this account may have to be held in check. But when, by the diligent use of the means now at their disposal, those who look for this further and distinct mark of recognition and protection, have proved themselves thoroughly worthy of it, it will, doubtless, be accorded them. In the meantime let the young learn with diligence and care, and the more matured and experienced practise honourably what they know, and the expectant watchers will not have to ascend the mount of observation many times ere they perceive the wished-for " little cloud, like a man's hand."

APPENDIX.

A.—AMENDED SUGGESTED RULES OF THE PROPOSED DENTAL SOCIETY.

1. This society shall be called "The Dental Society."
2. The object of this society shall be to consolidate members of the dental profession into one body, with the view of promoting the advancement of dental science by means of periodical meetings, correspondence, and otherwise.
3. All dentists in actual practice shall—subject to Rule 5—be eligible as members; each member to pay a subscription of £2, 2s. annually, or £21 in one sum as a composition for life. The assistants and pupils of practitioners may be admitted "associates" of the society upon the recommendation referred to in Rule 5, the annual subscription of each associate to be £1, 1s.
4. The council shall have power to confer the distinction of honorary membership.
5. Every person desirous of being admitted a member or associate must be proposed by two members of the society, according to the form annexed to these rules, which form is to be addressed to the council, with whom will rest the admission or rejection of candidates, and in case of rejection the council are not bound to give any reason for such decision.
6. The council shall have full power to eject any member or associate who shall do any act or thing to the discredit of the society, or annoyance of its members.

7. All payments to be made to the treasurer of the society, who shall make no disbursements without the authority of the council.

8. The affairs of the society shall be conducted by a council of management, to consist of a president, vice-presidents, a treasurer, secretary, and twelve others, to be annually elected by, and from among, the members of the society; one-half of which shall consist of members of the last year's council. Five to form a quorum.

9. The right of voting by proxy to be extended to country members, and at the election of council only.

10. Two members of the society shall annually be appointed to audit the accounts, and to report thereon at the annual general meeting.

11. An annual general meeting shall be held in January—at such time and place as the council may appoint—to receive the report of the council, to elect officers for the ensuing twelve months, and transact the general business of the society.

12. At every meeting of the society, or of the council, the resolutions of the majority shall be binding, though all persons entitled to vote be not present; and at such meetings the chairman shall have a casting vote, independently of his vote as a member of the society, or of the council, as the case may be.

13. Upon receiving a requisition signed by, at least, twenty-five members of the society, the council shall, within twenty-one days, call a general meeting of the members, giving a fortnight's notice, at least; the requisition, as well as the notice, to state in precise terms the object for which such meeting is called, and no business other than that of which notice is thus given shall be transacted at such meeting.

14. All information received shall be entered in books kept by the secretary for the purpose, which shall be open for inspection of members of the society.

15. No change shall be made in these rules, except at a general meeting of the members of the society specially convened for that purpose.

Form alluded to in Rule 5.

We   and   being members of the Dental Society, do hereby recommend   as a fit and proper person to be admitted a member of the society.

Signed {

Date,   18

To the Council of the Dental Society.

B.—COLLEGE OF DENTISTS OF ENGLAND—LAWS AND CONSTITUTION.

1. The title of this association shall be the "College of Dentists of England."

2. The objects for which the college is established are to unite members of the dental profession into a recognised and independent body, and to provide means of professional education and examination.

3. The college shall consist of fellows, members, honorary members, and associates—to be elected according to Rule 6.

4. The affairs of the college shall be conducted by a council of management, to consist of a president, vice-presidents, a treasurer, a secretary or secretaries, and a council of fifteen others—to be elected annually by, and from among, members of the college : two-thirds of which shall consist of members of the last year's council. Five members to form a quorum. The mode of election shall be as follows :—The chairman and two scrutineers having been appointed, the poll shall commence by each member personally delivering his balloting-paper to the chairman, who shall deposit the same in the balloting glass. The poll to remain open from seven to nine o'clock, when the chairman and scrutineers, attended by the secretary, shall retire, cast the poll, and sign the return. In the event of an equality of votes, the chairman shall have the casting vote.

5. The subscriptions to the college shall be as follows :— The payment of £21, in one sum, to be considered as a composition for life for fellows or members ; otherwise, an annual subscription of £2, 2s. to be paid by each fellow and member. The annual subscription of associates to be £1, 1s. Members shall pay a fee of £1, 1s. on entering the college, and associates a fee of 10s. 6d.

6. Every person desirous of being admitted a member or an associate must be proposed by two members of the college, and the candidate must be personally known to one of them. His name shall then be placed upon the list of candidates for

admission, and there remain for, at least, five weeks previous to the evening on which the ballot takes place, which shall only be when there are not fewer than twenty-five members present; and to secure election, two-thirds of the votes of the members must be in his favour. Fellows and honorary members shall be recommended only by the council.

7. The treasurer shall demand and receive for the use of the college all monies due or payable to the college, and shall keep full and particular accounts of all sums so received. An account in the name of the college shall be opened, and all monies deposited at a banker's to be appointed by the council.

8. No person combining any kind of business with the practice of the dental profession shall be a member of the college.

9. The council shall have the power to remove from the list of members and others those who may do anything to the discredit of the college or the annoyance of its members; but such persons shall have the right of appeal at a general meeting.

10. No person allowing his name to be associated with disreputable advertisements of any kind shall be a member of this college. And any member making a public exhibition of his diploma, or of any other document granted him by the authority of this college, shall have his name removed from the list of members.

11. The whole effects and property of the college shall be vested in the council of management for the time being.

12. An annual general meeting shall be held in January (at such time and as the council shall appoint), to receive the report of the council, to elect officers for the ensuing twelve months, and to transact the general business of the college.

13. At every meeting of the college or of the council, the resolutions of the majority shall be binding, though all persons entitled to vote be not present; and at such meetings the chairman shall have a casting vote, independently of his vote as a member of the college or of the council, as the case may be.

14. The council may at any time call a special general meeting, and they shall at all times be bound to do so on the written requisition of ten members, specifying the nature of

the business to be transacted. Notice of the time and place of such meeting shall be sent to the members, at least, fourteen days previously, mentioning the subject to be brought forward, and no other subject shall be discussed at such meeting.

15. The ordinary meetings of the college shall be held on the first Tuesday in each month, excepting the months of July, August, and September. The conduct of these meetings to be under the entire control of the council.

16. The council shall have the power to make bye-laws, fill up vacancies in their number, and transact the general business of the college.

17. No change shall be made in these rules, except at a general meeting of the members of the college, specially convened for that purpose.

AMENDED LAWS AND CONSTITUTION OF THE COLLEGE OF DENTISTS OF ENGLAND.

1. The title of this association shall be the "College of Dentists of England."

2. The objects for which the college is established are to unite members of the dental profession into a recognised and independent body, and to provide means of professional examination.

3. The college shall consist of members and associates. Honorary members may be elected in accordance with Laws 13 and 14.

4. The privileges of members shall consist in the right of voting at all general meetings, of attending other meetings, and all lectures and demonstrations which may take place at the college. Each member, whose subscription is not in arrear, shall also be entitled to a copy of the transactions of the college. Honorary members and associates shall have all the privileges of members, but shall have no share in the direction of the affairs of the college.

5. The affairs of the college shall be conducted by a president, vice-presidents, a treasurer, a secretary or secretaries, and by a council of nine others,* to be elected annually by, and from amongst, the members of the college. One-third of such council shall retire at the end of the year, but shall be eligible for re-election. The president, vice-presidents, and secretary or secretaries shall be *ex officio* members of the council. Any member of the college shall be eligible as a member of the council, on being proposed by five other members; such proposition to be sent to the council one month previous to the annual general meeting, and the names of such candidates shall be printed with the house list. The mode of election shall be as follows:—The chairman and two scrutineers having been appointed, the poll shall commence by each member present personally delivering his balloting-paper to the chair-

---

* This alteration not to come into operation until January 1860.

man. Country members, who have the privilege of voting by proxy, shall, if they exercise their privilege, send their proxy-papers, under cover, addressed to the chairman of the meeting. The chairman shall deposit all balloting-papers in the balloting box. The poll to remain open from half-past seven to nine o'clock in the evening, when the chairman and scrutineers, attended by one of the secretaries, shall retire, cast the poll, and sign the return. In the event of an equality of votes, the chairman shall have the casting vote.

6. The subscription to the college shall be as follows :— The payment of £21, in one sum, to be considered as a life composition; otherwise, an annual subscription of £2, 2s. shall be paid by each member. The annual subscription of associates shall be £1, 1s. Members shall pay a fee of £1, 1s. on entering the college, and associates a fee of 10s. 6d. All subscriptions shall be due on the first day of January in each year, and shall be payable in advance. Members and associates whose subscriptions are not paid within three months of the date on which they are due, shall forfeit the privilege of membership until the subscription be paid. If not paid within six months after it is due, the membership shall cease. The council shall, however, possess the power to re-admit the defaulting member upon paying his arrears, if they, in their discretion, think fit so to do, in which case the entrance fee will not be required.

7. The treasurer shall demand and receive for the use of the college all monies due or payable to the college, and shall keep full and particular account of all sums received. An account in the name of the college shall be opened, and all monies deposited at a banker's to be appointed by the council.

Laws 8 and 9 cancelled.

10. The names of new members shall be once advertised in the "Times" newspaper by the council at the expense of the college, within fourteen days after their election. Such new member shall also be permitted to advertise that they have been elected members in the local newspapers of their respective places of abode three times at their own expense. The following to be the form of advertisement :—

College of Dentists of England.

Mr.   of   was duly elected a member of the College of Dentists of England on the

Signed

Secretary or Secretaries.

Laws 11 and 12 cancelled.

13. Retired members of the profession may be elected honorary members of the college by the council.

14. Such members of the profession residing out of the United Kingdom, as may be considered eligible by the council, shall be nominated corresponding members of the college.

15. No person allowing his name to be associated with disreputable advertisements of any kind, circulating hand-bills, or exhibiting show-cases, boards, or placards, combining any other business or calling with that of a dentist, or acting for or assisting any person who combines any other business with that of a dentist, shall be a member or an associate of the college. And any member making a public exhibition of the diploma, or of any other document granted him by the authority of this college, shall have his name removed from the list of members.

16. The council shall have the power to remove from the list of members and others those who, in their judgment, may do anything to the discredit of the college, or the annoyance of its members; but members so removed shall have the right of appeal at a general meeting—such appeal to be made within one calendar month of the date of official notice to the offending member, otherwise the right of appeal will be lost.

17. An annual general meeting shall be held in January (at such time and place as the council shall appoint), to receive the report of the council, to elect officers for the ensuing twelve months, and to transact the general business of the college. Such annual meeting may be adjourned by resolution thereof from time to time, in case the business brought forward should, from any cause, not be concluded.

18. The council may at any time call a special general meeting, and they shall at all times be bound to do so on the written requisition of ten members, specifying the nature of the business to be transacted. Notice of the time and place of such meeting shall be sent to the members at least fourteen

days previously, mentioning the subject to be brought forward, and no other business shall be introduced at such meeting.

19. At every meeting of the college, or of the council, the resolutions of the majority present shall be binding (excepting only in the case referred to in Law 23); and at such meetings the chairman shall have a casting vote, independently of his vote as a member of the college, or of the council, as the case may be. Members of the college residing beyond twenty miles of Charing Cross shall be entitled to vote by proxy for the election of council and officers; and upon all questions at general and special general meetings upon a poll being demanded in writing signed by five members. In case of such poll being demanded, it shall be the duty of the chairman to name a convenient day and hour on which the poll shall be opened and closed.

Law 20 cancelled.

21. The council shall have the power to make bye-laws; but such bye-laws shall not contravene the spirit of the fundamental laws; fill up vacancies in their own number, and in any of the offices, and transact the general business of the college.

22. Every person upon being admitted a member or an associate of this college shall sign the following declaration :—

In consideration, of my being admitted a member or an associate of the College of Dentists of England, I hereby undertake to agree to, and abide by, the laws and the bye-laws of the said college.

(Signed)

23. The college shall not be dissolved unless two-thirds of the members shall vote for the dissolution.

24. No change shall be made in these laws except at a general meeting of members of the college specially convened for that purpose.

The following laws to become part and parcel of the constitution of the college :—

MEMBERSHIP.—*All dentists* in actual legitimate practice on the 20th day of April 1859, shall be entitled to become members of this college without examination. The council to determine all questions relating to legitimate qualification for membership by such practitioners.

Gentlemen who have not commenced practice as dentists on the 20th day of April 1859 shall be required to undergo an examination as to qualification to practise prior to being admitted members of this college.

The regulations for examination shall be under the entire control of the council.

ASSOCIATES.—The council shall have the power to admit as associates of the college, without examination, assistants of dentists, engaged as such, or qualified to be so engaged, on the 20th day of April 1859.

After the 20th day of April 1859, no person except those qualified as above, shall be admitted associates without passing an examination on dental mechanics. The nature of the examination to be determined by the council.

Associates of the college and *assistants* of dentists shall be eligible for membership upon passing the necessary examination.

CANDIDATES FOR THE LICENCE OF DENTAL SURGERY.

(Page 156.)

Candidates are required to produce the following certificates :—

1. Of being twenty-one years of age.
2. Of having been engaged during four years in the acquirement of professional knowledge.
3. Of having attended, at a school or schools recognised by this college, not less than one of each of the following courses of lectures, delivered by lecturers recognised by this college—namely, Anatomy, Physiology, Surgery, Medicine, Chemistry, and Materia Medica.
4. Of having attended a second winter course of lectures on anatomy, or a course of not less than twenty lectures on the anatomy of the head and neck, delivered by lecturers recognised by this college.
5. Of having performed dissections at a recognised school, during not less than nine months.
6. Of having completed a course of chemical manipulation, under the superintendence of a teacher or lecturer recognised by this college.
7. Of having attended, at a recognised hospital or hospitals in the United Kingdom, the practice of surgery and clinical lectures on surgery during two winter sessions.
8. Of having attended, at a recognised school, two courses of lectures upon each of the following subjects—viz., Dental Anatomy and Physiology (human and comparative), Dental Surgery, Dental Mechanics, and one course of lectures on Metallurgy, by lecturers recognised by this college.
9. Of having been engaged, during a period of not less than three years, in acquiring a practical familiarity with the details of mechanical dentistry, under the instruction of a competent practitioner.

10. Of having attended, at a recognised dental hospital, or in the dental department of a recognised general hospital, the practice of dental surgery during the period of two years.

N.B.—The students of the London schools are required to register the above certificates at this college; and special returns will be required from the provincial schools.

COPY OF MEMORIAL.

To the Queen's Most Excellent Majesty in Council.

(*Page* 163.)

The humble petition of George Waite, of No. 2 Old Burlington Street; Peter Matthews, 17 Lower Berkeley Street, Portman Square; James Merryweather, 57 Lower Brooke Street, Grosvenor Square; James Harley, 23A Davies Street, Berkeley Square; Somerset Tibbs, 58 Regent Street, Cheltenham; Norman King, 7 Bedford Circus, Exeter; and others, practising members of the dental profession:

Showeth,—

That, owing to want of recognised qualification, the profession of dental surgery in England does not hold that position which its growing importance demands.

That, owing to this want, students of dentistry often devote much time to strictly medical attainments, for the purpose of securing a medical degree, which time would have been far more usefully and beneficially spent in acquiring a practical knowledge of dental surgery; the consequence being, that when these students enter upon their professional career, they have still to learn all those practical details so essential to legitimate success.

That, certain members of the profession have long felt that it has become imperatively necessary that some educational course should be instituted; and believing that not only a general acquaintance with the principles of surgery, anatomy, and physiology, but also a special knowledge of such portions of these subjects as have particular reference to the region of the mouth, are absolutely essential to the duly-qualified practitioner, they have enrolled themselves as members of the College of Dentists of England.

That the board of examiners of the college has been constituted, a list of which is attached hereto.

That a Metropolitan School of Dental Science has also been established in connection with the college, for the purpose of affording systematised instruction in dental science, a list of the faculty of which school, and of the fees and other particulars thereof, is also attached hereto.

That the petitioners are desirous, on public grounds, and for the reasons above set forth, to obtain a charter of incorporation for the College of Dentists, under the title of " The Royal College of Dentists of England," such college to have the right and power to grant diplomas of proficiency to all candidates for membership.

And humbly praying that your Majesty will be pleased to grant the said charter of incorporation, and as in duty bound the petitioners will ever pray, &c., &c.

(Signed)

ABSTRACT OF ACT OF PARLIAMENT, TOUCHING THE GRANTING OF POWER TO THE ROYAL COLLEGE OF SURGEONS TO EXAMINE CANDIDATES FOR THE DIPLOMA OF LICENTIATE IN DENTAL SURGERY AND GRANT THAT DEGREE, DATED 23RD VICTORIA. 8TH SEPT. 1859.

AND WHEREAS by the Medical Act, made and passed in the twenty-first and twenty-second years of our reign, it is amongst other things enacted, " That it shall, notwithstanding anything therein contained, be lawful for ourselves by charter to grant to the Royal College of Surgeons of England power to institute and hold examinations for the purpose of testing the fitness of persons to practise as dentists who may be desirous of being so examined, and to grant certificates of such fitness."

AND WHEREAS, in order to provide for the due qualification of persons practising as dentists, it appears to us expedient that the said Royal College of Surgeons of England should have

APPENDIX. 399

power to institute and hold examinations for the purpose of testing the fitness of such persons, subject to the regulations and directions hereinafter mentioned. Now, KNOW YE, That WE of our especial grace and mere motion, at the humble petition of the said Royal College, have willed, ordained, constituted, and declared and granted, and by these presents, for us, our heirs and successors, do will, ordain, constitute and declare, and unto the said Royal College of Surgeons of England do grant in manner following, to wit,—

1. That it shall be lawful for the council of the said college to appoint a board of examiners for the purpose of testing the fitness of persons to practise as dentists who may be desirous of being so examined, and to grant certificates of such fitness. And it is our will and pleasure that such board of examiners be called the Board of Examiners in Dental Surgery, and consist of not less than six members, to be appointed as hereinafter mentioned, three of whom shall be members of the court of examiners for the time being of the said college, and the others of them shall be such persons skilled in dental surgery as the council of the said college shall from time to time think proper to appoint.

2. AND we do hereby authorise and require the council of the said college within six calendar months from the date of these our letters patent, to appoint three persons, being members of the court of examiners of the said college, and also three such other persons skilled in dental surgery as they may think fit, to be such examiners in dental surgery, who shall continue in office for such period, and shall conduct the examinations in such manner, and shall grant certificates in such form, as the council of the said college shall determine, and from time to time direct. And it shall be lawful for the said council of the said college from time to time, as vacancies shall occur in such last-mentioned board of examiners, to appoint any persons to fill up the same, nevertheless, so that the said board of examiners shall always be constituted as hereinbefore directed.

3. AND IT IS OUR FURTHER WILL AND PLEASURE, That the said college do admit all persons who shall be desirous of being examined as aforesaid, whether members of the said

college or not members thereof, to examination by the said board of examiners in dental surgery. PROVIDED, nevertheless, that such persons shall have attained the age of twenty-one years, and shall also have complied with such rules and regulations as to education as the council of the said college shall from time to time consider expedient.

4. THAT such reasonable fees shall be paid for the certificates of the said board of examiners in dental surgery as the council of the said college shall from time to time think fit, and by any bye-law or bye-laws direct. PROVIDED ALWAYS, AND IT IS OUR FURTHER WILL AND PLEASURE, That these presents shall not operate to create, or be taken or deemed to confer upon any person who shall obtain such certificate of fitness, as aforesaid, any right or title to be registered under the said Medical Act in respect of such certificate. IN WITNESS whereof, We have caused these our letters to be made patent.

Witness ourselves at our palace at Westminster, this eighth day of September in the twenty-third year of our reign.

By Her Majesty's command,

EDMUNDS.

ERRATUM.

In title, page 341, *for* Mr. J. Underwood, *read* Mr. T. Underwood.

www.ingramcontent.com/pod-product-compliance
Lightning Source LLC
Chambersburg PA
CBHW022111290426
44112CB00008B/636